NEW
MEANINGS
OF DEATH

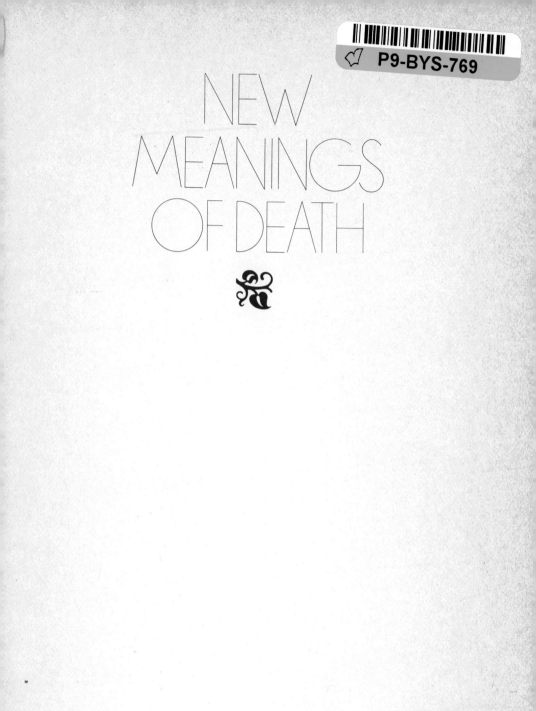

NEW MEANINGS OF DEATH

Herman Feifel, Ph.D.

Chief Psychologist
Veterans Administration
Outpatient Clinic
Los Angeles

McGRAW-HILL BOOK COMPANY
A Blakiston Publication

New York   St. Louis   San Francisco   Auckland   Bogotá   Düsseldorf   Johannesburg
London   Madrid   Mexico   Montreal   New Delhi   Panama   Paris   São Paulo
Singapore   Sydney   Tokyo   Toronto

NEW
MEANINGS
OF DEATH

234567890DODO783210987

This book was set in Baskerville by National ShareGraphics, Inc.
The editors were J. Dereck Jeffers, Elysbeth H. Wyckoff, and
Douglas J. Marshall; the photo researcher was Elysbeth H. Wyckoff;
the designer was Jo Jones;
the production supervisor was Dennis J. Conroy.
R. R. Donnelley & Sons Company was printer and binder.

The cover photo was taken by Elysbeth H. Wyckoff.

Library of Congress Cataloging in Publication Data
Main entry under title:

New meanings of death.

"A Blakiston publication."
Includes indexes.
1. Terminal care. 2. Death. I. Feifel, Herman.
R726.8.F44   1977   128'.5   77-460
ISBN 0-07-020350-4
ISBN 0-07-020349-0 pbk.

ACKNOWLEDGMENTS

The editor and contributors make grateful acknowledgment for the use of quotations in the text from the following works:

Lifton, Robert Jay, The sense of immortality: on death and the continuity of life, from *The Journal of the American Academy of Psychoanalysis,* 33:3–15, 1973.

Rosenthal, Ted, *How could I not be among you?* George Braziller, Inc. Reprinted with the permission of the publisher. Copyright © 1973 by Ted Rosenthal.

Frost, Robert, from "Birches" from *The Poetry of Robert Frost,* edited by Edward Connery Lathem. Copyright 1916, © 1969 by Holt, Rinehart and Winston. Copyright 1944 by Robert Frost. Reprinted by permission of Holt, Rinehart and Winston, Publishers.

Denver, John, "Around and Around." Used by permission. All rights reserved. Copyright © 1970 Cherry Lane Music Co., Englewood Cliffs, New Jersey.

Dickinson, Emily: "Death Is the Supple Suitor." Reprinted by permission of the publishers and the Trustees of Amherst College from *The Poems of Emily Dickinson,* edited by Thomas H. Johnson, Cambridge, Mass.: The Belknap Press of Harvard University Press, Copyright © 1951, 1955 by the President and Fellows of Harvard College.

Sassoon, Siegfried, "Counter Attack," from *Collected Poems.* The Viking Press Inc., New York, New York. Reprinted by permission of the publisher and G. T. Sassoon.

Berryman, John, "Dream Song 145" and "Dream Song 235" from *The Dream Songs.* Reprinted with the permission of the publisher, Farrar, Straus & Giroux, Inc., New York.

Plath, Sylvia, "Lady Lazarus," "Edge," and "Stings" from *Ariel.* By permission of Harper & Row, Publishers, Inc., New York. Copyright © 1963 by Ted Hughes.

Sexton, Anne, *Live or Die.* By permission of Houghton Mifflin Company, Boston, Massachusetts.

PHOTO CREDITS

*For Rebecca, Thelma, Harriet, Laurie
and all other givers and enablers of life.*

"We must learn to die before we can exalt existence."
Rabbi Abraham Joshua Heschel

CONTENTS

LIST OF CONTRIBUTORS

Jeanne Quint Benoliel, D.N.Sc.
  Professor of Nursing, Department of Community Health Care Systems, University of Washington, Seattle
Herman Feifel, Ph.D.
  Chief Psychologist, Veterans Administration Outpatient Clinic, Los Angeles; Clinical Professor of Psychiatry (Psychology), University of Southern California School of Medicine, Los Angeles
Charles A. Garfield, Ph.D.
  Research Psychologist and Assistant Clinical Professor of Psychiatry (Psychology), Cancer Research Institute, University of California Medical Center, San Francisco; Director SHANTI Project, San Francisco
David L. Gutmann, Ph.D.
  Chief, Division of Psychology, Northwestern University Medical School, Chicago; Professor, Department of Psychology, University of Michigan, Ann Arbor
Arthur Jaffe
  Businessman, Butler, Pennsylvania
Lois Jaffe, M.S.W.
  Associate Professor, Graduate School of Social Work, University of Pittsburgh; Psychiatric Social Worker, Irene Stacy Mental Health Center, Butler, Pennsylvania
Richard A. Kalish, Ph.D.
  Professor of Behavioral Sciences, Graduate Theological Union, Berkeley, California; Lecturer in Psychology, Department of Psychiatry, University of California, San Francisco Medical Center
Robert Kastenbaum, Ph.D.
  Professor of Psychology, University of Massachusetts—Boston

Orville E. Kelly
>Founder MAKE TODAY COUNT; Ambassador, Guideposts Associates, Burlington, Iowa

Myra Bluebond-Langner, Ph.D.
>Assistant Professor of Anthropology, Rutgers University, Camden, New Jersey

Daniel Leviton, Ph.D.
>Professor of Health Education and Director of The Adults' Health and Developmental Program, University of Maryland, College Park

Robert J. Lifton, M.D.
>Foundations' Fund Research Professor of Psychiatry, Yale University School of Medicine, New Haven

Howard C. Raether, J.D.
>Executive Director, National Funeral Directors Association, Milwaukee, Wisconsin

Robert E. Rodes, Jr.
>Professor of Law, University of Notre Dame, South Bend, Indiana

Dr. Cicely Saunders, O.B.E., F.R.C.P.
>Medical Director, St. Christopher's Hospice, Sydenham, England

Thomas L. Shaffer
>Professor of Law, University of Notre Dame, South Bend, Indiana

Edwin S. Shneidman, Ph.D.
>Professor of Thanatology, and Director, Laboratory for the Study of Life-Threatening Behavior, University of California at Los Angeles

Dr. Michael A. Simpson
>Consultant Psychiatrist and Physician, Senior Lecturer in The Academic Departments of Psychiatry and Medicine, Senior Research Fellow, Royal Free Hospital Medical School, London, England; formerly Assistant Professor of Psychiatry, McMaster University, Ontario, Canada

Robert C. Slater, L.H.D.
>Professor and Director, Department of Mortuary Science, University of Minnesota, Minneapolis

Avery D. Weisman, M.D.
>Professor of Psychiatry, Massachusetts General Hospital, Harvard Medical School; Training and Supervisory Analyst, Boston Psychoanalytic Institute, Boston

Laurens P. White, M.D.
>Associate Clinical Professor of Medicine, University of California at San Francisco

PREFACE

When McGraw-Hill approached me to update *The Meaning of Death* (1959), I was somewhat ambivalent. Beyond the demands it would entail, what "new" was there to add to such issues as love and death after 6000 years of recorded history? Everybody dies, even today, so what's new? Yet, I recalled this reasoning had not prevented my original efforts to impart life to *The Meaning of Death*. Besides, it was heartening to observe that many of the seminal concepts advanced in that book were now almost axiomatic in the thanatological domain. More relevant, perhaps, in picking up the challenge was my increasing understanding that knowledge tends to be dynamic and ever-changing, that information is filtered and retranslated as it moves through time. And, indeed, new perspectives are imposed on us in grappling with such current phenomena as the changing character and distribution of mortality, the growing secularization of death, the potential for sudden mass death. Most overriding for me, however, was the conviction that in the last analysis all human behavior of consequence is a response to the problem of death. It is the key issue in life. Hegel defined history as being "what man does with death." Hence, anything "more" or "new" in the field resulting from disciplined study, discerning experience, and compassion is worth a reading.

The animating perspectives and information in this book reflect the knowledgeability and acumen of a distinguished group of leaders representing such varying bases as medicine, psychology, anthropology, psychiatry, psychoanalysis, nursing, social work, education, funeral directing, and the law. We are also the beneficiaries of contributions from Lois Jaffe and Orville Kelly, both of whom are *in medias res*—wrestling with impending personal death.

Since the book does not attempt to encompass the panoramic realm of thanatology, such sectors as religion, philosophy, epidemiology, economics, and the humanities are touched only glancingly. The book does, however, provide the reader with clinical and empirical findings, horizons, and strategies pertinent for professional practice, existing conceptual frameworks, and public policy in the areas of dying, death, and bereavement. In more extensive vein, its information serves Everyman.

It is doubtful that humanity will vanquish death no matter how strong and wise we become. But if information and intelligence, along with faith, love, and art, can bolster us on the journey of life, it is the hope of the editor and contributors that some of the thinking presented in the book will help brace our steps. Life's ultimate meaning remains obscure unless it is reflected upon in the countenance of death.

I want to express my gratitude to Dereck Jeffers and Betsy Wyckoff of the editorial staff, Blakiston Publications, McGraw-Hill Book Company, for their cooperative efforts on behalf of the book.

Most of all, I want to acknowledge my obligation to the book's eminent contributors—seekers as well as discoverers.

Herman Feifel

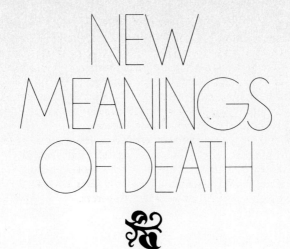

NEW MEANINGS OF DEATH

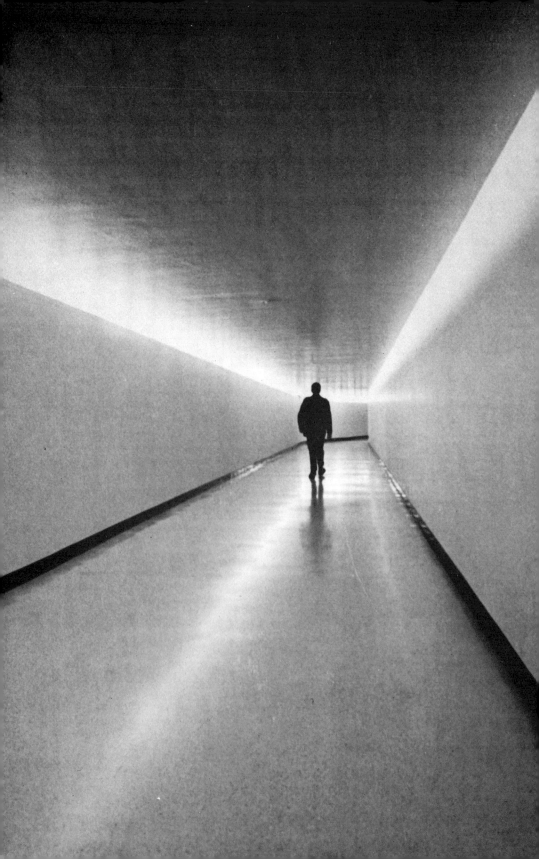

PART ONE
INTRODUCTION

1
DEATH IN CONTEM- PORARY AMERICA

HERMAN FEIFEL

People have spoken about life and thought about death since the beginning. Still, modern day discussion of death has never quite reached the major-league status of sex, sports, politics, or the weather. Nevertheless, there is no denying that surface consideration of death these days has become lively— almost chic—a surprising outgrowth of a culture portrayed as death-denying. There are a number of reasons for this development. Recent advances in innovative medical technology are altering the character of dying and compelling us to look more steadily at death. Blows from an impersonal technology are alienating us from traditional moorings, and weakening institutional and community supports. The consequences are increased loneliness, anxiety, and self-probing. It is a historic phenomenon that consciousness of death becomes more acute during periods of social disorganization, when individual choice tends to replace automatic conformity to consensual social values. Thus it was in classical society after destruction of the city-state and in the early Renaissance period after the breakdown of feudalism. Finally, ever since the day when the age of mathematical physics came to a climax at Alamogordo when a black cloud covered the sun and announced, "I am become Death—the shatterer of worlds," there has been a growing pessimism concerning the future of humanity.

Yet, despite these wellsprings of contact, Americans still approach dying and death warily and gingerly. As Woody Allen recently personalized it on his fortieth birthday, "I shall gain immortality not through my work but by not dying." A number of factors contribute to this state of affairs. Foremost among these, I think, is the fact that many of us no longer command, except nominally, conceptual creeds or philosophic-religious views with which to transcend death. People of the Middle Ages had their eschatologies and the sacred time of eternity. And although death portended judgment, it was accompanied by the possibility of atonement and salvation. Death was a door. More recently, with the waning of traditional belief, temporal man lived with the prospect of personal immortality transformed into concern for historical immortality and for the welfare of posterity. Today we are vouchsafed neither. With the advent of the H-bomb, physical science has presently made it possible for us all to share a common epitaph. Not only descendants and social immortality but history as well is being menaced. Time along with space can now be annihilated. Even celebration of the tragic will be beyond our power. Death is becoming a wall.

Further undercutting our capacity to integrate personal death is an impersonal technology which is steadily increasing fragmentation of the family and dismantling rooted neighborhood and kinship groups. Today, the family is essentially nuclear—composed of a husband, wife, and chil-

4

dren. No longer do we live in a community abounding with uncles, aunts, siblings, and cousins, and possessing homogeneous values. Consequently, when death intrudes into our lives, previously existing emotional and institutional supports to cushion its impact are absent.

Allied to this development is a spreading deritualization of grief, related to criticism of funerary practices as being overly expansive, irrelevant, and exploitive of the mourner's grief. An aftermath of this orientation is removal of an additional buttress which in the past bolstered many in the face of dying and death.

Another circumstance which has made death more difficult to confront is the gradual expulsion of death from common experience. Death has become a mystery to most of us. It is now a rare phenomenon for the average person to see an untreated dead person. A piece of domestic technology familiar in most nineteenth century households—how to deal with a corpse—has vanished. It is paradoxical that while direct exposure of children and young adults to dying and death is decreasing because of medical advances, dying and death are being given considerable but unrealistic attention in the gothic fantasies of horror films and in derivative TV renditions. These bring to our awareness disaster and battlefield deaths, but they are usually removed from the realm of feeling to that of impersonal statistics, black comedy, and fictive experience. Dying and death are now the province of the "professional," i.e., physician, clergyman, funeral director. Unfortunately, too many of them tend to use their professional knowledge as a buckler against unprotected encounter with death to bind their own anxieties. Accordingly, when the professional is called upon to blunt the edge of grief, to interpret death to family and survivors, he usually is unsuccessful.

Finally, in a society that emphasizes achievement and the future, the prospect of no future at all and loss of identity is an abomination. Death is seen as destroyer of the American vision—the right to life, liberty, and the pursuit of happiness. Hence, death and dying invite our hostility and repudiation. I submit that it is this outlook which, in substantial measure, lies behind our general negativity toward old age, herald of death.

In light of these vying and contradictory factors propelling us toward both accepting and denying death, it is understandable why ambivalence toward death is so characteristic of much of modern America's adaptation to death. Or maybe it is, as Avery Weisman has suggested, that we really are not that more accepting of death these days—it's just more difficult to hide from.

Unified and systematic findings are relatively sparse thus far in the thanatological field, but some commanding perceptions are beginning to take hold. What are they?

DEVELOPMENTAL ORIENTATIONS

It is becoming clear that death is for all seasons. It is not the restricted domain of the dying patient, elderly person, combat soldier, or suicidal individual. Children as young as 2 years of age are already contending with the idea of death. We have disabused ourselves of the fancy that sex is a happening that comes to life at puberty, as a kind of full-bodied Minerva emerging from Jupiter's head. In a similar vein, it is fitting that we now recognize the psychological presence of death in ourselves from infancy on. We have come to realize the mental hygienic aspects of being candid about birth (sex). Research studies and clinical experience direct that we do the same for the topic of death. We do not protect children by shielding them from the realities of death. We only hinder their emotional growth. This ban usually mirrors more the adult's and parent's own anxieties and apprehensions about death than the child's actual ability to handle the impact of death. Children are more capable of withstanding the stress brought on by their limited understanding of death than its mystery and implied abandonment. Further, recognition by children of the authenticity of death helps them make better sense of the world. Naturally, such aspects as individual differences, cultural context, method of explanation, and timing have to be considered. In broad perspective, what is truthful and helps sustain the reality-sense of the child will ordinarily prevent a child's adverse reaction to death.

At the other end of the chronological continuum—old age—it is manifest that the older person must joust not only with the possibility of body-image changes, beleaguered hopes, and the shrinkage of his or her social world but with the inescapable certitude of personal mortality. Ironically, we find that though many older persons want to share their feelings and thoughts about dying and death, they are frequently prohibited from doing so by our general reluctance to examine death. A net result is that too many elderly persons turn to regressive and inappropriate patterns of conduct in dealing with their fears, even hopes, about death. The periods of adolescence and middle age likewise share a strong consciousness about death (a more detailed discussion of death's perception throughout the life span will be found in Chapter 2 by Kastenbaum).

What is increasingly apparent is that disregard of the intellectual and emotional predicaments arising from self-consciousness about personal death, present in the mental functioning of the healthy as well as the sick, bars our access to a dominant gyroscope of individual and group behavior. As Kastenbaum has aptly phrased it, "Death is not just destination, it is part of our getting there as well."

CLINICAL MANAGEMENT

The forward march of medicine has had marked impact on the present character and duration of dying, at least in the more technologically developed countries. Major communicable diseases such as tuberculosis, influenza, and pneumonia are being replaced by more chronic and degenerative types associated with aging, notably heart disease, cancer, and stroke. Additionally, medical headway has lengthened the average time which now elapses between the onset of a fatal illness and death. This is bringing in its wake exacerbated problems of chronic pain, fear, dependency, loss of self-esteem, and progressive dehumanization for many persons.

Medical practice has also altered the locus of dying. No longer do most of us receive death in the privacy and security of our homes. Nowadays, we die in the "big" hospital, convalescent or nursing home, where our lot is often the death of a sickness rather than of a person.

There is expanded recognition of the psychotherapeutic value of open communication with the dying person. Seemingly, the unknown can be feared more, at times, than the most known dreaded reality. Further, clinical experience suggests that, for a goodly number of patients, information received about the seriousness of their situation can galvanize a "will to live" not available to them before. Untapped potentials for responsible and effective behavior as well as less depression and blame of others become evident. Additionally, honest and sensitive talk from physicians, nurses, and family about the gravity of the patient's condition tends to attenuate feelings of guilt and inadequacy not only in the patient but in professional personnel and family as well.

In truth, most dying patients do not expect miracles. What they ask for most of all is confirmation of care and concern. The summons is to help the person recreate a sense of significant being, to be an individual even though dying. The paradox in much of our current treatment is that at the very moment we enhance attention to the patient's physiological needs, we isolate the patient psychologically and socially. When efforts to forestall the dying process fail, professionals usually lose interest and transfer their motivation and resources elsewhere. After all, the saving of life is the paramount goal of the health professional. Therein is where the professional attains his emotional and financial rewards. In a corresponding vein, institutional structures dealing with death and dying seem to be more organized to meet anxieties and requirements of the helping professional than genuine needs of the dying person. A hospital's usual perception of operations and appropriate utilization of personnel classifies dying as a relatively ineffective and inefficient enterprise. The unhappy result is that the dying patient is often left to die emotionally and spiritually alone. We hardly tolerate his farewell.

In this context, I find it perplexing that so many professional colleagues still feel that truth and hope are necessarily mutually exclusive. Obviously, truth can be cold and cruel, but it can also be gentle and merciful. Deceiving disavowal and raw confrontation are not the only options in speaking about death. Indeed, if we were to act in the light of what we know about psychology and responsibility, we would follow a policy of first informing the adult patient about his or her diagnosis and plan for treatment. Then patient and physician would determine what to tell the family. The will, wishes, and integrity of the person should be a sine qua non in any decision making about the dying patient. In current parlance, the dying person needs to recapture his or her "civil rights." We should remember that although the dying do not possess much political or social clout, sooner or later we shall be *they*.

Fortunately, numerous nurses, physicians, the clergy, and other health professionals have not renounced the human, comforting, and emotionally sustaining aspect of their relationship with the dying patient. A superb application of this approach is exemplified by St. Christopher's Hospice in London, under the invigorating directorship of Dr. Cicely Saunders. Here, time is viewed as a matter of depth and quality as well as length. Being in a dying state does not veto respect for the sanctity and meaningfulness of life. The felicitous effect is a dying characterized by minimal physical pain, and a living until death—a *finis coronat opus* (the end crowns the work). The model that is St. Christopher's, hearteningly, is now being replicated in various parts of the United States and Europe. We must appreciate that the essence of dying extends beyond biology. It is a psychosocial as well as biological process, and the attitudes of physician, hospital, family, and friends all influence how the dying person feels and responds.

This leads to another facet of work in the area—the professional's own sensibilities about dying and death. Few undertakings are more emotionally exacting. Pain and death are themes not comfortably encompassed by theory and skill alone. Ministry to the dying is extremely difficult if we ourselves are not quite reconciled to the truth of personal death.

Lastly, the transition in expectations about life and death along with new alternatives available as a result of medical expertness (organ transplantation, hemodialysis) have brought with them awareness that social, economic, and legal, as well as manifestly medical, aspects are inherent in dealing with the dying experience. Communal and ethical relevancies loom large nowadays along with those of medicine and psychology. Adequate concern for the dying requires reassessment of existing social organizations and public policy responsible for health care and delivery.

THE SURVIVORS

The ache of death does not end with the death of a person. Its legacy of deprivation, void, sharpened sensitivity to our own transience, even stigma, is transmitted to family and friends— the "significant others." Grief and mourning tend to be too curtailed these days. Accumulated evidence indicates that there is a lot of mental-hygienic wisdom in the Irish wake and Jewish shiva. We are rediscovering that expression of grief is not a sign of weakness or self-indulgence. Rather, it is a normal and necessary reaction to loss or separation from a loved or significant person, and represents a deep human need. Funeral and ritual are important because they underscore the reality of death, bring the support and warmth of fellow human beings when needed, and provide a transitional bridge to the new circumstances brought about by the death of an intimate person.

In this regard, we are more alert to the fact that the positive by-products of mourning are enhanced when we allow room for expressions of anger, guilt, abandonment, even relief at times, along with the more accepted ones of privation, love, and idealization of the dead person, *de mortuis nil nisi bonum.* We are also learning that if we do not lament close upon the death of a loved one, we shall do so later on, only more discordantly. And, indeed, certain demonstrations of adolescent delinquency and significant increases in physical and emotional illness among bereaved persons have already been linked to a negligent mourning. There is the additional implication that avoiding grief is associated with rejecting it in others, a contribution of doubtful value in these days of callousness to human needs.

Two further findings are of importance. One is the phenomenon of anticipatory grief—grief which occurs even before the loss or death takes place. This can characterize the dying person as well as involved family members and professional personnel, and has functional as well as dysfunctional consequences. It is important to keep this dynamic in mind in understanding seemingly varying behaviors reported for family and health-care professionals facing the same death and dying. The second is that normal mourning, in most of us, lasts for at least 1 year after death. Even the more fortunate among us are usually bereft of support after the first month of a death. It is essential that community resources be available to mourners for at least that first year. Newly initiated widow-to-widow programs and similar enterprises are encouraging moves in this direction.

Overall, it is plain that we not truncate the grief and mourning process. The dead must die before we are able to redefine and reintegrate ourselves into life. And the greatest gift we can offer to the bereaved is to be with, not treat, them.

RESPONSES TO DEATH

The anguish of selfhood in contemplating death is not tolerable for most of us without resources, be they transcendental, inspirational, or existential. Major ways of establishing bearings with the idea of death have been religion, art, love, and intelligence. Choice has usually been determined by a confluence of such factors as life experiences, personality, cultural context, age, value-belief system, and level of threat. Unfortunately, knowledge of the specific interactive contributions of these variables is still not available to us in organized fashion. We do, however, possess glimmerings. For example, let us consider religious sentiment. Surprisingly, religious predisposition per se does not appear to be associated significantly with the strength of fear of death. Influence of cultural imprinting with respect to perception of death, at least in the United States, seems to be of a magnitude that subdues major differences in religious conviction.

An emerging datum of some salience is that the attitudes toward death of most persons reflect a kind of coexisting acceptance-avoidance orientation toward fear of death. The governing conscious response to fear of death is one of limited fear; on the fantasy level, one of ambivalence; and on the nonconscious level, one of outright aversion. This patterning appears to serve adaptational requirements, allowing us to maintain communal associations and yet organize our resources to contend with oncoming death. What is clear is that assessment of reaction to personal death must utilize a variety of outcome measures to capture differing levels of awareness. In the face of death, the human mind seemingly operates simultaneously on various levels of reality or finite provinces of meaning, each of which can be somewhat autonomous.

We are now more cognizant of the dissembling garbs with which fear of death can cloak itself. The depressed mood, insomnia, fears of loss, varying psychosomatic and psychological disturbances—all, at times, exhibit affinity to anxieties about death. In this regard, there is the suggestion of a possible tie between violent behavior and a person's ideas concerning death. Some of the violence of our times can be construed as an aggressive reaction to psychological death. An industrial society engenders feelings of impersonality in many of us. We find ourselves small cogs in a big unresponsive machine. Violence then becomes a means of revenging ourselves against a life which permits this alienation. We destroy presumably that which stands in the path of our attaining selfhood, identity. This conceptualization may have explanatory pertinence for presently prevalent intensified expressions of ethnicity—expressions which may serve as channels for conquering feelings of insignificance, i.e., symbolic death.

Violence can also be perceived as an active response to unmastered dread of death. The ideological attempt is made to transform death from an internal inevitability against which one is helpless to an external threat over which one has some control. Death is then understood as resulting essentially from the hostility of others, and violence is employed to vitiate or kill the person or institution seen as threatening injury or death. Mastery over death is gained symbolically by "killing" or "conquering" death. Additionally, violence supplies individuals with a type of ascendancy, or sense of triumph, in enabling them to decree when and under what conditions they can inflict injury, murder others, or kill themselves. Unhappily, if apathy is a retreat from life—a withdrawal from risk taking—violence is a striking out against death, an assertion of identity that devalues life even as it defies death.

We are no longer in a zealous partnership with God. The quality of sin has changed. When God and State are discerned as halting and enfeebled in punishing violence, and when the grave painfully symbolizes nothingness, the commission of violence and its meaning fall more actively into the bailiwick of self-judgment and criticism, with its potential for legitimizing violence. Herein may lie much of the irrational and absurd, so manifest and marked in the moral temper of our times.

If death were less of a stranger to us, it is conceivable that our compulsive need to extrovert fear of death and kill might be somewhat muted. Indeed, in contrasting manner, appreciation of finiteness can serve not only to enrich self-knowledge but to provide the impulse to propel us forward toward achievement and creativity. It was no less a person than Michelangelo who said, "No thought is born in me that has not 'Death' engraved upon it."

In the chapters that follow, the book's contributors bring to bear their scholarship and thinking to further advance our understanding of how death operates in and influences our lives.

REFERENCES

Ariès, P. *Western attitudes toward death: From the Middle Ages to the present.* Baltimore: Johns Hopkins, 1974.

Brim, O. G., Jr., Freeman, H. E., Levine, S., and N. A. Scotch, (Eds.) *The dying patient.* New York: Russell Sage, 1970.

Feifel, H. (Ed.) *The meaning of death.* New York: McGraw-Hill, 1959.

Feifel, H. Philosophy reconsidered. *Psychological Reports,* 1964, **15,** 415–420.

Feifel, H., and Branscomb, A. B. Who's afraid of death? *Journal of Abnormal Psychology,* 1973, **81,** 282–288.

Feifel, H. Religious conviction and fear of death among the healthy and terminally ill. *Journal for the Scientific Study of Religion,* 1974, **13,** 353–360.

Fulton, R., and Fulton, J. A psychosocial aspect of terminal care: Anticipatory grief. *OMEGA,* 1971, **2,** 91–100.

Glaser, B. G., and Strauss, A. L. *Awareness of dying.* Chicago: Aldine, 1965.

Gorer, G. *Death, grief, and mourning.* New York: Doubleday, 1965.

Jackson, E. N. *Understanding grief, its roots, dynamics and treatment.* Nashville: Abingdon, 1957.

Kastenbaum, R. Death and development through the life span. In H. Feifel (Ed.), *New meanings of death.* New York: McGraw-Hill, 1977.

Kübler-Ross, E. *On death and dying.* New York: Macmillan, 1969.

Morgenthau, H. J. Death in the nuclear age. *Commentary,* 1961, **32,** 231–234.

Parkes, C. M. *Bereavement: Studies of grief in adult life.* New York: International Universities Press, 1972.

Weisman, A. D. *On dying and denying: A psychiatric study of terminality.* New York: Behavioral Publications, 1972.

Weisman, A. D. The psychiatrist and the inexorable. In H. Feifel (Ed.), *New meanings of death,* New York: McGraw-Hill, 1977.

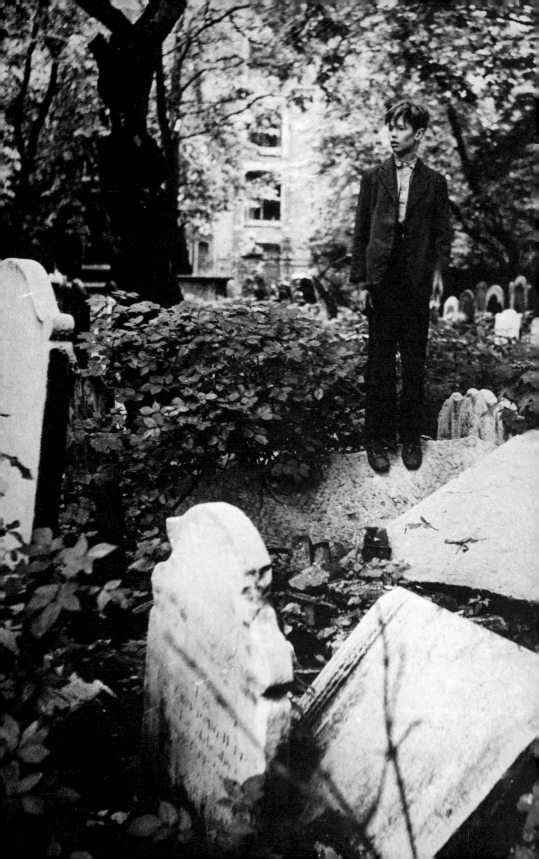

PART TWO

DEVELOPMENTAL ORIENTATIONS

2

DEATH AND DEVELOPMENT THROUGH THE LIFESPAN

ROBERT KASTENBAUM

The who-I-am that each of us knows intimately is a person in motion between points of entry and exit. Our origins are "back there," usually symbolized by the birth-event. Our terminus is "up ahead," the death-event. The fact that we are not called upon to fill out either our own birth or death certificates is a reminder that our lives are not only "bounded by a little sleep," in Shakespeare's phrase, but also bounded by public rituals that enclose our span of personal, conscious identity. None of us can remark, "Ah, I am about to begin," or, "There, I have concluded!"

We can think about beginnings and ends, then, but what we really *know* is being someplace in the middle. Fine: Let us violate most principles of organization and launch our inquiry into the relationship between death and human development in the midst of the life span.

THE MIDDLE: A GOOD PLACE TO BEGIN

Let us form in our minds the image of a person neither especially young nor especially old. This individual is in good health and has access to the basic necessities for survival. Birth and death both appear to be relatively distant points along the psychological horizon. If the person has a secret self-classification, it is probably as a youthful (if not strictly young) man or woman. But tomorrow the inner world might be transformed.

> The young man of whom I write inhabited a world that was unthinkable without him. . . . He felt a childish immortality within the day he occupied [p. 109].

This is the way Ben Hecht (1954) characterized the person he had once been.

> Neither literature nor reality awoke his sense of being mortal. His relatives began dying, friends collapsed and were shoveled into the earth, and he continued as unaware of death as if it were a language no teacher could bring to his tongue.
>
> Put beside that young man whose name and the remains of whose face I bear, I am quite a ghostly fellow. Not he who is long gone but I who still exist am more the spook. For his activities were solely part of living, mine are divided between living and dying. What he could not imagine, I think of a great deal of the time, and when it is not in my head it settles in my mood, and I can even feel it as a sudden brake on my laughter—the world without me—that strange, busy, and eerie activity from which I shall be absent [p. 109].

We cannot help but notice that this transformed person is living, mentally and emotionally, well beyond the habitation of the moment. Like the double-headed god, Janus, he is embroiled in both past and future. It is as though somebody has perished: either the young man he once had been or, as he chooses instead, something of the person he is supposed to be now. We would not be representing this man's private experience adequately if we persisted in seeing him as the "same" person who is moving in a fixed direction from birth to death. Whatever happened to that young man (as seen through the eyes of the older man) signaled a new beginning or "psychological birth" as well as a kind of death. But what did happen?

> I can recall the hour in which I lost my immortality, in which I tried on my shroud for the first time and saw how it became me. . . . The knowledge of my dying came to me when my mother died. There was more than sorrow involved. Her vanished voice echoed in my head and the love she bore me struggled painfully to stay alive around me. But my heart did not claw at the emptied space where she had stood and demand her return. I accepted death for both of us.
>
> I went and returned dry-eyed from the burial, but I brought death back with me. I had been to the edge of the world and looked over its last foot of territory into nothingness [pp. 109–110].

Just being born human and, therefore, mortal is not equivalent to the full realization of finitude. In the lives of some of us, the dawning of awareness takes on the character of both a new birth and a new death. "Farewell to innocence" might be too melodramatic a phrase, but it comes close to describing the phenomenon. A person can be as adult, worldly, and educated as a Ben Hecht and still lack the sense of his or her mortality. We are talking about more than a brittle intellectual understanding that death is inevitable. Perhaps a person does not become fully adult until death has been recognized as an authentic companion to life. Even in the middle of the life cycle, there are some of us who are well acquainted with grief and the taste of death, others whose orientation remains virginal. The difference cannot be discerned only by reference to the external events that have befallen a person but, rather, by what these events have given and taken away psychologically.

The middle-aged adult in our society has a relationship to life and death that relatively few people enjoyed in the past. He or she is more likely than his or her ancestors to have parents, grandparents, perhaps even great-grandparents, still alive. Similarly, he or she can anticipate generations of children, grandchildren, and great-grandchildren coming along during his or her life. The implications are many. The increased average life expectancy achieved during the first half of the twentieth century means that more people reach adulthood, but also that they do so with less personal experience of bereavement. A person might go a long way, then, before a life especially critical to him or her becomes the death that shocks and transfigures. This prolonged immunity to significant deaths is a phenomenon that some of us have taken for granted, unusual as it is from the historical perspective.

Furthermore, death has come to be regarded as somehow more "natural" for the elderly than for other persons. This attitude is so pervasive today that we have almost lost sight of the fact that through much of human history death was mainly the scourge of the young, and of the child-bearing woman. The shift in mortality from early to late in the life span for the general population has contributed to the constellation of thoughts, feelings, and attitudes many of us hold toward both life and death as we stand somewhere in between.

Whether or nor the reader, in company with Hecht, experiences his or her own life as "divided between living and dying," we have had enough preparation now to move through the life span in the more conventional sequence. Let us try to improve our understanding of what a person might have come through en route to middle age, and what might still lie ahead in the years as yet unexperienced.

IN CHILDHOOD'S HOUR

It is a celebration of life when a baby joins the family circle. Who wants to think of death at such a time? Yet the newcomer already has a partial biography, and even a "prehistory," in which death has played its part.

Death and Early Development

Month after month, year after year, a ripe ovum moves into position for possible fertilization. Each egg is a functional organic unit—that is to say, it is alive. But failure to advance to a new stage of development (the zygote, or fertilized egg) dooms the ovum to a few brief days of ripe existence. As a conservative estimate, more than 100 ova (potential persons, all) perish within a few days before a woman first becomes pregnant.

Spermatazoa die by the millions as short-lived potentials. The casualty rate is astronomical. Many ova and sperm perish in their states of incompletion for every pairing that results in a zygote.

The reasonable person in our culture will be swift to dismiss this wave of mortality that surrounds the occasional act of accomplished conception. After all, it is "normal." We could not accommodate ourselves to a situation in which every sperm or ovum actually became a human being. Furthermore, what dies is not a person as such, but a bit of protoplasm. We could convince each other that nothing much has happened when ovum and sperm die . . . but can it be said that no death has in fact occurred? Perhaps it is best simply to acknowledge and respect this phenomenon, and keep our values and rationalizations off to the side. The creation of a new human life does emerge from the context of *possible* life in which a vast number of potential individuals are terminated while still in their "makings."

Interpret it as we choose, life and death are close companions from the very start of our developmental career.

Psychobiological fact also undercuts our culture's tendency to emphasize the relationship between death and advanced age. The individual is at mortal risk from the moment of conception onward. True, lives that end prior to birth seldom are represented in the mortality rates that occupy computers and their tenders around the world. Although of concern to some health specialists, by and large prenatal death is not regarded as a significant social statistic. This bias draws our attention away from the actual continuous existence—and continuous risk—of the human from conception onward.

The newborn infant is already a survivor.

Hazards to life exist during the birth process itself, and the first few hours, days, weeks, and months of postnatal functioning. Each of us begins life in a state of relatively high vulnerability, and remains so for several years thereafter. Even the healthiest, most vigorous newborn depends upon consistent support from others to survive.

Early development is also accompanied by various forms of *partial death,* both physical and psychological. The umbilical cord, once a vital link to life itself, is sloughed off, dead and useless. Years later, the loss of each baby tooth is celebrated by the child as a tangible indication of growing up. But generations of tooth fairies have realized that they have the secret act of consolation to perform under cover of darkness. The coin placed beneath the pillow softens the loss both of a body part and of another link to the vanishing past of infancy and early childhood. Whether as conspicuous as the loss of a baby tooth or as subtle as the continuous supply of "fresh" dead cells to line the outer surfaces of the skin, the presence of dying-death processes accompanies the individual during his or her days of development as well as decline. Living tissues of various types develop, flourish, and die as part of the young organism's overall pattern of growth.

And one day the mother, passing along a crib and some outgrown baby clothes to a neighbor, notices her child running about, playing and shouting. She observes to herself: "There's my Big Boy: but where did my

Baby go?" This type of loss-in-the-midst-of-growth anticipates the middle-aged adult's own questing for vanished youth.

What is nostalgia, if not a mode by which the living pay homage to the personal deaths they have almost, but not quite, left behind?

The Child Discovers Death

What is the child's own orientation toward death? Here we come up against an attitude still prevalent in our culture: Children do not and, what is more, should not think of death. As adults we have the responsibility to protect our young ones from such a frightening and morbid topic—or so goes the usual reasoning. This chapter can provide little support for the parent who wants to go on believing that the normal child has little if any relationship to death, or that it is to the child's benefit when we engage in evasive maneuvers. The burden of the evidence is quite to the contrary.

Perhaps the first hurdle to get over is the assumption that children seldom think of death. Sylvia Anthony's pioneering study in England (1940; 1972) showed that death is a common topic for young minds. Subsequent experiences confirm this impression. Quite a different kind of research has revealed that the games children play and the songs and riddles they recite ring many variations on the theme of death. Games known in ancient Rome, the Middle Ages, and the Victorian age have been linked closely both with death and with the diversions of our own children (Opie and Opie, 1969). The cry, "Ashes, ashes, all fall down!" is one of the best known examples. The ring-around-the-rosies game was enacted by children who lived in the shadow of the plague hundreds of years ago. The extensive list of death-related games includes many variations on hide-and-seek. All players attempt to outwit or outfoot that person who has become "It," and whose lightest touch must be avoided. In some of its manifestations (such as "Dead Man Arise!"), the identification of "It" with a death personification could hardly be more obvious.

Sensitive observers often notice death-related themes conveyed through the speech, play, and artistic expressions of young children. Dolls die and are brought back to life. A baby sister tragically perishes in a crack-up between two matchbox cars, but the mommy, the daddy, and one's own self luckily escape without injury. A crayon drawing depicts grandmother as an angel singing in heaven (not always to the comfort of the still very-much-alive grandmother herself). A child does not have to be "morbid" or "abnormal" to think of death. Far more unusual would be the child whose curiosity has never been whetted by the mysteries of non-being and disappearance (Where did the moon go? What happened to that perfectly good ice cream bar I left out in the sun?), or the threat of separation (What if mother doesn't come back from the store?). One might have to assume that such a child has never seen a television shoot-'em-up, listened to headline news on radio, played war games with friends or toy soldiers, or looked at the "funnies" with their abundant slaughtering of "comic" characters. Furthermore, he or she never would have discovered that stamping on an ant or dismantling a worm does little by way of improvement—or even that flowers droop and petals fall.

It would be a full-time and ultimately futile job to shelter a child from death in all its manifestations, even within a society such as ours that has become famous for its virtuosity in trying to keep mortality out of sight and out of mind. Death forces itself into the child's world in many ways. The significance of a death encounter in childhood cannot be judged entirely on the basis of its outward dimensions. The demise of a pet animal, for example, can make a strong impact. "Old deaths" can evoke new thoughts and feelings, as when the child wonders about the relative whose photograph has been around the house so long, but who he or she has never met.

The death of people known and important to the child is an ever-present possibility. Each exposure opens a vast range of possible response. What happens depends to some extent upon who has died and what this person has come to mean to the child. But it also depends upon many other factors such as the circumstances that surrounded the death, how the news is communicated, how family and others behave (as distinguished from what they say), and how sensitive is the attention given to the child's several waves of thought and feeling about the loss.

Fortunately, much has been learned in recent years about the ways in which children are likely to respond when confronted with a significant death. One of the most important lessons is that early experiences with death can be associated with the life-style and problems that characterize the person many years later in adulthood. This possibility was examined by Herbert Barry (1936; 1949), whose clinical studies suggested that the death of a parent occurs with special frequency in the biography of adults who have major psychiatric problems. Numerous other studies followed, which tended to support Barry's conclusions. These studies have since been criticized on methodological grounds (e.g., Gregory, 1958). But more recent and sophisticated investigations continue to come up with the same basic conclusions. Beck et al. (1963), for example, found that depressed adults were more likely than nondepressed adults to have been orphaned during their childhood. Additionally, the degree of depression was stronger for those who had lost a parent before age 4. The significance of childhood bereavement upon adult development and behavior has since been confirmed by various observers, including the intensive case history study of Erna Furman (1974).

These studies should be interpreted properly. We cannot conclude that the death of a parent automatically condemns the child to an adult life of unusual grief and suffering. We cannot even conclude that bereavement is the most disturbing event that might occur in childhood; studies in progress on the effects of homes "broken" by divorce or seriously "bent" by marital strife could reveal important long-range effects as well. What we do learn is the significance of appreciating the impact of death upon the child well beyond the momentary shock. The boy or girl who is "taking it so well," or "doesn't seem to think about it at all," may well need more attention and support than appearances might indicate.

How best to assist the child when his or her world is invaded by the death of an important person is a question that has been explored elsewhere (e.g., Grollman, 1968). Most mental health specialists who have worked with bereaved children or their surviving parents probably would agree in general with the observations of Diane Becker and Faith Margolin (1967). After studying the ways in which surviving parents tried to help their young children after the other parent had died, Becker and Margolin were struck by the emphasis upon insulating, avoiding, and denying the finality of death. The parents discouraged questions and expressions of feeling. Becker and Margolin believe that quite the opposite course of action should be taken, based upon the child's natural curiosity about death and the need "to share memories, and to observe and share feelings with the adults in reaction to the death of a significant person."

Both the short- and the long-range effects of bereavement depend much upon the sensitivity and resourcefulness of those who remain in the child's world. This holds true for the deaths of significant people other than parents as well. What happens, for example, when a brother or sister dies? Cain and his colleagues (1964) discovered a variety of disturbed behavior patterns on the part of children who had lost a sibling through death. These included trembling, crying, and sadness, but also fear of physicians and hospitals. Some became afraid that they themselves might die at almost any time. A few suddenly appeared "stupid," did not seem to know their own age or to understand cause-and-effect relationships.

Guilt was one of the most frequent reactions, sometimes persisting for 5 years or more beyond the sibling's death.

> Such children felt responsible for the death, sporadically insisted that it was all their fault, felt they should have died, too, or should have died instead of the dead sibling. They insisted they should enjoy nothing, and deserved only the worst. Some had suicidal thoughts and impulses . . . this also being motivated by a wish to join the dead sibling. They mulled over and over the nasty things they had thought, felt, or said to the dead sibling, and became all the guiltier. They also tried to recall the good things they had done, the ways they had

protected the dead sibling, and so on [Cain, Fast, and Erickson, 1964, p. 743].

But precisely what is it that death "means" to a child? This is a significant question for its applied as well as theoretical implications. We are in a better position to support constructive patterns of personality development and help the child through difficult situations if we are well attuned to his or her characteristic ways of interpreting death-related phenomena.

In trying to determine how a particular child interprets death, we find several kinds of information useful:

Developmental level Very roughly, this can be translated into the question "How old is this child?" But rate of maturation varies considerably, and chronological age is only an approximate guide to the level of developmental functioning that has been achieved. Developmental level is an important consideration because it tends to establish the limits within which the child can comprehend *any* phenomena, whether or not related to death.

Individual personality Children as well as adults differ among themselves. Although developmental level is important, we would not want to overlook the contribution of individual personality to the child's interpretation of death. The "clinging" child and the one who is always "snoopy" and adventuresome, for example, are likely to shade the meanings of death somewhat differently. Whatever it is that makes a particular child distinctive or unique will also influence its way of interpreting death-related phenomena.

Life experiences The fact that death of a parent often is associated with problems experienced by the child later in life has already been touched upon. But many other life experiences also have the potential to bear upon the way in which the child interprets death while still a child. Prolonged separations from one or both parents, frequent changes of neighborhood by the family, illness, and many other life experiences can sensitize a child to death-related phenomena in various ways. The children of a funeral director, for example, grow up with different reference points with respect to death than do most other children. Usually we are aware only of extreme or dramatic differences in life experiences (e.g., death of a parent), but it is probable that many other life experiences also are influential in shaping the child's orientation toward death. We are not claiming that one kind of life experience is "better" than another as an influence upon death interpretations, but simply calling attention to the need for taking life experiences into account, instead of assuming that all children of a given age have taken the same view of death.

Communication and support How a child interprets death is also related to the general pattern of communication that has been established, especially with parents. It is a fortunate child who is part of a family that characteristically shares interests and concerns openly. The child who has participated in give-and-take on a variety of subjects, who knows that he or she really will be listened to, and that it is all right to say what is on his or her mind, is more likely to share death-related thoughts and feelings as well. Constructive patterns of communication and support tend to pay off in crisis situations. The family that seldom takes a child's views and sensitivities seriously will find it difficult to change its ways when all are confused and frightened in the midst of a crisis. A well-detailed example of this kind of situation is provided by the unfortunate Roscoe A., who is *Scapegoat* (Berman, 1973) of a family's inability to come to terms with death as thought or reality.

We will focus here on *developmental level* as a guide to the child's growing understanding of death. When concerned about a particular child, one would enrich the picture with knowledge of individual personality, life experiences, and the kind of communication and support that has been made available.

From the studies of Sylvia Anthony and others we know that death-related thoughts are common in childhood. Adah Maurer (1961) has argued from her observations that infants as young as 6 months of age already have an active mental orientation toward being and nonbeing. She points to the perhaps universal delight that infants take in playing "peek-a-boo" as demonstrating an attempt at mastery over forces of light and dark. From the beginning of its postnatal life, the infant alternates between waking and sleeping states as a matter of biological necessity. Soon, however, according to Maurer (1961),

> The healthy baby is ready to experiment with these contrasting states.
> . . . He replays in safe circumstances the alternate terror and delight, confirming his sense of self by risking and regaining complete consciousness. A light cloth spread over his face and body will elicit an immediate and forceful reaction. Short, sharp intakes of breath, vigorous thrashing of arms and legs removes the erstwhile shroud to reveal widely staring eyes that scan the scene with frantic alertness until they lock glances with the smiling mother, whereupon he will wriggle and laugh with joy. . . . To the empathetic observer, it is obvious that he enjoyed the temporary dimming of the light, the blotting out of the reassuring face and the suggestion of a lack of air which his own efforts enabled him to restore, his aliveness additionally confirmed by the glad greeting implicit in the eye-to-eye oneness with another human [pp. 201–202].

Close observers of infants and young children have noticed many behaviors that suggest a fondness for playing with appearances and disappearances, or comings and goings. It is not necessary to assume that very young children are thinking about death as such, or being versus non-being. It is enough to alert ourselves to the likelihood that the very young already are attuning themselves to some of the basic phenomena that eventually will become part of their mature conceptions of life and death. There is an emotional component here—the dynamics of separation and reunion. There is also a cognitive or mental component which could be of key significance for thought development in general, not just the development of death-related thoughts. Many students of human development have become interested in recent years in the earliest manifestations of mental activity, and how one stage of functioning leads to another. Probably the most influential writer on this topic has been Jean Piaget (e.g., 1954, 1972). One of the processes he has emphasized is the child's growing ability to appreciate constancy, stability. It requires much developmental progression before the child has a firm grasp of "object constancy," and can "conserve" relatively permanent features of reality. We have proposed elsewhere (Kastenbaum and Aisenberg, 1972) that to appreciate constancy requires the concomitant ability to appreciate nonconstancy. In other words, the child must interact cognitively with phenomena that vanish, go away for good, are of short or undependable duration, if it is to eventually form the concept of phenomena that are permanent and dependable no matter how or how long you look at them. Constancy has little or no meaning unless there is also the appreciation of nonconstancy. On this view, as soon as the infant or young child begins to develop a framework for interpreting reality, it is at the same time deeply involved in phenomena upon which the most abstract conceptions of both life and death are constructed. "Here-and-now," "now-and-then" (periodic phenomena), and "gone forever" are among the many distinctions the infant is just starting to master—but the start is there.

When children have developed to the point at which they can share some of their perceptions and thoughts with us through words, it is possible to learn much more about their understanding of death-related phenomena. Even a very limited vocabulary can express recognition of death. We have, for example, what appears to be a dependable report of an incident in the life of a 16-month-old boy (related by his father, a noted scientist). The youngster became alarmed when adult feet began to tread down a garden path—right toward a fuzzy caterpillar he had been watching. The foot did come down (unwittingly) upon the caterpillar. The boy studied its residue intently. Finally he said: "No more!" These two words—and the tone in which they were uttered—clearly communicated an appreciation for something of the cognitive and emotional reality of death. Incidents of this nature are reported with increasing frequency as we move up the chronological age ladder. The author has observed, firsthand, young children's encounters with death, and cannot escape the impression that they do recognize death to be "something special," even if they do not yet have all the words and thoughts to capture its meanings.

Come to think of it, wouldn't it be difficult to improve upon the 16-month-old boy's utterance if we were limited to a two-word statement? The youngster's "No more!" has a haunting similarity to the raven's message in Edgar Allan Poe's celebrated poem. The boy had not been reading Poe—more likely is the possibility that the poet retained since his own childhood the vivid impression that death, whatever else it might be, means "Nevermore." Certainly, it is common for adults to recall death-laden scenes when asked to produce an "earliest memory," or to go back to early childhood when asked to produce a death memory [see, for example, a pioneering study reported by G. Stanley Hall in his book *Senescence: The Last Half of Life* (1922)].

More detail regarding the child's gradual development of death concepts was provided by Marie Nagy's important study (1948; 1959). In this well-known investigation, she asked children ranging in age from 2 to 10 to express their thoughts in words and pictures. The findings suggested that children move through three stages of comprehension. The ages cited below are best considered as a guide, rather than a rigid set of norms:

Stage 1 (Until about age 5) There is much curiosity about death, focusing upon what becomes of the body, why the person is buried, etc. The dead are regarded as "less alive," not entirely devoid of sensation and functioning. Furthermore, the child has not firmly grasped the idea of finality. The fact of *separation* between the living and the dead does come across clearly to the child at this young age, and can be a cause of concern. Death is also seen as a state very similar to sleep.

Stage 2 (From 5 to about age 9) The child now comes to appreciate that death is *final*. This represents a big step forward in mental development—the idea that life does not go on and on just as it has been. The children interviewed by Nagy showed another interesting characteristic. They tended to think of death as a *person*. The death-person might be a frightening clown, for example, or a mysterious figure who makes his rounds in the night. Another feature of the children's death thinking at this developmental level was their belief that one could "luck out" and avoid death. Although death was seen as final, the clever or lucky person might not get caught. The personifications of death popular at this age perhaps helped children to protect themselves from the full implications of their realization that death is final. The death-person might be outwitted. In Nagy's words, at this age, "Death is still outside us and is not general."

Stage 3 (from ages 9 to 10 onward) Death now is understood not only as final, but as *inevitable* and *universal.* Everybody dies. One 10-year-old girl explained: "It is like the withering of flowers." The child realizes that mortality is a condition of life throughout the plant and animal kingdom, one's own self and loved ones not exempted.

Nagy's findings seem to have held up fairly well over the years, although in our own observations the personification tendency is not as evident. Perhaps cultural influences, always in flux, have much to do with whether or not a particular set of children selects personification as a major mode of death representation. A few other points are worth noting. Characteristics of children's thoughts and feelings about death can also be found in adolescents and adults—sometimes as playful expressions, sometimes as "slips" to a less mature level of functioning. We may add new conceptions of death to our repertoire as we mature and again new life experiences, but the earlier notions do not vanish completely.

There is an apparent conflict among different accounts of the young child's ability to appreciate death as final. Nagy's findings indicate that a firm conception of death is not achieved until age 9 or 10. Piaget has had surprisingly little to say about the child's conception of death. But his general view of mental development (buttressed by a large body of research) would seem to suggest an even later age range for the cognitive grasp of death's finality. Piaget's theory distinguishes a level of "abstract operations" (essentially, the ability to think about thought) that does not become well established until early adolescence or thereabouts. Until the person has developed these high-level mental processes, perhaps he or she cannot fully realize the finality and inevitability of death. Still again, we have the numerous observations of young children (belonging in Nagy's stage 1) who seem to recognize some of the prime characteristics of death.

These differences should not be reconciled too quickly; they suggest the need for more research, especially types of study that combine several methodologies. In the meantime, however, we suggest that what takes place is something of this nature:

Some (not all) children come to an early realization that life can become "No more!" Of these children, some also go on to the realization that death is inevitable, and will be their own personal fate. However, these realizations are achieved in a variety of concrete situations, when the child is ready for them. These are spontaneous acts of comprehension, often accomplished without the knowledge of adults. In response to direct questioning (as in a systematic study), the insight might not be forthcoming. One has to have the good fortune to be with the child when he or she is spontaneously "putting things together." Furthermore, the insights tend not to be binding or stable. This is attributable in part to the child's limited capacity to elaborate a firm conceptual network. In other words, few children possess the cognitive structure to maintain such "thunder-and-lightening" flashes of insight. But it is also likely that newly discovered death meanings seem to fade away because of their emotional impact. It is too much to live constantly with the feelings stirred up by early realizations of death. Adults have troubles enough in coming—and staying—to terms with death. Most children are likely to find the impact of death realizations too powerful to sustain in conscious thought on a thoroughgoing basis. This suggests that a child can show a keen grasp of death's essence from time to time—yet behave more typically as though death were reversible, a form of sleep, something that happens only to the aged, the wicked, or the unlucky.

We have much yet to learn about the child's discovery of death. It is likely, however, that the reality of early insights will have to be acknowledged eventually, as well as a complex and variable process through which the child works toward an adaptive network of death conceptions. The child's efforts to comprehend death are intimately related to his or her entire developmental pattern. It is by no means an exotic little sideline. Construction of reality (to use Piagetian language) requires also an appreciation of destruction, disappearance, loss, and endings. Additionally, one must appreciate *futurity,* where all that remains of our lives awaits us—but so does death. When a child's quest for understanding is disturbed, there are likely to be disturbances in the overall pattern of cognitive and personality growth. Should death take on the aura of overwhelming catastrophe (something that even big, strong adults cannot cope with or even talk about), then the child may be en route to long-standing problems in thinking about the future in general. We do not understand a child's core process of development without also understanding how he or she is progressing in comprehending the meanings of death.

"TOO YOUNG TO DIE"

"Tragic" and "untimely." These words are often used to describe the death of an adolescent or young adult. The routine use of these expressions gives us a clue to our society's ideas about the relationship between age and mortality. The young are part of society themselves, of course. This suggests that we attend both to the sociocultural and to individual-developmental orientations toward death if we hope to understand the meanings of death for young men and women. Furthermore, the actual nature and extent of death threats to the young should also be considered; otherwise, thoughts and attitudes are left floating about without clear reference points in what might loosely be called *objective reality.* We will begin with a few observations about mortal jeopardy for young adults.

Death Risks for Young Adults

The young person in the United States today has most of the statistics on his or her side in contemplating many years of life ahead. Take a 15-year-old, for example. Or, rather, take 1000 15-year-olds representing all their age peers throughout the nation. How many of these people are likely to survive at least long enough to become 16-year-olds? The statistical expectation (rounded off to the nearest whole number) is that 999 will make it. A girl of this age has only half the life-risk of the boy. On the average, only 1 girl of 2000 will fail to survive age 15, while the chances of a boy dying during his fifteenth year are slightly greater than 1 in 1000. Furthermore, the 15-year-old has an average life expectation of 57.7 years still to go. Again, the advantage is to the females (61.4 as compared with 54.1).

Let us sample the situation at a later point during the years of youth. Take age 25 now. Mortality odds remain quite favorable after a decade has passed. However, the risk of life has actually doubled throughout the intervening period. The mortality rate for all 25-year-olds is 1.5 per 1000, almost twice the rate for 15-year-olds. Females preserve their advantage. In fact, the discrepancy in mortality rates increases. At age 25, a male's probability of death during this year is double what it was at age 15, while a female's death probability has increased by only 58 percent over its former value. The long-term outlook remains good for both sexes. The hypothetical "average" 25-year old has 48.4 years ahead (females, 51.8; males, 45.1).[1]

Statistics such as these make some very obvious points:

1.   Youth, in the contemporary United States, is a period of time during which the expectation of death is rather low. (We are concerned here with the *objective* expectation, not individual interpretations of their prospects for survival.)

2.   Nevertheless, there *is* a mortality rate even at these favored ages. Statistics relentlessly inform us that some deaths must be expected among the young each year.

3.   The sex differences in mortality risk are clear-cut and consistent.

4.   The mortality risk increases appreciably within the limited age range of the young, even though it remains relatively low throughout.

The 15-year-old and the 25-year-old, then, although both "young," occupy somewhat different positions of life-risk, as do males and females at both points in time.

---

[1] These figures have been derived from information presented in Metropolitan Life's *Statistical Bulletin,* April 1975.

Death comes by many routes to the young, as to people at any age. However, two causes of death consistently show up as most frequent: accidents and suicide. Automobile accidents regularly head the list of fatalities in this age range. This fact introduces the realization that the leading cause of death among young Americans involves a behavioral-environmental interaction, rather than a biological disease hazard. This realization is intensified when we consider that suicide claims approximately another 4000 lives of those in the 15 to 24 age range every year (Cantor, 1975). Subtract automobile fatalities and suicide from the total, and the odds for survival among the young would increase markedly.

The statistical picture, although significant on its own terms, fades into the background when a particular young person dies, or is faced with terminal illness. Young men and women do suffer fatal heart attacks or contract life-threatening diseases. These "low incidence" occurrences often are of high impact, not only upon the afflicted individual but also upon those around him or her. Professionals in the health field frequently experience personal distress when called upon to care for a person who is "too young to die." Sympathy for the dying person may be intensified by the nurse's or doctor's partial identification with the patient. How many young student nurses, for example, have been "shook up" by encounters with attractive people of their own age who were losing the battle for life?

With these background considerations in mind, let us turn to the ways in which the young person and society relate to death at this developmental level.

Death Interpretations: Individual and Social

The adolescent and young adult are no longer limited to the relatively concrete thought operations of the child. Flights of abstract and imaginative thought are within the individual's power. Concepts of time, space, causality and, in short, all the basic ideas associated with a fully developed *mental apparatus* are in the possession of most people by the time they have entered well into adolescence. This, at least, is the picture suggested by the bulk of research and theory in mental development. It is consistent with the fact that many of the most remarkable achievements in science, mathematics, and the arts have been contributed by men and women in their twenties and thereabouts. This suggests that a young adult is as well equipped as anybody to understand death. An individual with subpar intelligence may not grasp some of the concepts necessary to understand death at any age. But at this age level it does seem reasonable to expect that a person of normal intelligence will have a well-formed set of ideas concerning the nature of death.

Nevertheless, there are important differences among young people in their death-related thoughts and attitudes. Personality or life-style differences are important here, as they were in childhood. Additionally, it is likely that young men and women differ in some ways in their orientations toward death, the woman's potential role as mother influencing her life-death relationship differently than the young man's potential role as father. (This impression, however, runs far ahead of the available data.)

Personality and sex differences are both influenced by cultural and subcultural patterns. It is not necessary for a cultural pattern to be intrinsically death-oriented for it to exercise an effect upon the individual's relationship to mortality. An important example is our society's encouragement of risk-taking behavior among men, especially the young. Anthropological observations could be used to make a case that young men tend to be high risk takers in most if not all cultures. Yet there seems to be an especially lethal interaction in our own society between cultural incitements for young men to "prove" themselves and the means that are popular and available for these activities. Hazardous use of automobiles, drugs, alcohol, and unnecessary risks in athletic competition are among the modalities of life-threatening behavior encouraged by the attempt to establish that one is not "chicken," and can do all that is expected to demonstrate masculine prowess (e.g., Haddon, Suchman and Klein, 1964; Kastenbaum and Aisenberg, 1972). As more young women move into activities previously dominated by men, there is at least the prospect for an increase in injury and death related to this risk-taking orientation.

Cultural attitudes toward war and violence also have considerable impact upon young adults. The person old enough to read these words will have registered some of the turmoil and conflict attendant upon this nation's involvement in Southeast Asia. Crimes of violence in our own cities have been another source of widespread concern over the past several decades. Young men often are the central figures in violent death, whether as "cannon fodder," to use the cynical term of an earlier generation, or as both perpetrators and victims of homicide. Thoughts about death among young adults have always been influenced by the prevailing cultural climate, including the peace-war status. Each new wave of young people therefore will have somewhat different orientations toward life and death, depending upon the particular form in which cultural violence has displayed itself. Even within the same generation, individual differences can be found in the response to the same life threats. Over the past few years there has been an obvious (if shifting) division in our society between war "hawks" and "doves." Actually, close inspection of response to previous wars will also reveal appreciable differences among the people most directly affected as well as the stay-at-homes. Even in our most "popular" wars, there have been some young people whose hearts and minds were not given over to bloodshed, and even in the most dubious military involvements, there have been some who could accept their roles without hesitation. Indeed, the fact that a person has experienced combat hazards does not in itself guarantee a "standard" orientation toward death. Many veterans of combat in Southeast Asia are still attempting to integrate these experiences with the life and death orientations they brought with them as young civilians.

Individual differences in death relationships within the same generation of youths can be demonstrated in a variety of ways. It is tempting to suppose, for example, that young adults will have much in common regarding their future outlooks because so much of their lives still lies ahead. When studies of time perspective are conducted, however, we discover major differences at the same age level, not only in *how* young people think of the future but in *how much* future they consider themselves to have. One such study combined time-perspective techniques with a "do-it-yourself death certificate" (Sabatini and Kastenbaum, 1973). Among other findings, it was evident that proportion of life remaining differed markedly within a population of college students. Just knowing that a person was of the current college generation therefore would not enable us to predict reliably that he or she envisioned death to be many decades away. These differences in subjective life expectancy have important implications. If we wish to understand differences in behavior and life-style between one young person and another, it might not be a bad idea to learn how they conceptualize futurity and death. The person who feels his or her life will end abruptly within a few years is likely to be on a different footing from the age peer who expects half a century or more to elapse before death must be faced as a personal issue.

We find differences again when (in the same study cited above) people are asked to indicate both how long they *expect* and how long they *prefer* to live. Three different orientations appear: those who are satisfied with the number of years they think they have coming, those who yearn for a longer life, and those who would prefer to die before their "time is up." We do not have to assume that every person has the identical reason for holding his or her particular orientation, or that this outlook necessarily will remain constant. Nevertheless, the ever-present minority of young people who express a preference for dying ahead of time require understanding on their own terms, and ought not simply be lumped with all in their age group when we feel like making generalizations. Similarly, when one young person accepts and another seeks to expand subjective life expectancy, we have another situation that invites our interest.

Still another dimension is revealed when we focus upon young people who have known the hard life of deprivation, discrimination, and economic insecurity (Teahan and Kastenbaum, 1970). Young adults regarded as representatives of the "hard-core unemployed" in a major metropolitan area were interviewed in depth, and their experiences in a new employment situation followed. One of the most striking findings was the common expectation for early and, frequently, violent death. As it turned out, those with the most constricted future outlooks (expecting a short, miserable life ending in violent death) were the least likely to hold on to the new jobs. The limited future outlook of the group in general seemed to be more characteristic of depressed elderly than "normal" young adults (except for expectation of violent modes of death). By 20 or 30 years of age, a person has already registered enough life experience to have developed a characteristic way of anticipating futurity and death. And it seems probable, as the studies cited here suggest, that characteristic ways of relating to futurity and death are also related to important patterns of behavior and decision making.

There is much more to the young person's relationship to death than we have been able to mention here. But it is time to move on—back to the middle of life, which was our beginning.

"RIPE IN YEARS"

Clichés about age are not limited to the young, of course; they follow us throughout the entire life span. One of the more sanguine clichés has it that "life begins at 40." This is actually a rather provocative statement. Historical fact would urge the opposite conclusion: life had *ended* by 40 for most men and women in societies previous to our own. If, then, there is something special about entering the fourth decade, this has been denied to most humans and is a rare privilege for us.

But what, if anything, is "special"? Probably the cliché centers around the idea that the experienced adult knows a lot more about life than he or she did in the flush of youth. The adult "knows his or her way around." For people who have made good use of their youthful experiences and remained physically vigorous, the cliché might be simply a fair description of their actual status. Perhaps, however, the cliché cuts deeper. Perhaps the person by midlife not only "knows," but "*really* knows." Assuming that the individual has actually *developed* and not simply put on years, this might be a new phase of enlightenment and perspective. Our own society seems to have very mixed expectations for the adult in midlife and after. A "purer" example of developmental expectations for the adult can be seen in the classical view of the life span within the Hindu tradition, still in evidence today within certain realms (Maduro, 1974). Youth was fine, but now a person is ready to become truly creative and establish a deeper relationship with the universe.

Appreciation of life's finitude might well be a core aspect of the adult's ripening. Although this appreciation comes relatively early for some individuals and, for others, late if at all, it could be that psychologically a person enters the second half of life *whenever* that appreciation is attained. Often this does occur during the middle years. The experience shared by Ben Hecht (1954) is not uncommon, although his gift of expression is distinctive. The youth "knows about" death; the older adult is more likely to sense death as intimate companion to his or her life, an intimacy that increases with the years.

There is a tradition in philosophical psychology (or, if you prefer, psychological philosophy) that argues that one *must* appreciate death keenly if one is also to appreciate life to the fullest extent. Freud (1915) is among those who have made this kind of observation. It is a proposition that does not lend itself easily to scientific investigation. Nevertheless, it does challenge our perspective and awareness. *"Maturity,"* whatever else it might mean, seems to imply a worked-out relationship to both life and death, and on both intellectual and emotional levels.

Death Sensitivity in Midlife

The adult of middle years continues to experience and cope with life in ways that have become characteristic of him or her through previous development. This, at least, is a reasonably safe general rule. But there are some background considerations that operate upon the sensitivities of most middle-aged men and women in our society.

More people now have both children and parents alive than ever before in history. But this fortunate circumstance is not without its psychological complications; it is one of the reasons why the individual's first personally relevant or disturbing death is not encountered until midlife. As a parent, the middle-aged individual is more apt to be stunned and disorganized today, should his or her child die: children are not supposed to die in these modern times. And as a child, this same middle-aged individual may find himself or herself unprepared for the death of his or her own parent. It had to come, of course—but longevity also has a way of fostering expectations that things will stay the same, parents will never die. The bare fact that the parent has lived *this* long sometimes provides psychological insulation from recognition of the eventual mortal move.

What happens when a middle-aged person loses a parent? This question has been relatively neglected, when compared with the attention given to the impact of parental bereavement upon young children. In general, our society does not encourage either an intensive display of grief or a prolonged period of mourning. This seems to be especially the case when the deceased is "only" and old person whose "time had come" anyway. But for the particular individual who is struck by the bereavement, the central fact may still be that it is his or her own mother or father who has died. It is a "big" death to this survivor, if to nobody else; yet society does not seem to understand or tolerate this feeling. The middle-aged parentally bereaved person therefore can find himself or herself in an isolated situation, under social pressure (and perhaps introjected personal pressure) to deny the significance of the loss.

Other dynamics are also possible, often combining in the same situation. Even though a full-fledged adult by external standards, a particular middle-aged person might still view himself or herself as subject to parental authority or domination. For years, there may have been the yearning to be free of this domination. The death of the parent can then arouse conflicting feelings of guilt and liberation—with still other powerful affects to follow when the individual discovers what it is like to function without the protective if constricting influence of the parent.

Death of a parent can also impel the middle-aged adult to cling more tenaciously to other people, often spouse and children. "How can you think of leaving me now?" This can be either the direct or the indirect message given by a bereaved parent when his or her own child prepares to leave home for marriage, college, or other reasons. What one might suppose would be taken in stride—the expected death of an old person—can have a strong impact not only upon the most immediate survivors, then, but also upon a larger network of individuals of all ages. Of course, the supposition that the death should be taken in stride would be but another example of an overly rational approach to death attitudes.

One other dynamic should be mentioned in this regard. The important people in our lives have differential life expectancies; i.e., some will live longer than others from this moment onward. We do not usually think about this explicitly, but most people can bring their own assumptions or expectations to mind when given the opportunity to do so. Using a procedure dubbed the "pecking order of death," it has been possible to obtain many clues to the private arrangements we make with death (Kastenbaum, in press). One of the most obvious findings relates to age. Most people anticipate that the oldest of their important people will be the first to die. This to-be-expected result is accompanied by some significant resonations. For example, there tends to be a sense of "rightness" about the sequence of expected demise. The individual really does not want anybody to die. But it is right for the oldest person to die first.

Although this death would be mourned, it would also be a source of (semisecret) comfort. The fact that Death calls the person "first in line" shows that It is playing the game fairly, faithful to the unwritten rules. The death of an old person can help to support the survivor's belief that a kind of rationality prevails. One's own turn will not be coming up for a while.

The situation is even more complicated, however. The death that comforts to some extent (because it is expected) also serves to reduce the distance between the survivor and his own moment of reckoning. Some people recognize that they have "added" other old or vulnerable people to their personal life-space after the oldest person in their lives had, in fact, died. This helped them to maintain a safe psychological distance between themselves and personal death.

These are just some of the inside-ourselves maneuvers that seem to become more frequent in midlife. We are seldom aware of these maneuvers, but can improve our self-knowledge with effort. The increasing intrusion of death, both in reality and in prospect, challenges the middle-aged person's ability to come up with psychological strategies for coping with the threat. It is questionable that investigators of death and development have enough knowledge yet to proclaim that one particular strategy is "normal" and another "abnormal." We are still early in the process of discovering how people do meet the emerging challenges of death in midlife with their cognitive, emotional, and social resources. It is possible, however, to form some idea of the relative value of these strategies by observing their consequences for the individuals who have used them.

The sensitivities of the person at midlife almost certainly are affected by knowledge that death is no longer uncommon at this age, as it had been when the individual was a youth. Examination of the mortality charts would disclose to him or her that the mortality rate has increased markedly, and will continue to do so. The chances of dying during one's forties are approximately twice as great as a decade previously, and will double again during the fifties. But a person does not have to be conversant with the broad statistical trends to recognize that friends, relatives, and colleagues in his or her own age group are starting to fall away. This phenomenon is not likely to increase one's sense of security. The person who has already developed a mature outlook on life and death may still have to adapt himself or herself to such disturbing observations. The stress is likely to be even more severe for the person who has managed to avoid mental-emotional confrontations with death until this time by reliance upon brittle defenses.

Another major source of stress derives from our society's emphatic preference for youth over age. As an "in-betweener," the midlife adult may anxiously interpret characteristic changes with age as signs that he or she is going downhill. Growing older is akin to growing deader in the minds and feelings of many of us. Two of the most obvious dimensions will be sufficient to illustrate this process. A woman might have developed much of her self-image around her "looks." Now she is alarmed that her looks are starting to "fade"—and that she is fading right along with them.

In its full-blown manifestation, this anxiety over physical changes in appearance resembles the desperation of the dying. "Heroic measures" may be undertaken to halt or reverse the process, or the individual might instead succumb to depression and resignation. She cannot bear to experience the partial death of the self that she has been nurturing for so long.

A parallel experience might be the fate of the man who has built much of his self-identity around exceptional physical prowess. A. E. Housman addressed a poignant poem "To an Athlete, Dying Young." But many athletes die young without benefit of death certificates. Although still in outstanding shape when compared with the general population, they cannot continue to compete successfully with other top athletes. The pitcher with a "dead arm" is simply an obvious and extreme example of the man who must come to terms somehow with the loss of a significant functional dimension of his total self. As a man or woman moves through the midlife period, many types of personally significant loss either afflict or threaten to afflict, some obvious, some quite subtle. Although still many years away from final cessation, the individual may already be experiencing losses that arouse intimations of mortality.

Some people do survive their own partial deaths. Many of us know a "lovely young thing" who blossomed into an even more complete and compelling person, or a "jock" who found the opportunity to develop his other resources only after paying last respects to his first profession. One of the midlife challenges encountered by many individuals is the need to replace or supplement who-I-have-been with who-I-am-still-becoming. Depending upon the person, this can be either a drastic or a reasonably harmonious transition. But this is the period in which a sort of *developmental death* seems to occur with the greatest frequency. The person holds on desperately to a youthful version of the self (or the image of same), and thereby impedes development of valuable new dimensions. This can be likened to a refusal to bury the dead. Or the person "buries the dead," and crawls in the grave along with the corpse. "That part of my life is over, and so I am over, too." This type of response does much to earn the middle years a reputation for dullness and stagnation. Continued development throughout the adult years is the alternative most of us would probably wish for ourselves and those we care about. Life span developmental psychologists are beginning to learn that perpetual development does indeed take place in the lives of some individuals, even if we do not yet know precisely why.

The main point here is that physical death has an important set of analogs in the psychological and symbolic spheres (Kastenbaum and Aisenberg, 1972). In the middle years of life many of us have to chart our own ways through deaths, near-deaths, and "rebirths" of the self.

Death Sensitivity in Old Age

One of the obstacles to understanding death sensitivity in old age is the fact that many people are supersensitive to being classified as "old" in the first place. There is ample reason for some sensitivity here. "Old" tends to be used as a put-down term in our society. It is a negative value judgment, then, mixed in with a straightforward classification. But is the classification really so straightforward? No, not really. For various purposes of convenience, "old" has been defined at certain chronological age levels. Age 65 is the most common point, but there are medical programs that consider a patient of 60 to be "geriatric," and population statisticians who argue that 75 is a more appropriate beginning point. The situation becomes even more complex when we move beyond chronological age and look instead at functional status. People have known for a long time, out of common sense, that one might be "old" at 40, another "young" at 80. Recent studies in gerontology tend to support this view (e.g., *International Journal of Aging & Human Development,* 1972). Much of what passes as the "natural" impairments of old age should be attributed instead to specific pathological processes that might be prevented or alleviated (Birren, Butler, Greenhouse, Sokoloff, and Yarrow, 1963).

Nevertheless, whatever cutoff points or language we choose to employ, it is fairly clear that the quality of life changes for many people with advancing age. Taking 65 as its arbitrary point, the Bureau of the Census reports that there are approximately 21,800,000 elders in the United States, more than 10 percent of the total population. Both the absolute number and the proportion of elders in the population are increasing. Women surviving into the later years of their lives already outnumber men by a considerable margin (12.8 to 9.0 million), and this differential will become even greater in the years ahead. By the end of the present decade it is anticipated there will be about 24.5 million elders in the United States, with women having an edge of 4.7 million.

Another basic fact about the older segment of our population is the prevalence of marital bereavement. One man in six is widowed, a rather high proportion. But much higher is the frequency of widowhood among women. About half of the women over the age of 65 today are widows. Although males do tend to die at an earlier age than females, the man who survives his wife is more likely to remarry than the woman who survives her husband. As we might expect, the older echelons within this population have an even higher prevalence of widowhood. Two-thirds of the women over 75, for example, are widowed.

Old age is that time of life, then, in which the familiar phrase "till death us do part" becomes a sharp-edged, insistent theme. Death takes one partner. The other is left to mourn, to get on with life as best as possible, and to contemplate his or her own eventual death. Furthermore, the deaths of the aged—as well as the deaths of everybody else—increasingly are taking place in institutional settings, usually hospitals or nursing homes. Add to this picture the well-known mobility of our society. Family members move here and there, taking advantage of opportunities to pursue their own life-styles. One major consequence of factors such as these is the fear—and sometimes the reality—of dying among strangers in a strange place.

Death intensifies the loneliness of the old person. The longer one lives, the more intimate companions one also outlives. The psychological implications can only be alluded to here: the reawakening of anxieties about separation and loss that have remained with an individual since early childhood, the fear that the few people still remaining in one's life may also be taken by death, the reduction in psychosocial support because many who knew and loved the old person are no longer on the scene, the concern that one might now be a burden on other people who have their own problems, instead of being strongly integrated into an effective kinship network. "I don't want to be a burden—on anybody!", many an elderly person has said. But the same person sometimes admits to himself or herself that "I don't want to be abandoned either!" Somewhat apart from the prospect of one's own death, then, the falling away of significant others is a powerful influence upon the thoughts, feelings, and actions of old people.

The old person who would prefer not to burden others may himself or herself be heavily burdened. The sorrow of bereavement can be experienced by both young and old. Under even the most favorable circumstances, it is usually a long and painful process. The old person is in particular jeopardy, however. He or she is likely to experience more bereavements (e.g., death of spouse). Before he or she has been able to "work through" the death of one loved person, another may also die.[2] Furthermore, there is less opportunity to find distraction through work or travel. Mandatory retirement, age bias in hiring, and the financial troubles afflicting many older people are among the factors here. Still again, both the physical and the psychological consequences of grief can be especially hard on the old person. Loss of appetite, insomnia, depression, and other common components of the grief response can have serious consequences for a person who is already growing enfeebled, who suffers from age-related health problems, who lacks the energy reserves of youth. It is for reasons such as these that we now speak of *bereavement overload* (Kastenbaum, 1969).

---

[2] In the author's opinion, it is questionable that a person ever truly "works through" the death of a loved one, although many people do "get on with life" and cover their wounds.

The *aging process* is sometimes blamed for all miseries that beset the old person. But, when we look closer, a host of specific stress and deprivation factors can be identified. The vulnerability to bereavement in the later years of life is among the most significant of these factors. Overloaded by grief, anybody would be likely to appear weary, grim, and withdrawn. Greater sensitivity to the burden of sorrow carried by many old people would be an improvement over the present tendency to dismiss all their problems as inevitable consequences of advanced age.

Personal mortality does not necessarily intimidate the old person. Studies reviewed by Munnichs (1966) suggest that many elders come to reasonable terms with their own finitude. This impression seems to be confirmed by most subsequent studies and clinical experiences. In one of our own clinical projects, only a few geriatric patients appeared obviously disturbed by death over a period of time, and these were people who were disorganized and alarmed in all spheres of functioning (Weisman and Kastenbaum, 1968). Most of the chronically ill elders in this study showed awareness of their situation, although they differed appreciably in their modes of adaptation. It was just as common for an old person whose death was in prospect to remain active as it was to withdraw and bring his or her affairs into final order. Both patterns usually were accompanied by clear awareness of impending death; different people selected different ways of living in the valley of the shadow.

Old people have many practical reasons to think about death. This sometimes is not appreciated by the younger people in their lives (including middle-aged children) who react as though *any* talk about death is "morbid" and distasteful. The old person may be concerned about the best way to distribute personal possessions to the survivors, about arranging for the type of funeral and burial or cremation that suits his or her value system, and about "saying goodbye" in a way that strengthens long affections and heals or resolves old hurts. Younger people sometimes are apprehensive that once an old person starts talking about death, there will be no stopping him or her. This is not usually the case. Death is a realistic concern of the old person, and he or she has a need to share his or her thoughts and feelings on this topic. After the opportunity to speak his or her mind and to entertain a relevant response, the old person is likely to go on to other topics, returning from time to time to death when there is something further to be said. *Obsession* with death is more likely to develop when there is nobody around who is willing to listen attentively to even a little "death talk."

The oldest Americans today are not only more numerous than in the past, but also, in general, healthier, better educated, and more aware of their rights. They are not less capable of contributing to society than younger people. Our emphasis here upon the old person's sensitivity to death is not meant to portray our senior generations as tottering on the edge of the grave. Indeed, many of our social institutions are having difficulty in keeping up with the vitality and innovations of lively people in their sixties, seventies, and beyond. Nevertheless, we do not really enter into the developmental situation of the older person unless we are willing to consider his or her relationship to death. Even the youngest reader of this page is likely to become an old-timer eventually, and to cherish the days remaining. A mature appreciation of death will illuminate both old age itself and the decades that many of us will pass through en route to that developmental destination.

THE DESTINATION AND THE GETTING THERE

Some of us glory in taking life day by day. Others of us interpret each hour's markings in terms of a long-range framework or outcome. Our personal styles have much to do with what both life and death mean to us, as perhaps this chapter has indicated. Yet certain basic conditions of life tend to affect us all, whether we are present-, past-, or future-oriented. These conditions include the general attitudes and the hazards to life that are prevalent in our culture. The constantly changing characteristics of our own physical and psychosocial selves interact with cultural forces from life's inception through its cessation.

What we hope to have conveyed on these pages is an empirically informed view of life's relationship to death throughout the entire life span. There is much more to be said on this topic, and meanings and facts both require periodic monitoring as time goes on. One of our key concerns has been to indicate that death is one of the central themes in human development throughout the life span. Death is not just our destination; it is a part of our "getting there" as well. Death-relevant thoughts, experiences, and circumstances always accompany us. Many educators persist in touching upon death as though it were a special property of the aged. This approach both distorts the total life situation of the old person (which is not totally absorbed in death by any means) and introduces a false sense of insulation around earlier phases of the life span.

The particular kind of "destination" that death might be for an individual also deserves serious consideration (Kastenbaum, in press,). Both the individual's interpretation of death and the specific circumstances under which it eventually occurs are likely to influence the nature of death-as-destination. Furthermore, our ideas about this destination may change appreciably during the course of our maturation and life experiences. It might be useful to remind ourselves that a person does not have to regard death as destination at all! The outcome of a fully actualized life perhaps is that fully actualized life itself. The life has an end point, to be sure. But that is quite a different emphasis from focusing upon the death itself as destination, negation, or culmination of the developed self.

In our own experience, we have been most impressed with the kind of person who seems to live fully within both the moment and the life span. The life-death counterpoint enriches this person, whether young, middle-aged, or elderly. The "destination" and the "getting there" are integrated into the individual's total relationship with life and death. Perhaps this is a worthwhile model not only for those of us who seek to understand the relationships between death and development, but also for the person who wants to "take himself along" throughout the long journey of human identity through the life span.

REFERENCES

Anthony, S. *The child's discovery of death.* London: Routledge, 1940.

Anthony, S. *The discovery of death in childhood and after.* New York: Basic Books, 1972.

Barry, H. Orphanhood as a factor in psychosis. *Journal of Abnormal and Social Psychology*, 1936, **36**, 431–438.

Barry, H. Significance of maternal bereavement before the age of eight in psychiatric patients. *Archives of Neurology and Psychiatry*, 1949, **62**, 630–637.

Beck, A., Sethi, B., and Tuthil, R. Childhood bereavement and adult depression. *Archives of General Psychiatry*, 1963, **9**, 295–302.

Becker, D., and Margolin, F. How surviving parents handled their young children's adaptations to the crisis of loss. *American Journal of Orthopsychiatry*, 1967, **37**, 753–757.

Berman, E. *Scapegoat.* Ann Arbor: University of Michigan Press, 1973.

Birren, J. E., Butler, R. N., Greenhouse, S. W., Sokoloff, L., and Yarrow, M. R. (Eds.) *Human aging: A biological and behavioral study.* Washington, D.C.: U.S. Government Printing Office, Publication No. (HSM) 71–9051, 1963.

Cain, A. C., Fast, I., and Erickson, M. E. Children's disturbed reactions to the death of a sibling. *American Journal of Orthopsychiatry*, 1964, **34**, 741–752.

Cantor, P. The effects of youthful suicide on the family. *Psychiatric Opinion*, 1975, **12**, 6–13.

Freud, S. Thoughts for the times on war and death (1915). In *Collected Papers* (vol. IV), London: Hogarth, 1953, pp. 153–172.

Furman, E., *A child's parent dies.* New Haven: Yale, 1974.

Gregory, I. Studies of parental deprivation in psychiatric patients. *American Journal of Psychiatry*, 1958, **115**, 432–442.

Grollman, E. (Ed.) *Explaining death to children.* Boston, Beacon Press, 1968.

Haddon, W., Suchman, E. A., and Klein, D. *Accident research.* New York: Harper & Row, 1964.

Hall, G. S. *Senescence: The last half of life.* New York: D. Appleton & Co., 1922; reprinted: New York Arno, 1972.

Hecht, B. *A child of the century.* New York: Simon & Schuster, 1954; reprinted: New York: Ballantine Books, 1970.

International Journal of Aging and Human Development. Functional age. 1972, **3,** (2) (whole issue; various authors).

Kastenbaum, R. Death and bereavement in later life. In A. H. Kutscher (Ed.), *Death and bereavement.* Springfield, Ill.: Charles C Thomas, 1969. Pp. 28–54.

Kastenbaum, R. Is death a life crisis? In N. Datan and L. Ginsberg (Eds.), *Life-span developmental psychology: Normative crises and interventions.* New York: Academic, in press.

Kastenbaum, R., and Aisenberg, R. B. *The psychology of death.* New York: Springer, 1972.

Maduro, R. Artistic creativity and aging in India. *International Journal of Aging and Human Development,* 1974, **5,** 303–330.

Maurer, A. The child's knowledge of non-existence. *Journal of Existential Psychiatry,* 1961, **2,** 193–212.

Munnichs, J. M. A. *Old age and finitude.* Basel, Switzerland: S. Karger, 1966.

Nagy, M. The child's view of death (1948). Reprinted in H. Feifel (Ed.), *The meaning of death.* New York: McGraw-Hill, 1959, 79–98.

Opie, I., and Opie, P. *Children's games in street and playground.* London: Oxford, 1969.

Piaget, J. *The construction of reality in the child.* New York: Basic Books, 1954.

Piaget, J. *The child and reality.* New York: Basic Books, 1972.

Sabatini, P., and Kastenbaum, R. The do-it-yourself death certificate as a research technique. *Life Threatening Behavior,* 1973, **2,** 20–32.

Statistical Bulletin (Metropolitan Life). Expectation of life in the United States at new high. April 1975, **56,** 8–10.

Teahan, J., and Kastenbaum, R. Future time perspective and subjective life-expectancy in "hard core unemployed" men. *Omega,* 1970, **1,** 189–200.

Weisman, A. D., and Kastenbaum, R. *The psychological autopsy: A study of the terminal phase of life.* New York: Behavioral Publications, 1968 (*Community Mental Health Journal* Monograph 4).

3

MEANINGS OF DEATH TO CHILDREN

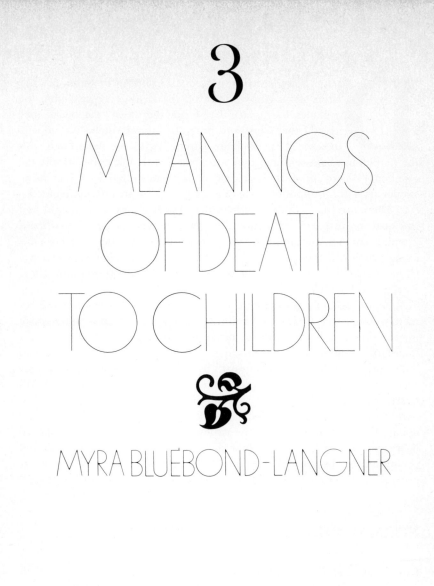

MYRA BLUEBOND-LANGNER

Death is very much a part of the fantasy thoughts of children. It is also a part of children's everyday life—the games they play, the stories they hear, the books they read, the television programs they watch, the movies they see. Yet American parents today are more open with their children about sex than they are about death and dying. While the question "Where did I come from?" is being answered with increasing candor its natural opposite "Where am I going?" is steadfastly avoided.

There are times, however, when the subject of death in general and this question in particular cannot be ignored—when a pet dies, when a grandparent dies, and, most tragically, when the child himself or herself is dying. Ironically, these are the times when the greatest efforts are expended to shield children from the facts of death and dying (Grollman, 1967; Karon and Vernick, 1968).

As with sex, efforts to dismiss or evade a child's questions about death merely compound the trauma. Failing to provide the child with adequate information leaves the child to puzzle out the mysteries of death on a foundation of ignorance and confusion. Adult avoidance of the subject can only lead the child to interpret death as a most terrible, awful, and fearsome event. The problem before us then is how to deal with the child's questions about death without creating more problems for the child or for ourselves, who are often equally troubled by the subjects of death and dying. This chapter examines the various meanings of death to children. More specifically, it considers how the concepts of death are formed and communicated by normal as well as terminally ill children, and suggests general guidelines for talking to children about death.

NORMAL CHILDREN AND DEATH

Researchers agree that age is an important factor to be considered in assessing a child's understanding of death. How important a factor it is, and in what sense it is important, is open for discussion.

For some time Maria Nagy's research (1959) on children's views of death was accepted without question. Many supported her proposal that a child's ideas about death are formed between the ages of 2 and 9 (Jackson, 1965; Kliman, 1968; Cook, 1973; Zeligs, 1974). Nagy argued that the child's ideas of death develop in three stages. Each stage is marked by a different view of death and correlates with a particular biological stage of development.

The child who is less than five years of age does not recognize death as an irreversible fact; in death he sees life. Between the ages of five and nine, death is most often personified and thought of as a contingency. Only at the age of nine and later does he begin to view death as a process which happens to us according to certain laws [pp. 80–81].

Children under 6 years of age view death as a "type of departure or sleep." Life continues, only under changed circumstances. The deceased eat, breathe, think, and feel, only in the confines of the coffin. Nagy feels such statements indicate that children under the age of 6 do not recognize death as final. Death is simply a type of separation.

By the time children reach the age of 7 they see death as an irreversible but not necessarily inevitable process, at least as far as they themselves are concerned. Death exists, but remains remote. Children either imagine death as a separate personality or identify it with the dead.

It is only when children reach the age of 9 or 10 that they conceive of death as both an inevitable and an irreversible process. Death is part of the life cycle of all living organisms, including their own.

Some scholars have questioned the universality and universal application of Nagy's findings to children of all cultures, pointing out that her analysis was based on the study of postwar Hungarian children. Grollman (1967), for example, suggests that future investigators consider the role of social, economic, and cultural background in children's concepts of death and dying. The research of McIntire, Angle, and Struempler (1972), Rochlin (1967), and Schilder and Wechsler (1934) bears out Grollman's concern.

McIntire et al. (1972) found that unlike Hungarian children, American children tend to "cast aside fantasy" and focus on "organic decomposition" as early as age 5 and in some cases as early as age 3. Also the personifications of death which dominate the descriptions of death given by Hungarian children between the ages of 5 and 9 rarely appear in those given by American children of the same age (McIntire et al., 1972; Schilder and Wechsler, 1934).

The work of McIntire et al. and Rochlin demonstrates the need to examine variations within cultural groups. While children from lower socioeconomic groups are more likely to cite "violence as the general and specific cause of death," middle-class children are more likely to cite "disease and old age" as the general cause, and the "arrest of vital functions" as the specific cause of death. These variations apparently reflect differences in the experiences of the children. Children from lower socioeconomic backgrounds have "repeated exposure to death and chronic illness," whereas middle-class children are more familiar with "all of the death delaying tactics of modern medicine."

While differing in no essential way from Nagy's model, Kastenbaum and Aisenberg (1972) assert that any model of children's views of death, regardless of how many variables it considers significant, should begin with the period shortly after birth, not as late as age 3. They state that "highly abstract and well verbalized expressions are beyond the toddler's range," but that does not mean that the child has no ideas about death, about "nonbeing." The work of Adah Maurer (1966) also indicates that "there are many ways by which the young mind can enter into a relationship with death." As we have seen in other areas of cognitive research with children, for example, religious concepts, sexual awareness, language acquisition, grave interpretive errors can be made when the investigator attributes meanings to children's behaviors on the basis of adult understandings, or when he or she assumes that a child's inability to verbalize indicates lack of knowledge or an inability to conceptualize the material.

All the models that have been discussed thus far, and used in related studies of children's concepts of death, are essentially developmental, age-graded models. They share the tacit assumption that at some point in the maturation process (some researchers argue that it occurs as early as age 3, others as late as age 9), the child casts aside "immature," "childish," "fantasy-type" explanations, for more "mature," "adult," "scientific" conceptions of death.

If we extrapolate from statements made by researchers in the area (Nagy, 1959; Rochlin, 1967; Morrissey, 1965; among others), it appears that mature is often associated with some lay notion of scientific (that is, not religious, an emphasis on biological process) and immature with fantasy. In other words, as the child grows up, his or her view of death changes from a notion of death as a reversible process not unlike sleep in another place, the result of being caught by the "bogey-man" or "death-man," to a view of death as an irreversible, universal event, a consequence of living, the result of physiological processes, age, or disease.

Problems arise in this regard when one examines the full spectrum of responses adults give to questions like "What is death?" "What happens when you die?" "Are you going to die?" While the adult's immediate response is to the effect "Of course, everyone dies," or "It's part of life," answers one would consider mature or scientific, further scrutiny of these replies reveals concepts that heretofore have been attributed only to children under 9 years of age. Kastenbaum and Aisenberg, for example, report that adult descriptions of death are replete with macabre images. Personifications of death as gentle comforter, grim reaper, wrinkled old woman, and gay deceiver are not uncommon. In fact their work as well as my own preliminary studies with adolescents and college students (Bluebond-Langner, 1976) suggest that similar thoughts are present in all adults, in all cultures, at all times.

Kubler-Ross's (1969) work with terminally ill adults is also relevant in this respect. She demonstrates that even among patients who are able to conceive of themselves as dying, there is preoccupation with death as the ultimate separation and a tendency to portray themselves as going on to another life after death. Patients paint themselves into scenes where God takes them into the splendor of heaven. These are views of death which most other researchers ascribe only to children under 7.

Major differences between adult and child views of death appear to be stylistic. For example, when children talk about life after death, the deceased is in the coffin; adults place the deceased in heaven or hell. Granted, it may be his or her soul, but this soul is anthropomorphized to the extent that we cannot distinguish it from the deceased himself or herself. These differences can be attributed to differences in religious education (the child under 6 years of age has had little if any formal religious instruction) and verbal sophistication.

While differences in imagery can be readily explained, how do we explain the apparent similarity in conceptualization in American children and adults? And for that matter, are we certain that the similarity exists? And if there are existing differences between adult and child conceptualizations of death, are these differences the result of a developmental process that can be linked to age or the result of other factors?

Some researchers (Jackson, 1965; Zeligs, 1974; Cook, 1973; and Kliman, 1968) claim to have duplicated Nagy's findings, and consequently support the universal application of Nagy's model to children of all cultures. They argue that there is a difference between an adult view of death and that of a child, and that these differences can be attributed to age and maturity. Other scholars (Grollman, 1967; Morrissey, 1965; Rochlin, 1967; McIntire et al., 1972), however, report that their data contradict part, if not all, of Nagy's model. Their data can be interpreted as support for conceptualizations that contradict the age-graded, developmental model and emphasize other variables (for example, social and cultural background and experiences) over age.

Transposing these two position statements into questions to focus further discussion, we now inquire: Do children's concepts of death develop with respect to age, with newer, more "scientific" explanations replacing "fantasy" explanations? Or, are all views of death present at all times in one's development; and does the particular account of death that one gives at any one time reflect not so much age as intellectual and social experiences and psychological concerns and circumstances at the time the question is asked; and does the forum of such expression even belie the conception?

Formulation of an alternative model to the age-graded, developmental model came to me as a result of work with terminally ill children (Bluebond-Langner, 1974, 1975a). I was faced with two problems. First, how could I account for the fact that all the children, ages 18 months to 14

years (the majority between 3 and 9), like any other children before diagnosis, came to know not only that they were dying but also that this was a
final and irreversible process from which there was no escape when—
according to Nagy and others—even if a child could discern the prognosis,
he or she would not necessarily see death as final and irreversible. Second,
why had I discovered that they knew and others had not (Bluebond-
Langner, 1975a).

The solution to both problems lay in a consideration of factors that
those who had studied normal and terminally ill children's views of death
had overlooked, namely, such aspects as experiences, temporal concerns,
life circumstances, and self-concept at the time the question is posed.
These factors determined not only the information the child had but also
what he or she would say, and how he or she would express it.

As a result of many findings with terminally ill children, I began to
wonder if the same thing might also be occurring in normal children. That
is, what children tell you about their view of death reflects their experiences, concerns, circumstances, and self-concept at the time of interview. If
this were the case, it could explain the contradictions in the literature
concerning normal children's views of death and help establish important
guidelines for talking to normal children about death.

TERMINALLY ILL CHILDREN AND DEATH

For a long time it was assumed that terminally ill, preadolescent children
were neither concerned with nor aware of their diagnosis. A lack of questions about their condition and the possibility of death, coupled with "an
air of passive acceptance and resignation," were taken as evidence of a
lack of concern about the diagnosis and lack of knowledge of the prognosis
(Richmond and Waisman, 1955). More recent studies claim that while it
is possible for certain children to become aware of their prognosis, it is
probably due to the peculiar circumstances in which they find themselves,
for example, cancer hospitals (Agranoff and Mauer, 1965; Geist, 1965).
Even in these cases, however, death was not considered to mean the same
thing to children as to adults (Natterson and Knudson, 1960; Solnit and
Green, 1963; Morrissey, 1965). In essence, Nagy's model, based on inter-
views with normal children, is applied to terminally ill children; that is,
the terminally ill child's view of death is seen as no different from that of
a normal child of the same age.

Impact of the illness, the experiences, concerns, and changes in self-
concept that follow in its wake are not discussed and do not appear to have
been considered as significant variables. My research with terminally ill

	1	2	3	4	5
Diagnosis	"It" is a serious illness	Names of drugs and side effects	Purposes of treatments and procedures	Disease as a series of relapses and remissions (– death)	Disease as a series of relapses and remissions (+ death)

FIGURE 3-1   Stages in the process of the acquisition of information.

children indicates that it was the failure to consider these variables as well as a tendency to equate children's overt expression with their conception, to attribute meanings to children's behaviors on the basis of adult understandings, that led these investigators astray; that kept them from discovering, as I did, that terminally ill children not only become aware of the fact that they are dying but also conceive of death as adults do.[1]

The leukemic child's acquisition of information about his or her condition is a prolonged process involving experiences in the disease world and changes in self-concept. The stages in the process of the acquisition of information are represented in Figure 3-1.

The child first learns that "it" (not all the children know the name of the disease) is a serious illness. By the time he or she reaches stage 2 the child knows which drugs are used when, how, and with what consequences. Arrival at stage 3 is marked by an understanding of the special procedures needed to administer the drugs and additional treatments that may be required as a result of the drugs' side effects. The child knows which symptoms indicate which procedures and the relationship between a particular symptom and procedure. The child sees each procedure and each treatment as a unique event. It is not until the child reaches stage 4 that he or she is able to put the treatments, procedures, and symptoms into a larger perspective, the cycle of relapses and remissions. The child sees that one can get sick over and over again in the same way and that the medicines do not always last as long as they are supposed to, if at all. But it is not until the child passes to stage 5 that he or she realizes that the cycle is finite, that it has an end, and that end is death. The child learns that there is a finite number of drugs and that when these drugs are no longer effective, death becomes imminent.

As children pass through the five stages in the acquisition of informa-

---

[1] The discussion which follows is taken from my dissertation *Awareness and communication in terminally ill children: Pattern, process, and pretense,* which was based on a study of 40 terminally ill children in a large, Midwestern metropolitan teaching hospital. Among the problems I pursued and summarize in this paper are: How do terminally ill children become aware of the fact that they are dying? What do dying and death mean to them? And how do they communicate these views?

dx	1	2	3	4	5
Well	Seriously ill	Seriously ill, but will get better	Always will get better	Always ill, but will never get better	Dying

FIGURE 3-2 Changes in self concept.

tion, they also pass through five different definitions of themselves. These parallel shifts in self-concept are represented in Figure 3-2.

In order for the child to pass through these stages in the acquisition of information and changes in self-concept, certain significant events have to take place. The child passes from diagnosis to stage 1 almost immediately after the parents learn the diagnosis. He does not pass to stage 2 until he has been to the clinic four times, spoken with other leukemic children during these visits, and his parents are told that he is in a remission. The first relapse provides the experience that moves the child to stage 3. He remains at stage 3 until experiencing several more relapses and remissions. Shortly thereafter the child passes to stage 4. It is not until he learns of the death of a leukemic peer that the child moves to stage 5.

If these events do not occur at the appropriate time, the child does not pass to the next stage. For example, if a child is at stage 4 and another child does not die, he does not move to stage 5. By the same token, if a child is at stage 2 and another leukemic child dies, he does not pass to stage 5. Information is cumulative; the child can integrate certain information only if he has the necessary requisite information. Without the requisite information, the child cannot integrate new information to come to a new conclusion.

As you may have noted, age and intellectual ability have not been mentioned as factors in a child's coming to know that he or she is dying. They are not significant. What is significant is the ability to integrate and synthesize information—an ability which is not age-related, but experience-related. The role of experience in developing awareness and, as we will see later, in determining forms of communicating that awareness, also explains why age and intellectual ability are not related to the speed or completeness with which the child passes through the stages. There are 3- and 4-year-olds of average intelligence who know more about their progress than very intelligent 9-year-olds. The reason for this is that the 9-year-olds may still be in their first remission, have had fewer clinic visits, and hence less experience. They are only aware of the fact that they have a very serious illness. A more detailed examination of the passage through each of the five stages is beyond the scope of this paper. Still, from the above discussion, we can at least begin to see the role experience, concerns, and self-concept play in a child's coming to know that he or she is dying.

Let us now turn to the role these variables play in the child's view of death, as reflected in behavior at stage 5. The passage from stage 4 to stage 5 can take place in a very short span of time. For example, one child on hearing the news of another child's death quickly assimilated all the information he had and came to the conclusion that he himself was dying.[2]

Tom   *Jennifer died last night. I have the same thing. Don't I?*

Nurse   *But they are going to give you different medicines.*

Tom   *What happens when they run out?*

Nurse   *Well, maybe they will find more before then.*

Most conversations follow the same general format, regardless of what the other party to the conversation may say. The child usually opens the conversation by mentioning either an individual who has died or someone who is in danger of dying. In the next statements the child attempts to establish the cause of death by either asking a question or stating a hypothesis and assessing the other party's reaction.

Scott   *You know Lisa.*

Myra   *(Nods)*

Scott   *The one I played ball with. (Pause) How did she die?*

Myra   *She was sick, sicker than you.*

Scott   *I know that. What happened?*

Myra   *Her heart stopped beating.*

Scott   *(Hugged Myra and cried) I hope that never happens to me, but . . .*

Having established in his own mind the cause of death, the child ends the conversation by comparing the deceased to himself.

If the child has recently discovered his or her prognosis, he or she can, when making the comparison, call attention to how he or she is different from the deceased.

Benjamin   *Dr. Richards told me to ask you what happened to Maria.*[3]

Myra   *What do you think happened to Maria?*

Benjamin   *Well, she didn't go to another hospital or home.*

Myra   *She was very sick, much sicker than you are, and she died.*

---

[2] This is not surprising, for as Kastenbaum and Aisenberg (1972) have pointed out, "The tendency for the child's cognitive pendulum to swing back and forth makes it natural for him to replace, 'He is dead,' with 'I am dead.'"

[3] Dr. Richards had not told him to ask other people. Later he told me that he used her name so that people would feel obligated to tell him.

Benjamin *She had bad nose bleeds. They packed her. I had nose bleeds, but mine stopped.*[4]

If children have been aware of their prognosis for some time, they may, like Mary, talk about how they are like the deceased.

Occupational Therapy Student *Mary, what should I do with these? Mary? (Holding up the paper dolls that Mary and I had worked on.)*
Mary *Put them in their grave, in the Kleenex box. Let me do it. Bring it over here.*
Occupational Therapy Student *(Brings the Kleenex box and the dolls over to Mary and puts them on her lap).*
Mary's Mother *Well, that's the first thing you've offered to do since the doctors said we could go.*
Mary *I'm burying them. (Carefully arranges each doll between two sheets of Kleenex.)*

Thus, while Benjamin's speech about Maria and Mary's doll burial are both conversations wherein the child discloses his or her awareness of the prognosis to another, Benjamin's conversation is more typical of a child who has just become aware of his or her prognosis, whereas Mary's is more typical of a child who has been aware for some time.

There are children who for a variety of reasons (a discussion of which space does not permit) feel that they cannot speak freely about the awareness of their prognosis, even with people they trust. Such children will not engage other people in a conversation about the prognosis and/or another child's death. They will simply state their awareness and terminate the interaction. For example, one child announced, "I'm not going to school anymore," and turned over on his side refusing to speak to me. Another child blurted out to his brother, "I won't be here for your birthday," and crawled under the sheet.

In breaking these statements down for analysis, we see that they accomplish the same thing as disclosure conversations. To say, for example, "I'm not going to school anymore," is to say, "I'm not like other children, I am different."[5] All other children must go to school. When you are dying

---

[4] Benjamin asked everyone he saw that day what happened to Maria. Later when I asked him why he asked everyone he said, "The ones who tell me are my friends. I knew Maria died. I saw the cart come for her. They told everyone to go in their rooms. I wanted to see if you were really my friend."

[5] Many of the doctors took statements like this and the one that follows as an indication of the child's awareness of his or her impending death.

or dead, you do not have to go to school anymore. Or, another example, "I won't be here for your birthday," is a way of saying, "I will not be around here. I'm leaving this earth."

It is also interesting to note that disclosure statements are a telegraphic form of the disclosure conversation. By that I mean, while the content varied slightly, the same three parts were represented. The statement began with an announcement of a death, but it was one's own. The cause of death, the illness itself, was not established in detail but implied. And one's own status was compared to a normal living child's, rather than to a leukemic's.

One notes that in all the examples given of disclosure of awareness of prognosis, there are no references to heaven. Heaven was part of only one child's view of death, a Spanish-American child, who asked, "Do children play in heaven?" When her mother told her they did, she responded, "Good, now I can play with Julio and Jorge (two Spanish-American children who had died)."

The other children never took death further than the grave. Grave imagery was far more prevalent than heaven imagery. The child's view of death was expressed in terms of what he would miss on earth (for example, birthdays, TV programs, school), rather than what would be waiting for him in an afterlife. The child was concerned with leaving this world, people, and things he knew, not with going to another world.

Other indications that a child knew he or she was dying and what dying meant included: a marked fear of wasting time; avoidance of discussions about the future; preoccupation with death and disease; death imagery in play, art, and literature; anxiety about increased debilitation; concern that things be done immediately; establishment of distance from others through displays of anger or silence. True, each of these behaviors reflects a particular view of death which can be grouped according to the categories established for different ages by Nagy (1959), namely, death as separation (ages 3 to 5), death as the result of intervention by a supernatural being (ages 5 to 7), and death as the result of a biological process (ages 7 to 9). More significant, however, is the fact that all the children, regardless of age, displayed many of these behaviors and views of death simultaneously. For example, a 5-year-old terminally ill child saw death not only as separation but as an irreversible process as well, a view Nagy and others argued would only be found in 9-year-old children. Before examining why a child displays one behavior or one view of death on one occasion, and another on other occasions, let us consider these behaviors and the views of death they reflect in more detail.

The view of death as ultimate separation is poignantly revealed in children's displays of anger. The children stated, and adults agreed, that these displays helped everyone to prepare for the final separation. For example, when I asked Jeffrey why he yelled at his mother he replied, "Then she won't miss me when I'm gone." When I repeated this to his mother she said, "That's right. Jeffrey knows that if he yells I'll leave. He yells so I can have an excuse for leaving. He knows I can't take it."

The tendency to view death as a separate personality, or more commonly with these children, to identify death with the dead, was revealed in two significant ways. First, as we have noted, the child comes into awareness that he is dying through a comparison of the deceased with himself. Second, there is great reluctance to mention the name of the deceased child or to play with his toys or toys brought by the deceased child's mother—as if death were somehow contagious.

These "magical, fantasy" views are coupled with very real, "scientific" views of death. As Tom's conversation so dramatically illustrates, death would come when the drugs "ran out." Following this, his conversations about drugs and their side effects diminished. This was not surprising since the child now realized that the drugs were not the answer he and his parents once thought them to be. Likewise, little reference was made to one's condition or progress. What was there to say? There were only indications of further deterioration, of closeness to death.

To these children, death also means no future; consequently, conversations about the future declined noticeably. The future was limited to the next holiday or occasion. At the same time, the child also tried to rush these holidays and occasions, to bring them closer to the present. For example, one child asked for his Christmas presents in October; another wanted to buy a winter coat in July. In June, several of the children at stage 5 asked the physicians if they could go back to school in September. Even the doctors who doubted that a child could know his or her prognosis without being told regarded these actions as indications that the child was suspicious, and perhaps even probing for information about how much longer he or she had to live.

The child knew that holidays and events had a new significance for parents as well. A child would often talk about the ways a particular holiday or occasion used to be celebrated and the way it was celebrated since he or she had become ill.

> On my birthday now I get to pick what I want to do. . . . My birthday this year comes on a Tuesday.[6]

---

[6] This statement was made 4 months before the child's birthday. The child died a few weeks later.

I get more Christmas presents now than before I got sick. My sister gets the same, she's not sick.

The child no longer spoke about former long-range goals and plans. He never again mentioned what he was going to be when grown-up, and became angry if anyone else did. One child, who when first diagnosed said he wanted to be a doctor, became quite angry with his doctor when she tried to get him to submit to a procedure by explaining the procedure and telling him, "I thought you would understand, Sandy. You told me once you wanted to be a doctor." He screamed back at her, "I'm not going to be anything," and then threw an empty syringe at her. She said, "OK Sandy." The nurse standing nearby said, "What are you going to be?" "A ghost," said Sandy, and turned over.

Children's lack of interest in future plans does not reflect a lack of interest in the passage of time. Children are concerned about the time they have left. They will often push themselves to get things done. They will also get angry when people take too long to remember things, to answer questions, to bring things to them. The parents and staff often commented on such behavior. "They demand because they know time is short." "It's as if they know that if they wait too long, they might be dead by then. They're not just being difficult, Mary included. That child knows something."[7]

Children often verbalize their fear of wasting time directly. When they want something and people do not move right away, they will often say, "Don't waste time," or, "We can't waste time." For example, one day after clinic, Andy's father was talking to another parent in the clinic waiting room. Andy wanted to leave. Pulling on his father's sleeve, he said, "Don't waste time." The father looked at him and said, "I'm just talking," and continued talking to the other parent. Andy with some urgency in his voice then exclaimed, "We can't waste time." This is not the usual way a 5-year-old gets his father's attention when he wants to leave a place. While his intent was not necessarily to communicate the fact that he would soon die, he was, even in such seemingly unrelated moments, expressing his awareness of his condition and what it means—time is short.

Time takes on a meaning not usually found in children this age. Time is not endless, as it is for most children, as it once was for these children. These children are having their time cut short. They are dying and they

---

[7] Mary was a demanding child who never directly said anything about her prognosis. Those who did think that she was aware of it based their claim on her demanding behavior. They felt it just was not a matter of being spoiled, as she "does it now with all of us. It used to be just for her mother's benefit. Now it's because time is running out and she knows it."

know it. Death and disease are constants in their lives. Images of death fill disease-related as well as non-disease-related thoughts, play, and conversation. All is seen in terms of death, disease, and dying.

Children's decision to display one type of behavior over another, to present a particular view of death, reflects not only their experiences but also their understanding of the circumstances of the interaction and their concerns at the time. Interaction often takes place in a mutual pretense context (Glaser and Strauss, 1965). Among the many rules which must be followed if mutual pretense is to be maintained are: avoid dangerous topics, focus on safe topics, and help individuals to take leave if it appears they will break down and shatter the pretense. Behaviors such as avoiding discussion of the future and one's condition and displaying anger so that people about to break down will leave, reflect adherence to these rules. Children cooperate with the pretense, lest they be left alone, abandoned, a fate they fear "worse than death."

Other concerns that motivate behavior revolve around the physical aspects of dying and separation. When children first learn their prognosis, they are most concerned with the physical aspects of dying, especially mutilation, pain, and direct cause. This is closely revealed in conversations that occur immediately after another child has died. As time passes and they internalize the prognosis, their concerns shift and their behavior changes. They are now more careful to observe the rules of mutual pretense and prepare for the final separation by distancing themselves from others.

In conclusion, terminally ill children of all ages come to know that they are dying in terms heretofore thought only to be possible in children over 9. Their views of death and dying as revealed in their behavior reflect their experiences, concerns, and circumstances at the time of the interaction. To these children (regardless of age), death and dying are mutilating experiences, bringing in their wake separation and loss of identity. Death is part of the disease cycle, and the life cycle as it has become for these children. It is a final and irreversible fact of life.

If this multifaceted view of death is possible for terminally ill children of all ages, might it also be possible for normal children of all ages? After all, these children were like other children before they were diagnosed. They did not suddenly become imbued with wisdom beyond their years (much as we might like to think or believe). In this vein then, I now turn to a consideration of normal children's views of death with particular attention to the nature of their view of death and the experiences, concerns, and circumstances that affect it.

STUDYING TERMINALLY ILL CHILDREN'S VIEWS OF DEATH FOR UNDERSTANDING NORMAL CHILDREN'S VIEWS OF DEATH

On the basis of my research on terminally ill children's views of death and preliminary work on normal children's views of death, I would propose that all views of death (that is, death as separation, the result of intervention by a supernatural being, an irreversible biological process) are present at all stages in one's development. The particular view of death that a child presents at any one time reflects his or her social, psychological, and intellectual experiences and concerns at the time of the interaction. Hence, it is not surprising that children of 5 speak of death as separation, as that is what they are most concerned with. Much of their time is spent in first separations (for example, parents leaving for work, going to school). Children have difficulty working through the feelings of these temporary separations, let alone the final separation of death.

Seven-year-olds, with their newly developed sense of individuality and independence, view death as a remote possibility, at least as far as they themselves are concerned. If death comes, it will be because they have been overcome by a greater force (Nagy, 1959). Fascinated by the macabre, as evidenced in play, jokes, and stories, these children personify death.

By the age of 9 children are expected to be able to separate the "fantasy" world from the real world. Science is beginning to be emphasized in school. They are called upon to conduct experiments, to make observations, and to give scientific explanation for their work. When they give an explanation of various phenomena (for example, death, sex, birth), they follow the same pattern. The fact that they are able to discuss death as a biological process does not necessarily indicate that they do not also see death as 5-year-olds do, i.e., as separation or as the result of forces beyond their control, or even as something that will happen to them. Similarly, this characterizes 7-year-olds, for whom we have documented evidence that they see death not only as the result of supernatural forces but also as a final, irreversible biological process, more specifically the result of old age or disease (Rochlin, 1967; McIntire et al., 1972). What has led previous investigators (Nagy, in the case of normal children; Richmond and Waisman, in the case of terminally ill children) astray is their tendency to equate what children say with what they think; to allow what is on the forefront of their mind to stand for all that is in their mind.

In conclusion, then, the key to discovering what death means to normal children is the same as that for discovering terminally ill children's views of death—examination of the variables of social, psychological, and intellectual experiences and concerns, circumstances of the interaction, and employment of methods that get at those variables. This should be the guide for future research on normal children's views of death. I would argue that this approach will further our understanding and help us to resolve the contradictions in the literature regarding normal children's views of death.

While systematic study following the aforementioned guidelines has not as yet been conducted, there is a strong suggestion from the work of Rochlin (1967), McIntire et al. (1972), Bluebond-Langner (1975a and 1976), Kastenbaum and Aisenberg (1972), among others, to warrant consideration of these variables in formulating new guidelines for talking to children about death. It is to this pressing task that I now turn.

TALKING TO NORMAL CHILDREN ABOUT DEATH

Given that children have some conception of death at least as early as age 2, that the possibility of their own death or that of a loved one through accident or disease or aging is ever-present, and that the ideas children have about death affect their emotional, psychological, and intellectual development, it is important to talk with children about death (Kastenbaum and Aisenberg, 1972; Jackson, 1965). The death of a loved one should not be the child's first experience with having to talk about or deal with a particular death (Furman, 1974).[8] Opportunities should be taken early on. Events in everyday life—the death of a flower or pet—may provide such an opportunity.

Preparing and conducting a ceremony for a dead pet can act as a springboard for discussion of a child's ideas about death and what he or she thinks is appropriate behavior. For example: Should one cry? Should one be buried or cremated? What would you want for yourself or someone you loved? Why? What do you think happens when you/someone dies? In other words, the preparation and event of the funeral can be done in a modified form of play therapy. The child has an opportunity to try on, to rehearse some of the emotions and behaviors he or she will experience with a loved one: denial (The animal will come back), guilt (Maybe I did not take good care of the animal), sadness (I miss the animal), anger (Why did the animal leave me?), crying, replacement (Can I get a new one?). This

---

[8] Furman (1974) found that bereaved children who had discussed death before a parent died fared better than those who had not.

by no means implies that the death of a pet is equal to or will have the same impact as the death of a loved one. It only suggests the value of such an experience, if not for the child, at least for the adult, so that when and if a loved one dies, the adult has an idea of the direction of the child's thinking.

Whether one is discussing the death of a pet or a loved one, there are certain things to bear in mind, many of which have already been suggested by the previous discussion of children's ideas of death. For purposes of this chapter let us focus on discussions surrounding the death of a loved one, as this is probably the most difficult for all concerned.

When a loved one dies, children may in some sense feel responsible. Children often believe they have magical powers and by wishing someone dead, as children are wont to do, they have caused that person's death (Furman, 1974; Kastenbaum and Aisenberg, 1972). Care must be taken to recognize that children may be feeling this and the accompanying guilt that results, and to stave it off at the outset through careful and appropriate explanations of how the person died. Remember that children look for cause (Grollman, 1967). They ask "why" questions early on in their development. They will supply a cause even if you do not, just as they will integrate the experience the best way they know how, whether you discuss it with them or not.

Children's knowledge of what questions and behaviors you accept, their past experiences, what death means to them cognitively and affectively, all will profoundly influence their behavior at the time. They may know that death means the end of life, whether they express it or not, but what is really bothering them, and hence what is coming out, is their fear of being deserted. In loss, they sense separation. Reassure them, directly as well as indirectly, through use of soothing tones and touching behavior, that they will not be left alone or abandoned.

When discussing death with children, create an environment that allows them to express their thoughts and feelings. Your tragedy is not theirs. You all may have lost, but you each have lost differently and as such react differently. Just as children can have the same concept of death as adults but express it differently, so too they can have the same feelings but show them differently. This problem came out quite clearly in the case of certain siblings of terminally ill children. Mothers became disturbed when the siblings responded to news of the death with expressions of, "Good, now I can have all his toys." Later it came to be realized that this was the siblings' way of expressing anger with the deceased for leaving them (a feeling shared by the parents), of holding on to a part of the deceased (a desire of the parents as well), and also of expressing all the long-suppressed hurt at being neglected by the parent (a guilt felt by the parents).

There are some definite no's, all of which can be avoided if you know where you are. This does not mean that you have to accept death or even be composed when talking about it—just be aware of your own feelings and thoughts. Do not tell children fantasies even you do not believe. Heaven is appropriate only if you or the children believe in it. In either case, however, remember this is an abstraction that children may not understand or may internalize very differently. Avoid the use of images of death as sleep or a trip, lest children become afraid of these things. Similarly, do not tell children God wants good people.

As with discussions about sex (where many of the same rules apply), one conversation is not enough. Children want to know different things at different times. Respect and be aware of what children know. They have many ideas, however right or wrong. Above all, take your cues from the children, answer what they want to know, what they are asking about, in their terms.

TALKING TO TERMINALLY ILL CHILDREN ABOUT DEATH

Much of what has been said about talking to normal children about death also applies to terminally ill children. But there are points that bear restatement or special consideration. First, we must not overlook the problem that it is a long time before children become aware of the fact that they are dying. They ask different questions and have different concerns and needs at different stages in their illness. Briefly, when children are first diagnosed, they are concerned about the serious nature of their illness, about the fact that they are sicker than they have ever been before. When they begin to achieve a remission, they want to know about the drugs used in treatment and their side effects. They are interested in the fact that while they have been ill, they are now recovering. When children experience their first relapse, old doubts return. They wonder if they will always be sick. They try to learn everything they can about every procedure they have to endure. When they suffer further relapses, they ask questions about the chronic nature of their illness. They want to know if and when the suffering will ever end. At such a time the death of a friend may provide the information they need. They may realize that like their friend, they too will die.

I mention these earlier stages because, if the adult is going to help children, he or she must recognize not only where children are at but also where they are coming from. While knowledge of the prognosis and open acknowledgment of it may be in the forefront of our minds, it is not necessarily uppermost in children's minds. They have a lot of living, living with dying, to do. They are concerned with that living, and only later, with dying. And even then, as we will see in a moment, they are concerned with dying in terms of the living.

In addition, while children want to express their awareness, they do not want to do so at the risk of being left alone. They know that direct expression of awareness could cost them the companionship of those they want near them, their parents. So to assure their continued presence, they practice mutual pretense. However, the fact that children do try to communicate their awareness also seems to indicate that they are interested in sharing their knowledge with other people. Therefore, I would suggest that the best approach to psychological management of terminally ill children would be one that allows a child to practice mutual pretense with those who feel most comfortable in that context, and open awareness with those who feel most comfortable in that context. One should not use an either-or approach in these cases any more than in the case of sex.

If you are the person with whom the child practices open awareness, listen to what he or she says. Take your cues from the child. Answer only what is asked, in the child's own terms. Remember, children will honor whatever rules you set up. They benefit most when questions are responded to in their own terms, when they are helped to do what they want—reveal to some, conceal from others—and be what they are—children aware of themselves, their needs, and the needs of others.

REFERENCES

Agranoff, J. H., and Mauer, A. M. What should the child with leukemia be told? *American Journal of Diseases of Children*, 1965, **110**, 231.

Bluebond-Langner, M. I know, do you?: Awareness and communication in terminally ill children. In B. Schoenberg et al. (Eds.), *Anticipatory grief.* New York: Columbia, 1974.

Bluebond-Langner, M. *Awareness and communication in terminally ill children: Pattern, process, and pretense.* Unpublished doctoral dissertation, University of Illinois, 1975. (a)

Bluebond-Langner, M. Field research on children's and adults' views of death. Fieldnotes, 1975. (b)

Bluebond-Langner, M. Field research on children's and adults' views of death. Fieldnotes, 1976.

Cook, S. *Children and dying: An exploration and a selective professional bibliography.* New York: Health Sciences, 1973.

Furman, E. *A child's parent dies.* New Haven: Yale, 1974.

Geist, H. *A child goes to the hospital.* Springfield, Ill.: Charles C Thomas, 1965.

Glaser, B., and Strauss, A. *Awareness of dying: A study of social interaction.* Chicago: Aldine, 1965.

Grollman, E. A. Prologue. In E. A. Grollman (Ed.), *Explaining death to children.* Boston: Beacon Press, 1967.

Jackson, E. N. *Telling a child about death.* New York: Channel Press, 1965.

Karon, M., and Vernick, J. An approach to emotional support of fatally ill children. *Clinical Pediatrics*, 1968, **7**, 274–280.

Kastenbaum, R., and Aisenberg, R. *The psychology of death.* New York: Springer, 1972.

Kliman, G. *Psychological emergencies of childhood.* New York: Grune & Stratton, 1968.

Kubler-Ross, E. *On death and dying.* New York: Macmillan, 1969.

Maurer, A. Maturation of concepts of death. *British Journal of Medicine and Psychology*, 1966, **39**, 35–41.

McIntire, M., Angle, C., and Struempler, L. The concept of death in Midwestern children and youth. *American Journal of Diseases of Children*, 1972, **123**, 527–532.

Morrissey, J. Death anxiety in children with a fatal illness. In H. J. Parad (Ed.), *Crisis intervention.* New York: Family Service Association of America, 1965.

Nagy, M. The child's view of death. In H. Feifel (Ed.), *The meaning of death.* New York: McGraw-Hill, 1959.

Natterson, J., and Knudson, A. Observations concerning fear of death in fatally ill children and their mothers. *Psychosomatic Medicine*, 1960, **22**, 456–466.

Richmond, J. B., and Waisman, H. A. Psychologic aspects of management of children with malignant disease. *American Medical Association Journal of the Diseases of Children*, 1955, **89**, 42–47.

Rochlin, G. How younger children view death and themselves. In E. A. Grollman (Ed.), *Explaining death to children.* Boston: Beacon Press, 1967.

Schilder, P., and Wechsler, D. The attitudes of children toward death. *Journal of Genetic Psychology*, 1934, **45**, 406–451.

Solnit, A., and Green, M. The pediatric management of the dying child: Part II, the child's reaction to the fear of dying. In A. Solnit and S. Provence (Eds.), *Modern perspectives in child development.* New York: International Universities Press, 1963.

Zeligs, R. *Children's experiences with death.* Springfield, Ill.: Charles C Thomas, 1974.

4

THE COLLEGE STUDENT AND DEATH

EDWIN S. SHNEIDMAN

The college student is—by virtue of his or her time of life (typically about 20 years of age) and his or her place in the world (in a setting of ideas and stimulation, books and learning)—in a highly dramatic, life-expanding situation. College life, for most, is exciting. Thus the threat of death, which does nothing but diminish and annihilate, is, especially for a college student, a dramatically devastating trauma. It is the essence of the wrong event at the wrong time, the worst of winter's blasts in the summer of life, terribly premature, horribly out of season with life's flow, the most dire occurrence at the most inauspicious moment.

Independent of our democratic pretensions, we tend not to be egalitarian about death, and perhaps rightly so. We mourn the death of a young gifted person, a beautiful person, more than that of an old person, a wicked person, or even an ordinary person. And, in general, we mourn the death of a college student—at the threshold of full adult life, trained, bright promise unfulfilled—more than any other.

The raw facts are illuminating but not reassuring. United States statistics about college-age death (U.S. Department of Health, Education and Welfare, 1970) inform us that in 1969 the percentage of the total population between 15 and 19 years of age was 9.1, between 20 and 24 years, 7.8; in 1968 the reported number of all deaths in the United States was almost 2 million (1,930,082); the percentage of deaths for the 15- to 19-year-old and the the 20- to 24-year-old group was each around 1. The mortality rates (per 1000 in that age group) were 1.1 and 1.4, respectively. Those years are obviously a time of life—except for death in war—when death is an event of relatively infrequent occurrence. As to the reasons for death, the four leading causes of death in the United States for ages 15 to 24 for both sexes are accident, homicide, malignant neoplasms, and suicide. The school years are obviously a time of life when the threats to life itself are not so much from internal disorders of the soma, but rather from threats by others in the environment and from imprudencies from within the self.

In every life, the decade of the twenties, from the late teens to age 29, is the time of life which, for many, is a make-or-break era (Shneidman, 1971). That is a time when one has to stand on one's own two feet and face the world. In another setting (Shneidman, 1967) I have discussed three types of crises as they relate to time of life: one, called an *intratemporal crisis*, which occurs within a time of life such as adolescence or middle age; a second, called an *intertemporal crisis*, which occurs as one turns the corner from one stage of life to another, e.g., the crisis of moving from being a child to becoming an adolescent, or from being an adolescent to becoming an adult, involving the trauma of moving through life; and a third, called an *extratemporal crisis*, which relates to those crises which are out of phase with one's time of life. The latter describes the individual who is, so to speak, developmentally precocious, way ahead of his or her own years, too mature, an old person in his or her teens; or, conversely, those crises which happen to persons who are "retarded" in the sense of being immature, almost childish, infantile, too young for their years. Obviously, optimal movement through life implies that one develops as one is pushed along by inexorable time. In *Pierre,* Melville says, "Oh what quenchless feud is this, that Time hath with the sons of men." And so it is that we are pushed willy-nilly, screaming, kicking, sometimes willing the obligatory, not only from day to day but from birthday to birthday and from decade to decade. College students can have all of these three types of personal crises.

College time is a fulcrum point; college commencement is both an ending and a beginning. The college student's view of his or her relationship to death is essentially that of a person far removed from death, and yet at that time when life and love and death are all highly romanticized. The romanticization of death—death as lover, death as special, death as arcane, death as heroic—is a separate and fascinating topic (Shneidman, 1973). The very topic "death and the college student" implies that there are stages in the human life cycle; infancy, childhood, young adolescence, a time for college, adulthood, etc. And further, it implies that one's basic orientations and attitudes to the topic of death and to one's own death change and develop (and sometimes even mature) as one moves through life's time. The most widely recited statement of this apparently ubiquitous fact about the stages of life is Jacques's speech on the seven ages of man in Act II, Scene vii of *As You Like It.* ("All the world's a stage, and all the men and women merely players.")

In our own century, a number of psychologically oriented authors have elaborated on or explicated this archetypal theme. On first appearance the most simple (but perhaps, on reflection, the most profound) opinion is that of C. G. Jung (1933). He propounds a two-phase view: That life is made up of an upward movement toward that moment when one perceives his or her own mortality (somewhere usually in middle age) followed by a second stage of life, in which the primary task is to prepare for one's own death. This turning point in life can be called the "noon-day" of life. It is essentially a "watershed" view of life. Charlotte Buhler (1961) discusses the various stages in the course of the human life cycle; Gerald Heard (1963) writes of the five ages of man; Ernest Schachtel (1959) speaks of the important periods in what he calls the "human metamorphosis"; Harry Stack Sullivan (1953) talks about the developmental epochs in the human life cycle; and there are others.

Perhaps the best known twentieth-century explication of the stages of life is Erik Erikson's (1963) conceptualization of the development of human personality in eight hierarchical psychosocial or psychosexual stages, a scheme which implies that one needs successfully to resolve one stage before going on meaningfully to the next stage. In puberty and adolescence, the fifth stage, the core issues revolve around identity versus role confusion; in young adulthood the issues are intimacy versus isolation.

In relation to intimacy versus isolation, one is reminded of Francis Bacon's thought that to love is to give hostages to fortune. The alternative however is isolation, not risking, not daring, not investing, not loving—hoping not to be vulnerable. For most of us the risk of being vulnerable and suffering loss seems more desirable than to be lonely, loveless, and to live a life that is essentially barren and arid. Hiram Haydn (1974), in talking about his great friend Henry A. Murray, said: "Never to have been in love is never to have lived fully; never to have had a friend about whom one feels the way I have described constitutes an equal deprivation of life." Death is the irreversible stopping of the living interaction with all those loves and relationships. It is what Melville's anguished Captain Ahab cries at the death of the Parsee in the penultimate chapter of *Moby Dick:* "Gone?—gone? What means that little word? What death-knell rings in it, that old Ahab shakes as if he were the belfry."

COLLEGE STUDENT ATTITUDES TOWARD DEATH

Recently I wrote an article on death for a popular psychology journal, *Psychology Today* (1970), which included a 75-item questionnaire on death and then, several months later, published the results of the questionnaire findings. The single biggest surprise in the results was the sheer volume of responses. Within a month of the original article more than 30,000 readers returned the death questionnaire (and more than 2000 of them sent substantial letters with their replies), breaking the record set by previous questionnaries in that journal on the topics of sex, violence, and drugs. For the 1971 report I chose a random sample of 500 responses—a sampling of about 1 in 60. This present section is a first report on the 90 college students included in that sample of 500—18 percent of the initial sample, and representing around 5400 college students among the 30,000 respondents.

America's current attitude toward death is deeply ambivalent: awe of death and an attraction to death; risking death and loving life; wanting happiness and behaving in self-destructive ways; regarding death as taboo and insisting on a new permissiveness to talk about it; an obsession with The Bomb and a deep concern with spiritual rebirth. We live in a death-conscious time, in which people, the center of their own world, boldly assert that they are not psychologically degradable.

Views of death have undergone radical changes in the last few generations—perhaps the first major radical changes since the seventeenth century of Descartes. The Cartesian view of death is tied to a view of the individual as essentially a biological vessel, subject to the whims of fate or fortune. Death is one such whim. The Cartesian philosophic spirit necessarily implies a fatalistic view of life.

The results of the death questionnaire unequivocally demonstrate the demise of fatalism. Contemporary college students—and perhaps most twentieth-century people—have made themselves the center of their own universe, and have put themselves back into their own death. They recognize death and dying as aspects of living. Thanks primarily to Freud, college students see the individual as playing conscious and unconscious roles in his or her own fate. Most students believe in the possible influence of psychological factors on death; 96 percent either "firmly believe" or "tend to believe" that psychological factors can influence or even cause death, and half believe that most persons participate consciously or unconsciously in their own deaths.

Many elements go into shaping people's views of life and death and the part they play in either by their own volition. The usual experiences with death in America have changed dramatically over the last two generations. It used to be that almost everyone, by the time of adolescence, had personally witnessed a death, usually at home, of some loved one—a baby brother or sister, a mother or father. Today most dying is done in hospitals, largely out of sight, and always under formal institutional regimen.

The interface between religion and death is especially fascinating. Numerous studies have shown that nominal religious affiliation is not enough to understand religious conviction. But we asked for "religious background," which allowed us to see that people's religious environment, whether they accept or reject the tenets of their faith, whether they stay with the church of their parents or leave it, certainly affects many of their attitudes toward death. Important in most current attitudes toward death is one's own estimate of his or her religiosity. Among college students the "antireligious" are twice as numerous as the "very religious"—a sharp difference from the total *Psychology Today* sample.

While most of the antireligious college students say that religion plays no role in their own attitudes, a substantial number report that religion has significant impact on them, apparently pushing them away from the traditional religious outlooks on death. Students who consider themselves not hostile to organized religion are less likely than the antireligious to attribute a very significant role to religion.

If religion does not play a significant role in forming attitudes toward death in this secular age, what does? Introspection and meditation, say over one-third of the students. Given another choice and asked to apply the influences to their own deaths, about one-third reinforce their first choice by selecting existential philosophy as the most important influence. They mention Camus and Hesse often.

If we put together attitudes at various ages in reference to beliefs, we find—with no great surprise—that attitudes toward death change as one matures. Typically, religious beliefs become more secular or scientized. One then sees death simply as the end of life. The typical childhood conception of death is in terms of an afterlife, which for most involves ideas of heaven or hell (57 percent), but by young adulthood, the percentage of individuals who believe in an afterlife as their primary view of death has been cut almost in half to 30 percent. From late adolescence on, the largest single percentage see death simply as the final process of life. Consistent with this view, the most distasteful aspect of death for college students is that "one can no longer have any experiences."

The findings of the questionnaire point to the fact that over the past generation or two there has been a tremendous secularization of death. Nowadays people die ascetically in antiseptic hospitals rather than aesthetically in their homes. The physician has replaced the priest; the doctor is today's magician who has the power to extend life, our new escort from this vale of tears. The funeral industry directs the forms of mourning, ushering us from burial to bereavement.

Historian Arnold Toynbee (1969) has written that death is essentially a two-person affair, involving both the survivor and the decedent. He further asserts that if a married person truly loves the spouse, that person will wish the spouse to die *first,* so the spouse will be spared the anguish of bereavement. Student respondents to the death questionnaire divide on this issue: 17 percent say yes and 23 percent say no; most (60 percent) are undecided. The reasons they give for yes and no responses are about equally divided between selfish and selfless reasons. One is reminded of what Lord Nelson is reported to have said as he lay dying aboard the *Victory:* "The pain is so great that one might wish oneself dead, but one would like to live a little longer, too." As ambivalence is the keystone of life, so is it a characteristic of death.

One 20-year-old college student wrote about the death questionnaire: "If I pass this test do I get immortal life as a prize? Think what a bummer that would be. Fear of death puts a little excitement into life. R.I.P."

COLLEGE STUDENT CONCEPTUALIZATIONS OF DEATH

It is as true nowadays as when Professor Henry Murray wrote, one short generation ago (specifically in 1949), "that the American of today has no compelling religious belief, no certainty of a moral order, no articulate philosophy, no heart's vision that demands aesthetic utterance." Are contemporary college students a generation adrift? We have seen that they do not think about death more often than most people, and we are not surprised, as we reflect upon it, that when they are asked to write about death, they are able to do so in a rather sensitive and articulate way. In the *Psychology Today* study, most college students viewed death (as did most of the respondents) as "The end; the final process of life" (26 percent) and were most distressed (36 percent) by the notion that death meant that they could no longer have any experiences, that it was a stopping of the mind's introspective flow—a rather twentieth-century psychological and phenomenological view of "cessation."

A group of college students (enrolled in a course on death and suicide) were asked: "What does death mean to you? How do you conceptualize your own death?" The following quoted paragraphs are a sampling from among hundreds of responses. Here are a few:

Death means the end of consciousness. Like dreamless sleep, like before birth—no memories. Nothing. The body decays, its elements become part of the earth so when one dies he gives back to the earth.

Life is accidental, but I cannot understand the concept of myself. What makes the peculiar accident of my mother and father called *me*, feel like *me* and not like my brother? Because of this, I'm not sure that I don't believe in reincarnation if not of the soul. Then the possibility that a random collision of atoms will create another me who thinks and feels.

The part of *me* which conceptualizes cannot conceptualize "not conceptualizing," therefore it is impossible for me to think of my own death without removing myself to a pin point of time and observing, not-me—and in this act my conceptualization faculty is still present. (Male—age 21)

Another:

Death signifies the termination of all meaning your life has begun to assume through careful working through of your ideas. It comes, and it drops one into a void from which he can never return. It destroys all which one held of any worth, of any value whatsoever. It robs one of his life. But it also provides a cease-fire, an escape from the almost unendurable suffering to which one has submitted, an oblivion, an out at last. Death is a long, long sleepless sleep. One returns to nothingness, and then it is as if one had never existed. It makes all of one's efforts to confront himself, to confront the world, to confront the passage of time—so stupid, in retrospect (not that the dead person is able to indulge in retrospection), so futile, so worthless, so absurd. Death is the crowning absurdity to a pathetically meaningless life anyway. (Female—age 21)

Another:

I'm not really certain that I've formed an absolute idea of death. I see death as something very *final* and permanent. It is the end of what I know now as existence. I cannot conceive of non-existence. When I try to picture my death, even though I no longer have a body, *I* am still conscious and I am still myself. Yet, when I try to think of it rationally, it only seems reasonable that when I die, that is the end. It's just a part of the natural cycle of the whole life-decay process. Man is a product of natural selection and the fact that he is able to worry about death and must create for himself consolations of after-life is his way of accepting what is for every other creature a part of living.

Another way of explaining it is that in nature, a flower, for ex-ample, blooms and then eventually dies and all its material remains decay and it's gone. Then the next spring another flower blooms from the same bud and so life and flowers continue. But the flower that followed the first flower was a different flower; the first flower is gone and while every year there will be a flower, that first flower will never *be* again. (Female—age 18)

A sizable number of student reflections touch on what is, in its poten-tial magnitude for human destruction, the most impactful manner of death in history: megadeath—the possibility of killing millions in the flash of a moment.[1] I have been led by my students to believe that the haunting omnipresence of The Bomb underlies, in some sinister but discernible way, much of the malaise, disenchantment, and incivility of youth in our time, reflecting a breakdown of national and international morality which has been "the story of their lives." As one student said: "The Bomb lives!" by which he meant that, at some surface or deep level of consciousness, the specter of nuclear destruction hangs in the air like an unmovable cloud.

---

[1] No serious student of mass murder by the state in our time can afford to miss reading Gil Elliot's searing book *The Twentieth Century Book of the Dead* (New York: Ballantine Books, 1972), a volume which lists the 110 million people killed by government action since 1900. Further, better to understand the *secularization* of death in this century, it is useful to compare current attitudes with the religious aura that surrounded death in another "death-laden" time, specifically during the great plagues of the mid-fourteenth century, as fascinatingly described in Philip Ziegler's *The Black Plague* (Middlesex, England: Penguin Books, 1969).

THE COLLEGE STUDENT AS DIRECT VICTIM

The majority of college-age deaths—55 to 60 percent—are related to accidents. They are sudden, ugly in their emotional impact, traumatic for the survivors, shocking. But youth is a time for risk taking and "accidents can happen." It is difficult (and perhaps unseemly) to compare the abrasiveness of one kind of death with another, but death from cancer seems to be an especially burdensome death for the survivor—and, of course, for the benighted victim. To die of cancer in one's teens or twenties, in college, seems a particularly "unfair" and tragic thing. One then dies over a period of time, sees oneself growing sicker and weaker, slipping toward death, experiences the anxious concern of loved ones, and is usually the living (but failing) object of frantic medical efforts.

The following case involves a college student who was feeling rather poorly, couldn't quite diagnose his own symptoms, went to his physician, and was sent by his physician to a hematologist who diagnosed him as having acute myelogenous leukemia. This young man, a student in a local university, was, when first seen by me, a patient in the university hospital. His doctor requested that I see him because of his cantankerous behavior on the ward, his shouting at nurses, his swearing, and what the doctor described as his "bitchy behavior." When I first saw him, he was sitting up in bed, behaving in a rather feisty and imperious way to the others in the room. I greeted him at the outset by saying that I had heard that he had been misbehaving. He seemed to like that approach, and we hit it off quite well from the beginning. In my own heart I decided to see him because I felt that he was in for a rough time, and with his own defenses and alienating behavior, he might turn people away from him and have an unnecessarily psychologically painful death. I began to see him almost every day, alone, just he and I. It developed that he was an only child, his father was dead, and his relationship with his mother for the past several years could be characterized as a running verbal hostile fight. The content of our sessions grew more serious as he became increasingly ill. He sobered and matured enormously within a matter of weeks, and without any leading on my part, chose to talk openly about his impending death.

The session reproduced below (with some minor editing) is one recorded with his knowledge and reproduced here with the permission which he willingly gave before he died. It is several weeks after the first meeting. At this time he was quite ill, extremely weak, physically wrung out, and painfully aware of his downhill course. He died about a week after this session.

ES *The nurse told me that you had a bad night.*
ST *Yes, it has been pretty bad lately. I am giving up. I want it to be over. I*

don't expect any miracles anymore. It is going to be a slow process. Maybe not so much a painful process but a slow process. I would like to get out and then I would also like to get to sleep and die. I don't know what to say. I am just tired. I woke up this morning and I was really frightened, just saying "Dear God, dear God, what am I going to do?" But dear God, dear God doesn't answer.

ES   *Were you really frightened?*

ST   *Yes. Really frightened.*

ES   *What was it fear of?*

ST   *Of the unknown and of another day. Dr. Shneidman, if there was a way that I could end it now, I would do that. It is taking so long. I don't have much patience I guess.*

ES   *I am sure this is a trial for you in many deep ways, including that one.*

ST   *How do you do it?*

ES   *There is no easy way. You endure it, and then if you are lucky, you can look back on it. I wish I could give you some nice moral, common sense statement.*

ST   *I'm scared. You said you would say what death was. You said it was something I wouldn't know anything about. If I can only be sure that it would be peaceful. Will it be peaceful?*

ES   *I can practically guarantee it.*

ST   *This is so important. It is almost more important than anything else that it be peaceful.*

ES   *I am convinced of that.*

ST   *My mother still wants to believe that maybe something can happen. I suppose I do also.*

ES   *So do I.*

ST   *My mother has become so important.*

ES   *In what ways have your relationships with your mother changed in the past few weeks? They have obviously changed.*

ST   *I have loved her. I have let myself love her without feeling that she was going to emasculate me. I have let her love me. I have let her be a mother. She has been so beautiful. I get more comfort from her than from anybody else.*

ES   *Do you think it took your illness for that to happen?*

ST   *I don't know. I know for me it has, because now there is no reason to be wary of her castrating tendencies because she really means well for me. She brings me such comfort. She is so selfless. Crying is not supposed to help, yet it hurts when you get a fever, and you sweat a lot which is what I do. Life is so. . . . I don't know.*

ES   *In what other ways have you changed?*

ST   *It is a hard question. I don't know if I could be honest because I could say one thing now, but if it happened, I might do something else. For one thing, I would be very wary about all health things. I think I would know myself a little better, a lot better. I would look upon myself as a much better person. I think I would be less concerned about my physical appearance, although I don't think I would ignore it. I think I would be less selfish, more concerned with trying to get the most out of every day. If there was a God, if there was somebody that knew, that I could pray to to perform this miracle, I would be most thankful, and I would show it in every way I could. The idea of recovery is so farfetched, so unreal. I don't have a chance. I want to live so much, I do. I don't want to die now. Right now, all they think about is getting me out of the hospital for a few days and then taking me back in, doing as good a job as possible of keeping me alive as long as possible, which is something I really don't want to do, because if it's over, isn't it over? Isn't that the natural way? My mother keeps saying to take each day as it comes, but it is extremely difficult. I had a lot of trouble doing that before. I am having even more trouble doing it now. I went to bed last night after listening to you talking about it, I went to bed feeling good. It was very comforting, but then I woke up this morning, and I was in this terror, just like I need constant reassurance that I have been a good person and that there is someone there to love me. They told me I had a really good chance. They have tried everything. Now a perfectly good person with an awful lot to give is going to die. A young person is going to die. His death is going to be senseless. Do you fear death?*

ES   *Of course.*

ST   *I was just wondering about somebody who is more or less a specialist in the area of death, how he felt about it.*

ES   *I am as human as anybody. There are different levels of me just as there are different levels of you. I think I am very close to you. Like you, I don't like illness, pain, inactivity, uncertainty, death.*

ST   *I feel peaceful now.*

ES   *I will come to see you tomorrow.*

ST   *I hope I will still be here.*

What is to be noted in the above exchange is not so much the focus on any single affective state, but rather the wide panoply of human emotions which is displayed in this relatively brief session. To list some of them, we can note his anguish, his puzzlement, the thread of hope and yearning beyond realistic probability. Also, his diffuse anger at "dear God" who doesn't answer his pleas and prayers, his resignation, his despair, his fantasied escape. And more than this, "irrational," simultaneous presence of seemingly contradictory emotions. That is the way the death scene is played. It is not a series of discrete feeling states, displayed cleanly, seriatim; rather it is a confluence and a booming flux of cries and whispers of simultaneous hope and hopelessness, of yearnings for help and declarations of helplessness. All these zigs and zags occur on an essentially downhill curve of which the person himself or herself often has some deep presentiment. The task of the clinical thanatologist is made both more painful and more tolerable by the fact that in practically every case "all" that he or she needs to do is to be with the dying person, close by, even touching hands, and responding to the needs of the person to talk about any topic as that person moves into death.

One more vignette: At the beginning of one of my courses on death and suicide I was approached by a lovely young woman who, although she was animated and obviously bright (and was, as I learned after her death, a member of Phi Beta Kappa), seemed to be somewhat ill. For one thing she wore bandaids on each of her fingers. During our first conversation I asked her what was wrong, to which question she responded by telling me that she had scleroderma—a disease with an often-fatal outcome. I puzzled aloud as to whether or not she ought to take the course, but when she said that she would really like to try and if it became too onerous in content she would drop it, I consented to let her enroll. I came to know her rather well. She completed the course, but within a few weeks entered the hospital fighting for breath and died of her disease within a matter of days. In her hospital room she said to me: "I badly don't want to die, but most of all I don't want to die badly." She was a remarkable and fine person. Her husband has given me portions of her diary and his permission to reprint these excerpts written a few weeks before she died.

> I've just experienced several days of deep depression, full of morbid thoughts of death and illness. The thing that disturbs me about such depressions is my uncertainty as to their generation and cause. If they are psychochemical or endocrinological in origin then I can dismiss them much more easily than if I believe they are the upwelling of some great hidden angst. Are they the maudlin, morbid reflections of a chemically unbalanced brain? This is somewhat of an alienating idea, those thoughts aren't *me*, they're just my body acting up. Having read more deeply into existentialist ideas lately it's intellectually somewhat emotionally repugnant to me to alienate my "inner self." But with such thoughts of death, decay, the aging in my own body and mind, my love for Bob and my pain at eventually leaving him— all inevitably *true*—(I can't dismiss them as fantasies). I can't live happily. Solomon says life isn't meant to be happy, but I'm thinking that I prefer the delusion if such feelings as I have are the alternative.
>
> I'm sitting outside in the patio. The sun warm and a tiny bit burning on my back, the sky blue and clear, the air fresh and just tinged with the smell of perspiration that always accompanies sunbathing, the birds twittering music from somewhere, distant car horns. It's hard to concentrate on being anguished! So I'll stop and enjoy being, now.
>
> Barring the accidents that we all are subject to, a woman my age would see herself comfortably in young adulthood, with a long future. Conversely someone with "6 months to live" would know that . . .

but I am constantly aware—afraid that each day may bring the accident, or asphyxiation or choking, or pneumonia that could be quickly fatal. Will this reaction be uneventful, save for discomfort on my part due to my illness? Or will it end in disaster?

Too, I don't know whether I am a "normal" appearing person or not. I thought I was with perhaps a few unusual signs—short fingers, mouth open. Now I feel that (someone made some comment on this last night) I don't appear normal to others and a great ego defense is down. Am I sick? Am I well? What am I capable of doing? What *should* I do? What do others think I should do? When will I have to admit I can no longer make it to school for a few hours each day, three or so days a week? What can I do then? When will it happen? I (like probably everyone else with a problem) feel that it's especially cruel for me—to appear to be healthy and to be so weak as to not be able to walk a block or so without panting and stopping. Death is so close and yet, possibly so far away.

THE COLLEGE STUDENT AS SURVIVOR

As often as a college student is direct victim, another college student (lover or spouse) is the targeted survivor-victim of the death. Grief and mourning in one's teens and twenties for a contemporary is a heavy burden that comes out of season. To be a widow or widower in college is an especially cruel life blow. Melville's Redburn says: "Talk not of the bitterness of middle-age and after life: a boy can feel all that, and much more, when upon his young soul the mildew has fallen. . . . Cold, bitter, cold as December, and bleak as its blasts, seemed the world then to me; there is no misanthrope like a boy disappointed, and such was I, with the warm soul of me flogged out by adversity." These lines begin to approach what the death of a college spouse can do.

There are some especially good recent publications on bereavement, chief among them Parkes's *Bereavement* (1972) and Glick, Weiss, and Parkes's *The First Year of Bereavement* (1974). One of the main findings of these studies seems to be that widows and widowers of any age (20 through 80), compared with matched nonwidowed individuals of that same age, suffer a higher rate of morbidity (serious illnesses, hospitalizations, accidents, physical complaints, and psychological distress) and a higher rate of mortality. Bereavement is a serious state, amounting almost to a life-threatening illness. Being a survivor-victim is being a person at risk.

The following is part of a recorded interchange between me and the college student widower of the young woman whose words I have just quoted. The portions of verbatim text fill in the details and tell us many things about the burden and the course of grief in a college student survivor.

ES   *Now to start with, your relationship with Edith was unusual in that you knew she was ill from the beginning.*

R   *That's correct, I first met her 10 years ago, she was 18. I was talking with this friend saying I'd really like to meet a girl who was intelligent and particularly knew something about music, particularly Bach. And she said she knew a girl and gave me her name and phone number; so I called her up, it was a blind date and that was that. It was just after her illness had been diagnosed and her parents, if I remember correctly, told me about it . . . when they saw that we were becoming serious, after we had been courting for some time. And I really didn't know exactly what the disease was, I mean as far as life span was concerned.*

ES   *Did they tell you the name of the disease?*

R   *Yes.*

ES   *Did you look it up?*

R   *No. As I think of it now, I wonder why I didn't try to find out more. Maybe I was afraid. I don't know. I knew her life would be shortened, but I don't think I really allowed myself to think about it or to find out exactly what it was. It was terminal about 8 years after. I have thought about it, because it seems to me strange of my not pursuing it. She was the first girl I guess I really had a good meaningful relationship with, and I think I might have been very frightened to find out the truth. But I didn't want to know. . . . We went to Europe in the summer 2 years before she died, and when she came back, she had some sort of bronchial thing that never cleared up. And when we saw that we realized it was kind of a significant thing. She would draw the same sort of conclusion and talk about it. The fact that she was not getting better, that the disease was progressing along its course. I'd see things and realize that it was true, but then I'd sort of block it out, trying to deal with the right now. . . . The more I think of it, the more I really realize I think I blocked a tremendous amount out.*

ES   *Her death was not totally unexpected to you. When she came into the hospital, she was struggling and failing. You knew she was in serious physical trouble. This is a delicate question. Please tell me how you were told that she had died, and then what happened?*

R   *The doctor that had been attending her told me when I came in that morning to see her, and he brought me aside. He took me somewhere. I think he gave me a tranquilizer. He was a resident. I was extremely impressed with him. I was probably in shock, but I remember the clear thing I did feel was some sense of relief that I don't have to wait any longer. That incredible waiting that I realized I had been going through was suddenly over. But then there was this, I don't know. . . . I went home alone from the hospital, alone, really alone. I really don't recall what happened the rest of the day. I think that a good friend of ours stayed with me that night. I was feeling very freaked out. I must have gone around for maybe a week or so before I really began to feel the loneliness and her loss. I finally stopped running around taking care of everybody, and really felt the mourning, really felt her loss.*

ES   *What did that mourning feel like?*

R   *I wouldn't know how to describe it. It's a feeling inside of having an incredible emptiness. I felt sort of at a loss, kind of wondering how my life was going to continue. How it possibly could go on. Everything sort of like disintegrated. Sort of like a piece of me just was kind of lost.*

ES   *Did you have certain patterns or habits of expectations, of wanting to talk to her or expecting to see her?*

R   *Yes, that happened a few times. I'd look at a doorway, maybe to the bedroom from the living room, and expect her to come walking through.*

ES   *What helped the most?*

R   *I don't know that there's any one thing that helped me the most. Perhaps Susan, probably has helped a lot. Even though it was after a year, she forced me to the issue of dealing with Edith, really moving her out of the apartment, and started showing me things. About 6 months after Edith died, I went around and grabbed everything that had anything to do with her and put them in boxes and shoved them in the closets; but still Edith was in the closet. She was still there. We moved things round the apartment to make it different. I started doing some of those things, but she just kept saying that she really felt it wasn't her place, that it was still Edith's. She wanted it to be hers. So she did force me a great deal.*

ES   *Did you get rid of all her things?*

R   *Oh no. As a matter of fact we have some pottery that Edith had made that we use, that I had never thought of using before.*

ES   *Do you sleep in the same bed that you had before?*

R   *Yes, but I've moved the bed in the room and I sleep on the other side of the bed.*

ES   *Advertently?*

R   *Yes. I did that purposely.*

ES   *Does Susan know that you made these changes?*

R   *I've told Susan that the bed used to be in a different location, and I never made anything of it. I did this about 6 months after Edith died, before I met Susan. I did a few things, painted one of the walls, and a few things like this, rearranged the furniture. But there was still the other thing. It was very hard for me to commit myself to Susan. This was a big problem. This is over 2 years now. We've been married for several months and had been going together for 2 years. I took all that time to make a commitment.*

ES   *Why was that?*

R   *I don't know. I searched in myself a lot for what it was. And I wasn't really able to grab it. I'm sure that part was really there. A part of it was the holding on. I'm sure that was also a large part of it. I don't think it was until Susan and I were married that we went through all the boxes in the closets, took all the stuff, and decided either to throw it away or use it, to get it out of the closet, literally and figuratively.*

ES   *Did you make any inquiries as to Susan's state of health? Did you ask her, for example?*

R   *Susan is very healthy. I don't recall. I might have asked her, but I'm conscious of the fact that I certainly noticed her health. She's also younger than I am by a few years, and I thought of that. You know what that means. I think part of that means that I don't want to live longer. I don't. I don't want her to die before I do. I'm sure that's there. I'd be surprised if it weren't. . . .*

ES   *I knew Edith and then I knew you. How did that work out?*

R   *Well, I think I came to you. I'm not sure if it was because you knew her. I think that was part of it, because you did know her and you knew me through her. But I think it was because of you yourself. I felt you were the type of person who could help me.*

ES   *In what way?*

R   *I can't recall, whatever, but I think that some of the things that you said at the time helped me, helped to alleviate my desperation that I felt. A few times I did come in I was feeling pretty desperate. Completely kind of lost and floundering. But that worked out.*

THE COLLEGE STUDENT AS THANATOLOGIST

Admittedly, a college course on death is still a somewhat unusual curriculum offering. Yet in the last few years there has been a pleasant proliferation of courses on this topic at universities throughout the country. These courses are typically well subscribed and typically described by the students as an exceptionally rich college course experience (Shneidman, 1974, 1976).

What is most rewarding in teaching undergraduate courses on death is the growth that one sees in students in the brief interval of a semester. One hears often from them that the course—the reading, the video and audio tapes of dying persons, the plays (i.e., *Quiet Cries*), the guest speakers, the lectures, the afterlecture rap periods—has helped them personally in their wrestlings with the notion of death (and in other aspects of their lives also), and more than occasionally one hears that the course has pointed them toward a decision to enter the helping professions, specifically, to work with dying persons.

In relation to death, the college student can also be a helper, giving succor to dying persons and to their loved ones. Rather than attempting to describe a college student in this role, I asked a young man (who attends one of my training seminars on thanatology at the UCLA Neuropsychiatric Institute) to write of his own feelings and experiences related to thanatological work.[2] Here is his brief report:

I am a graduate student in Clinical Psychology, in my 20's, currently (1975) doing my internship year at the UCLA Neuro-Psychiatric Institute. A large portion of my program is taken up through my work on the Psycho-Somatic Liaison Consultation Service where I am assigned to the Medical and Surgical/Oncology Service. I requested this particular service specifically because of special circumstances in my own life and because of a large and significant gap in my training as a clinical psychologist. These two factors above all others, I believe, have led me to seek out intensive training in the area of Clinical Thanatology, i.e., psychotherapeutic intervention into the lives of those with life-threatening illnesses.

The personal life stress event which started me on this unusual training path was the unexpected terminal cancer diagnosis of my mother. Ten years previous to my mother's illness my aunt (her sister) had died a physically and psychologically agonizing death from cancer with my entire extended family, excluding my mother, determined to keep the reality of her illness from her, and from themselves as much as possible. I was determined from the moment of learning my mother's diagnosis that she would die what I later was to hear labeled as "an appropriate death." At the time I had no label, no understanding of how to deal with it, but I vowed to myself that I would learn at the earliest opportunity.

It is now a year since my mother died and I am partially on the way to learning how to cope with death from a professional and even hopefully a personal standpoint. I have been involved in a training program heavily weighted toward intensive clinical involvement which has included intensive supervision as well as a didactic and case oriented seminar on psychotherapy with the dying.

My primary interests are in the areas of the functioning of social systems and especially in the dynamics of the family unit. These, I have found, fit well into my thanatological work. I am primarily concerned with the impact of a terminal illness on the nuclear and extended family system. I participate in family therapy on the unit and have started a multiple conjoint family therapy group where

---

[2] I wish to thank David Wellisch for writing this report at my request and for permitting me to use it in this chapter.

several family units meet together (without the ill members of their families) to cope with their problems collectively. All of this is not to minimize my concerns for the individual who is bedridden with a life-threatening illness, but to assure psychological support reaching the "survivor-victims" who are also caught up in the wake of the illness.

I work a large number of hours with the nursing and medical staffs. This is largely done in group contexts on a formal basis. I meet with each shift of nurses in a separate group, because each shift is a dynamically different interpersonal working system with its own strengths, deficits and problems. I also meet with the medical staff weekly in "psychosocial rounds." This is a time, on an overt level, when each patient's psychological and social realm is considered, but covertly, on a process level, it is a time when medical staff can ventilate feelings about their patients which depart from the usual medical protocol. The most meaningful interchanges for me with medical and nursing staff are the hallway conferences which are spontaneous in nature and are times when real feelings and creative thoughts are generated toward the "person" part of the patients and their families.

I never before have needed as extensive a personal support system for myself as I do now in relation to my work in thanatology. I rely heavily on my two hours per week of individual supervision as well as a group seminar which often becomes a supportive milieu. Lastly, I rely on the support of my wife who is a continual source of solace in this taxing work which I do sometimes bring home and carry with me more than occasionally.

What is of keen interest to me is how this "job description" is necessarily infused with personal feelings and personal reactions. We are given more than subtle clues to the "psychodynamics of occupational choice," and we see the importance—the vital necessity—of meaningful "support systems" for a person involved in the psychological abrasive reactions that thanatological work invariably engenders.

VICTIM AGAIN: POETIC CODA

Any communication written by an individual of college age in the dramatic context of the real possibility of imminent death always mirrors a poignant situation—an urgent reaching across words and pages in which one party is desperate and the other is powerless. The Berkeley poet and perennial student, Ted Rosenthal, who was dying of leukemia in his early manhood, wrote for himself and for the world in the poetry he composed in the torment of his figurative night. "Night poems written in anger," he called them. Below are the concluding lines of his posthumous *How Could I Not Be Among You?* (1973), addressed as an anguished cry to any individual—in this case, *you*, the reader— who will have survived him.

> *Though you may find me picking flowers*
> *Or washing my body in a river, or kicking rocks,*
> *Don't think my eyes don't hold yours.*
> *And look hard upon them*
> *and drop tears as long as you stay before me*
> *Because I live as a man who knows death*
> *and I speak the only truth*
> *to those who will listen.*
>
> *Never yield a minute to despair, sloth, fantasy.*
> *I say to you, you will face pain in your life*
> *You may lose your limbs, bleed to death*
> *Shriek for hours on into weeks in unimaginable agony.*
> *It is not aimed at anyone*
> *but it will come your way.*
> *The wind sweeps over everyone. . . .*
>
> *Step lightly, we're walking home now.*
> *The clouds take every shape.*
> *We climb up the boulders; there is no plateau.*
> *We cross the stream and walk up the slope.*
> *See, the hawk is diving.*
> *The plain stretches out ahead, then the hills, the valleys, the meadows.*
> *Keep moving people. How could I not be among you?*

REFERENCES

Buhler, C. Meaningful living in mature years. In R. W. Kleemeier (Ed.), *Aging and leisure.* New York: Oxford, 1961.

Elliot, G. *The twentieth century book of the dead.* New York: Ballantine Books, 1972.

Erikson, E. *Childhood and society.* (2nd ed.) New York: Norton, 1963.

Glick, I. O., Weiss, R. S., and Parkes, C. M. *The first year of bereavement.* New York: Wiley, 1974.

Haydn, H. *Words and faces.* New York: Harcourt, Brace & Jovanovich, 1974.

Heard, G. *Five ages of man.* New York: Julian Press, 1963.

Hinton, J. *Dying.* Baltimore: Penguin, 1967.

Jung, C. G. *Modern man in search of a soul.* Trans. by W. S. Dell and C. F. Baynes. New York: Harcourt & Brace, 1933.

Lifton, R. J. *Death in life: Survivors of Hiroshima.* New York: Random House, 1967.

Melville, H. *Redburn.* New York: Harper & Brothers, 1850. (Numerous reprints).

Melville, H. *Moby Dick.* New York: Harper & Brothers, 1851.

Melville, H. *Pierre, or the ambiguities.* New York: Harper & Brothers, 1852.

Murray, H. A. Introduction. Herman Melville's *Pierre, or the ambiguities.* New York: Hendricks House, 1949.

Parkes, C. M. *Bereavement.* New York: International Universities Press, 1972.

Rosenthal, T. *How could I not be among you?* New York: George Braziller, 1973.

Schachtel, E. *Metamorphosis.* New York: Basic Books, 1959.

Shneidman, E. S. Sleep and self-destruction. In E. S. Shneidman (Ed.), *Essays in self-destruction.* New York: Science House, 1967.

Shneidman, E. S. The enemy and death questionnaire. *Psychology Today,* August 1970, 37–41, 62–72.

Shneidman, E. S. Death and you. *Psychology Today,* June 1971, 43–45, 74–80.(a)

Shneidman, E. S. Perturbation and lethality as precursors of suicide in a gifted group. *Life-Threatening Behavior,* 1971, **1**, 23–45.(b)

Shneidman, E. S. (Ed.) *Death and the college student.* New York: Behavioral Publications, 1972.

Shneidman, E. S. *Deaths of man.* New York: Penguin, 1973.

Shneidman, E. S. (Ed.). *Death: Current perspectives.* Palo Alto, California: Mayfield, 1976.

Sullivan, H. S. *The interpersonal theory of psychiatry.* New York: Norton, 1953.

Toynbee, A. *Man's concern with death.* New York: McGraw-Hill, 1969.

U.S. Department of Health, Education, and Welfare. *Facts of life and death.* Washington, D.C.: U.S. Government Printing Office, PHS Publication No. 600, 1970.

Weisman, A. D. *On death and dying.* New York: Behavioral Publications, 1972.

Ziegler, P. *The black death.* Middlesex, England: Penguin, 1969.

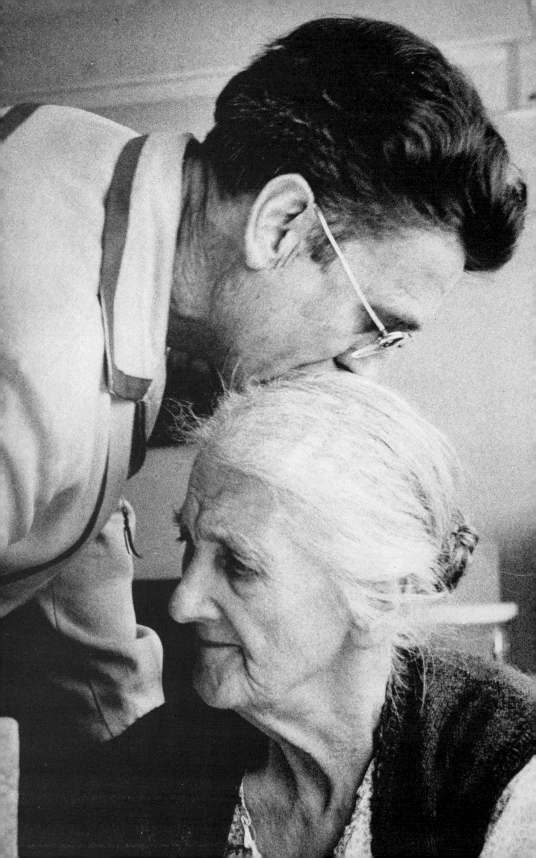

PART THREE

CLINICAL MANAGEMENT

5

DEATH AND THE PHYSICIAN: MORTUIS VIVOS DOCENT

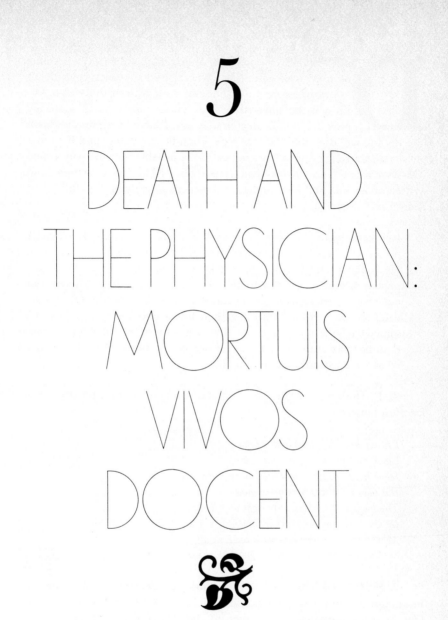

LAURENS P. WHITE

Death will affect you, and although it seems unbelievable, it may well affect me. My attitude toward your death will never be quite the same as it is toward my own, but it will be affected by the context in which I view my own death. The degree to which I have incorporated death into my life will directly affect the way I handle my dying, and if I am a physician, nurse, clergyman, friend, or lover, it will affect the way I deal with you when I am involved in your dying. Many have thought and written about this problem, perhaps none more directly and usefully than Seneca in letters to Lucilius:

> Rehearse death. To say this is to tell a person to rehearse freedom. A person who has learned how to die has unlearned how to be a slave. He is above and beyond the reach of all political power. What are prisons or bars or warders to him? He has an open door. There is but one chain binding us in fetters and that is our love of life. There is no need to cast this love out altogether, but it does need to be lessened somewhat so that in the event of circumstances ever demanding this, nothing may stand in the way of our being prepared to do at once what we must do sometime [p. 72].

A. E. Housman (1936) put a similar thought in more poetic, if less forceful, language:

> *I to my perils of cheat and charmer*
> *Came clad in armour by stars benign.*
> *Hope lies to mortals, and most believe her,*
> *But man's deceiver was never mine.*
> *The thoughts of others were light and fleeting*
> *Of lovers meeting or luck, or fame.*
> *Mine were of trouble and mine were steady*
> *So I was ready when trouble came* [pp. 15–16].

A good deal of our problem in dealing with death must be related to its unknown, and perhaps unknowable, quality. Our fear of our own death may be exacerbated by our reaction to and fear of the death of someone for whom we care. Professor Jacob Needleman (1969) went to the heart of the matter when he wrote:

> The first step in regarding another as mortal is to acknowledge with all of our being that we do not know what a person is or what death is, but that we have fears about these things and a contradictory view

of reality that goes hand in glove with those fears. This awareness of our own ignorance and fear would be, if we are to believe Socrates, the beginning of wisdom. The hasty flight from this awareness either into philosophical presumption, religious sentimentality, or dogmatic faith in the Cartesian natural science would be the reversion to ignorance. And what good can come from ignorance [p. 736]?

Caring for a patient who is going to die has all the elements of threat, failure, and helplessness which we so often associate with the process of dying itself. It is not surprising that this should be so, because in the process of caring for a person there is, to a greater or lesser degree, some identification with his problem as well as with his personality. To the physician engaged in such a dyad the impending or threatened death of a patient may be even more of a threat than it might be to someone else, for the physician tends to have a greater fear of death than does the ordinary individual. It is the purpose of this essay to look at some of the things which are involved in patient care, including some of the fantasies which contribute to the difficulty, and to propose some changes in the physician's concept of his or her role which might go some distance toward resolving them.

PHYSICIAN-PATIENT RELATIONSHIP

There are probably very few relationships as satisfying to all those involved as the relationship between a competent surgeon and a patient with acute appendicitis who is in pain and threatened with serious illness. To the surgeon the role of rapid intervention, diagnostic astuteness, reassurance, and then curative action reassures his need for a sense of mastery, a sense of involvement, and a need for validation of his success. To a patient who is in pain, with considerable apprehension, and an awareness that things have gone very wrong indeed, a most important need is for someone to make things right. He can't do it alone, and the patient is aware that he depends on someone else. When a brief and definitive operation is done, the patient's dependence is short-lived, although no less real, and he is rapidly restored to the ranks of those who are able to maintain an independent life and make their own decisions. The patient's need for action is met by equal need on the part of the physician to act, and ordinarily there are no complications involved in this sort of a relationship. Each participant has a defined role, and each one's conception of that role can be validated in a short time.

In contrast, the doctor treating a patient who is not going to get well and the patient with a fatal illness have changes in their roles which may be difficult either to acknowledge or to accept. This is probably especially true for the physician who, from his training and from his need, may still consider his role to be that of curing the patient, but who, by the current definition of dealing with the patient with incurable disease, is not going to have his efforts climaxed by cure, or the survival of the patient. It is, therefore, clear that if physicians cannot change their ideas about their roles as physicians, they are going to feel frustrated and on many levels a failure because of their inability to cure dying patients. This sense of failure on the part of physicians is very real, and I cannot think of any way in which the death of a patient can be regarded by physicians as a reassurance of their sense of mastery. The death of a patient not only affects their human feelings, but also magnifies their feelings of impotence, ineptness, and even guilt. If the physician makes a negligent mistake in treating a patient, and is aware of the mistake, he should feel guilty. (It is, perhaps, fortunate in one sense that we probably don't recognize most of our medical mistakes.) Ironically, however, the physician may feel guilty and incompetent upon the death of a patient even when performance and judgment, viewed by himself and others, have been of the first order. As I will discuss further, this sense of guilt and incompetence appear to be related to the fantasy that the physician should be able to cure all diseases and endow all patients with eternal life.

It is obvious that one immediate solution to this problem, which would delight us all, is for a new cure to be found for some specific disease that could make us feel successful and could avoid a lot of suffering. Short of that happy outcome, a more practical approach to the problem is to change in some way our concept of what our job as physicians may be. I will get back to this point later.

A QUESTION OF SEMANTICS

Words are toys of the mind, but like toys they may condition the way in which we think about things. Years ago, the Ford Foundation published a series of records on semantics and the extent to which the words we use condition our feelings and understanding of things. This record pointed out that, in the United States and to a great extent in England and the Anglo-Saxon countries, when children misbehave, they are admonished to "be good, don't be bad." In France, in contrast, when children misbehave, they are admonished to "soi sage," be intelligent. In Germany, the admonition is to "get in line." In Scandinavian countries, the warning is "var shnell," be kind. In Southwestern America, in the Hopi Indian tradition, the child is told "that is not the Hopi way." One can imagine that this sort of use of words conditions the way in which people growing up in these backgrounds think of their misbehavior. In San Quentin prison, when death row existed and prisoners sentenced to death had to be moved for any reason, the prisoner was shackled and conducted by two guards down the endless corridors of the prison, and the word went in front of him "dead man coming." There can be little question that such a shout would condition the reactions of those hearing it, whether they be guards, inmates, or the "dead man" himself.

To an extent which I can't calculate, the use of the word *terminal* to describe a patient must have a great role to play in the way in which we regard such a patient, as does, of course, the word *patient* itself. In your home you are a human being with whatever that implies to you and me, whereas in my office you are a patient. To some extent this defines you in my mind and me in yours. Hopefully, your role as a patient can be as little restrictive as possible, but, obviously, if you are seriously ill, you are more of a patient and have given up more of your independence than somebody who requires no medical care at all. Add to this the notation *terminal,* and not only does your condition become further defined in my mind but so do some of my feelings about what can be done for you and what can be done by me. Now, it is obvious that if I die today, I am terminal at this minute. The fact that I don't feel terminal has nothing to do with my terminality, and it can be seen in this rather simpleminded way that terminal as applied to an individual really means someone who dies shortly. Terminal really doesn't mean someone who I say is going to die, because I am so often wrong. Therefore, it seems important to me to make this distinction and for physicians to avoid the loose use of the word *terminal,* with all of the implications it has on an emotional level both for the doctor and for the patient.

THE PHYSICIAN'S ATTITUDE

Since so much that happens in the relationship between doctor and patient depends on the doctor's attitude, it is worth spending some time examining this. At the outset, it seems important to emphasize that we are all going to die. Even if a cure for cancer of the lung appeared tomorrow, this would simply mean that one reason for death had been eliminated, not that death itself had disappeared. It was no more than 100 years ago that medicine could accomplish so little that there would have been no need to emphasize that the role of the physician was not to cure patients; this was often a goal, and when it occurred, always a pleasure, but it, by no means, defined what the role of the physician was. As medical skills have increased and the medical armamentarium has been considerably enlarged, the cure of some diseases has become a reality. It's probably worth emphasizing that the prolongation of life which has occurred in the last 2000 years has come mostly from preventive medicine, not from curative medicine, from preventing illness, not from curing it. It is, however, our ability to cure some diseases that has created the problem for physicians which is so acute at the moment, namely, the inability to cope effectively with one's role as a physician when the patient does not get well.

It is argued by those of a trivial turn of mind that if the goal of a physician is not the cure of the patient, then the physician isn't trying very hard. Nothing could be further from the truth, assuming that we are speaking of physicians of good character and good will. When the goal of the physician is not cure, but rather care, more attention may be paid to what the patient really needs, rather than what the physician really needs. I am by no means unconcerned about the physician's needs, but want to set them in a frame of reference where they make some sort of sense in terms of what is possible with the patient. If the physician's main need is to care and to exert his best professional skills to provide the patient with optimum care, this may obviously be accompanied by the patient improving, or even getting completely well, and such a result is a delight to both participants. It may, in the event that the patient fails to get well, allow the physician to continue to give that concerned and loving care which ought to be every patient's right, without feeling that he is a failure, and without a feeling of complete loss of mastery in a complicated situation. It is the sense of mastery which appears to be at the heart of the problem.

A physician who feels that he can cure lung cancer in July 1976 has simply had too little experience with patients with lung cancer to be considered an expert. For a physician confronted with a patient with lung cancer, to state to the patient that nothing can be done is really to acknowledge a loss of the sense of mastery, because what he is really saying is that nothing can be done to cure the patient, and what the patient is hearing is that nothing can be done at all. It is from this sense of frustration and defeat on the part of many physicians that patients, faced with a complex and life-threatening illness, and given no support from their physicians, seek out magic and quack remedies offered by those unscrupulous or merely ignorant "healers" who recognize the importance of offering something to a desperate person. It is a profound fault on the part of medical professionals that so much of the time their feeling of impotence leads them to reject the patient, who in desperation then turns to these unscrupulous practitioners for the emotional, and often magical, support that seems to be needed. In such a situation, if a physician can acknowledge that the patient can't be cured, but that his job goes far beyond curing a patient to caring for him or her, and that caring for a dying patient can be important, rewarding emotionally, and helpful in a variety of ways, then he has done a great deal to support a patient in this difficult time. It is a curious anomaly that in this relationship it appears to be the doctor who is unable to accept his real role, rather than the patient who is unable to accept his fatal diagnosis.

I am convinced that one of the main reasons why most doctors are doctors is that they are convinced that in any relationship with doctor and patient it's the patient who is going to do the dying. There must be some level of resentment of this situation on the part of many patients, and I have heard often enough a patient saying, "I just wish you had my disease, not I." Nonetheless, the patient seems to have less trouble accepting the potential outcome of his or her illness than the doctor does accepting his or her inability to change that outcome. Therefore, the obvious suggestion is that physicians change their concepts of their role, particularly with patients with what are currently fatal diseases. The role of physicians should, therefore, be one of caring for patients, providing both expert technical care and the involved, concerned human care for another individual. This means helping patients to live as long as they can live comfortably, and helping them through the process of dying when that becomes inevitable. It means not abandoning patients because they are dying, not abandoning them because we conceive of them as terminal, or conceive of them as being already dead.

TECHNOLOGY AND DEATH

Curiously, our technology has allowed us to become trapped in a dilemma about prolonging life. This concerns the ability of physicians to maintain certain physiologic parameters of life after an individual has reached a point in illness or injury where useful or enjoyable life appears to be over. We are all aware of patients who have been kept "alive" by the use of respirators, IV fluids, and repeated cardiac defibrillation or massage. There is no question of the value of thse heroic measures in certain cases of cardiac arrest, chest injury, or shock. It is the application of these life-prolonging methods to someone whose life seems to be over which raises difficult, but proper, questions. Our lack of clear-cut answers may be related to at least four problems: (1) Our technology is so recent that we have had only a brief time to try to think out, and even to feel out, answers. (2)

Our definition of death is in the process of changing, in part because of our technology, and increasingly is being thought to center on "brain death" and not on the former parameters of absent heart beat and respiration. (3) No definition of death is going to satisfy everyone, and we can all share the awareness of the difficulty of being absolutely certain as to when a person is really dead. We accept our fallibility and shudder at the responsibility of working within its strictures. (4) The responsibility for making the life-death decisions we now face is very harsh.

When I listen to lay groups discussing this issue, I am struck with the frequency with which physicians are blamed for "keeping people alive," or for "using people as guinea pigs." This blame we must accept, because our technology has created the problem, and created the real fear in many minds that after all chance for meaningful life has passed, people may be kept indefinitely "alive" at the hands of the medical profession. Perhaps we should appreciate the compliment implicit in this appraisal of the power we physicians have, with so much work, recently acquired. Most physicians, are, however, deeply concerned with ways of making appropriate decisions as to the use of this power. Its use involves very difficult decisions about life, about when a patient is beyond recovery, about when a brain is truly dead. These decisions are to be made by people who are usually quite aware of their fallibility and their weakness. We must also admit that many physicians do regard their role as being able to prolong life, any life, for as long as possible and with whatever means are available. I cannot condemn any person dedicated to that goal, and it is within that framework, and at the hands of those workers, that our dilemma is created. It is vital, however, to be absolutely clear about the distinction between prolonging life and prolonging the process of dying, when the latter means simply the temporary postponement of the cessation of heartbeat and respiration by mechanical means after the brain, the essence of the individual, has ceased to function. Perhaps we might leave it that this is an area which requires much open thought, an area in which many points of view have merit, and which is too important to be resolved solely by physicians.

In California the recent passage (1976) of the Keene Bill (AB 3060) has directly tackled this problem. This measure provides an individual with the legal right to leave written instructions for his family and physicians that, in the event of illness preventing him from expressing his wishes or illness which makes recovery unlikely, he does not wish to allow or to undergo extraordinary measures to prolong his life. We, in California, are waiting to see the effect of this bill. It clearly represents a response to the nightmare of the Quinlan case, as well as an effort to assure the patient of some control over his dignity and destiny.

DISCUSSING DIAGNOSIS WITH PATIENTS

One of the ways in which physicians may help patients is by treating them as individuals of unique worth to whom we owe not only our best efforts but our honesty. By this I mean that all patients should be told in as direct and open a way as possible our conception of the facts as they relate to their illness. By facts, I mean diagnosis by name, and discussion of prospects in detail. By in detail, I do not mean in the most frightening or antagonistic or ominous way possible, but in as straightforward a way as possible. I also think this should probably be done on more than one occasion, because so often patients hear selectively, and they should probably have the opportunity to discuss our idea of reality as it relates to them as often as they want to. Some patients won't want to even once, but these are definitely in the minority. Other patients, of whom it might be said that such a discussion would hurt them irreparably, would probably not hear anything they didn't want to hear. All of us who are involved in this practice are aware of numbers of patients who, after extensive discussions of diagnosis and its implications, appear to be completely unaware of their diagnosis. By the same token, we are also aware of patients whose doctors have told them nothing, who are intimately aware of their diagnosis and its implications, and who in kindly fashion do not trouble the physician who seems unable to talk to them about these unhappy details. It appears to be almost an axiom that patients may know either much more than we have told them or much less, and that the only thing they can't stand to hear from us is a lie. When we are unable to talk to them about their disease, just as when their families are unable to talk to them, they really have nowhere to turn. The isolation of illness is then compounded by our clear instructions that it is not to be talked about. Our unwillingness to talk about someone's disease and his or her feelings about it is not consistent with giving good care.

Another important element in discussing diagnosis with patients is making sure that the family is involved in such a discussion. If a patient knows one thing and the family another, communication is diminished by at least that amount. Discussions with the family are vital, but I make it a point to try not to discuss diagnosis and prognosis with the family without the patient being present. In this way everybody knows at the same time what everybody else knows, but, more importantly, everybody knows that everybody knows, and that different stories are not being given to different people. There probably are a few people who don't like, or perhaps can't tolerate, this sort of discussion, but they are certainly a tiny minority, and in my experience, and that of many others, if they can't tolerate it they will quickly forget that such a discussion ever took place.

THE ROLE OF DENIAL

It is important to discuss the role of denial in patients with serious or fatal illnesses. It is equally important to recognize that denial exists in the professionals of the helping professions as well. We are all aware of moments in our lives when we have refused to admit the reality of something displeasing. There must be many more moments when our denial of reality blanks it completely from our awareness. Some people seem to have more of this tendency or capacity than others, and a few, who deny our form of reality, have various psychiatric diagnoses attached to their problems and their lives. In general, it would seem that denial is not adaptive or helpful as a way of dealing with problems. Most of us have come to view denial as a bad thing, and to see those persons who use denial as making some sort of error. A long series of patients, who have taught me so very much else, have also convinced me that denial is not necessarily a mistake, particularly in patients who face certain grim realities. This is probably true because denial is so variable, both in its degree and in the time span it occupies.

Many years ago a patient gave me a phrase, an understanding, and a gift which have been central in my life for 25 years. His name was Charles Young, and the gift beyond my repaying. He was dying of melanoma, early in middle life, riddled with metastases which were apparent to him, and not responding to the ineffective drugs then available. He was concerned about the effect upon American life of the then Senator Joseph McCarthy, and one day told me he thought he'd fly to Washington and assassinate McCarthy, saying, "Before they could even get me on trial, I'd be dead." Then, with an enigmatic smile, he added, "You know, Laurie, I know I'm dying, but I don't really believe I'm dying." In these simple words he gave me an answer to the enigma of denial, and in truth, a solution for dealing with it. Since then, I haven't felt any great need to "deal with it" in most cases. I can deal with the patient, being as truthful as I know how to be, and the denial which is built into the patient will enable him or her to deal with the truth. A very few people seem to look disease and death steady in the eye, using little denial. For them, withholding the truth would seem to be an obscene trickery, unlikely to deceive for long. At the other extreme are those few individuals who may follow a detailed discussion of their diagnosis and prognosis by asking if someone could tell them what is wrong with them. In short, it appears that the great majority of humans have a degree of denial which is appropriate to them; that this denial is consistent with the ways in which they have dealt with other problems and realities in their lives; and that it forms an integral, if occasionally variable, part of the way they deal with illness, and if necessary, with impending death. From the point of view of the medical professional, therefore, denial on the part of the patient can often be used as an ally or a strength. It allows some of our errors of commission or omission to escape too much notice.

Hackett and Weisman (1969) have studied the knowledge held by groups of patients about their diagnosis and prognosis. They found interesting differences in their sample, with almost all patients with heart disease having been given detailed information about both factors, but with only 7 of 20 cancer patients so fully informed, although 10 others had been given some information. Of even more interest, however, was their observation that only 9 of 20 patients with heart disease were fully aware of diagnosis and prognosis, even though nearly all had been told, and that 10 of 20 patients with cancer, not all of whom had been told, were aware of diagnosis and prognosis. A similar study has been done with children with leukemia, where a massive effort to screen the children from awareness of the facts of their cases was carried out, without any apparent effect on the children, 96 percent of whom were aware of what was happening and what it could mean to them.

And what of denial on the part of the health professional? How many hundreds of times have women found lumps in their breasts, and asked their physicians to do something, only to be told it was nothing serious. In San Francisco only 60 percent of internists and family physicians will perform Pap tests on their female patients, although this test can be lifesaving in detecting cervix cancer at a curable stage. Similar refusal to perform sigmoidoscopy can be cited. It is clear that a great deal which can be done for early diagnosis of cancer is not being done. It is my view that laziness is not the reason, but rather an unwillingness to find something unpleasant. It may be a vestige of the old fear of the herald bringing bad news to the emperor. It may relate to our identification with the patients, and our fear that similar tests might produce bad news in ourselves. Certainly very few physicians and nurses get checkups, annual physical examinations, or other routine measures which might help in early diagnosis, or lead to preventive steps. And this unwillingness, in the light of what we know, largely stems from denial. In opposition to this I must cite the very large number of physicians who have stopped smoking, which is certainly a lifesaving step. I recently, however, had a call from a man who smoked heavily, and who had asked his physician if he should stop. The physician said there was no need, since by having a chest film every 6 months, an early cancer of the lung could be picked up and cured, in the event it occurred. Such is clearly not the case in a disease with an overall cure rate of less than 5 percent, even in so-called "early cases," and it turned out that the particular physician was also a heavy smoker. I advised the man to quit both cigarettes and that physician, because denial on the part of the professional was affecting the advice he gave. I'm sure there must be times when this is true for us all.

One of the main reasons for having these matters openly discussed is encompassed in what I'll loosely call "the will of the patient to resist his illness." No one has been able really to define this well, or to produce any data that confirm this view, but many have the impression that patients who fight their disease may outlive those who give in easily. Ignorance of what one has, even assuming that it will persist, is certainly no basis for fighting it. A well-informed patient might be expected to be in a better frame of mind to fight than one who does not recognize the realities that he or she is facing.

This recognition of "reality" is a complex, and probably central, issue for those threatened with early death. Denial certainly operates at any level of such awareness, but an ability to acknowledge, if not to accept, the reality of one's condition, may be of great importance in dealing with it.

During the great slaughter of people in the German concentration camps, the German technicians developed and carried out an ingenious series of deceptions to screen the victims from the reality of their impending execution. Speed was essential, calmness and ruthless efficiency important, but the main ingredient in the success of so much killing was an unwillingness on the part of the victims to imagine, or to accept, their fate. Starved, beaten, terrified, dehumanized, in strange surroundings, the victims can hardly be criticized for their failure to resist. The same behavior was seen in Russian soldiers, Dutch Jews, American pilots. No resistance was ever offered during the entrance into the camps, when so many were immediately gassed and cremated. All the resistance, when it happened, came from groups within the camps who had discovered what their fate would be and who had decided to fight for their lives. One will never know whether such a fight ever took place in the pure death camps, such as Belsec, for no one survived to tell of it. At Treblinka, Sobibor, and Auschwitz, groups did organize, did plot, and eventually did fight. At Treblinka, where over 800,000 were slaughtered, 400 fought, and 45 survived.

Elie Cohen, a physician who survived Auschwitz and has written about it in Eric Boehm's *We Survived*, described his delusional thinking upon entering the camp. Knowing of its purpose, and of his likely death, he convinced himself that, as a physician, he was likely to be spared because the Germans might need physicians. Rabbi Leo Baeck, the chief rabbi of Berlin, was a prisoner at Theresienstadt in the so-called "privileged" camp/ghetto. When the decision to move the Jews to Auschwitz for gassing was made, he found out what was in store. He decided to withhold the information from the others, reasoning that "to live in the expectation of death by gassing would only be the harder." Although the Germans deported most of the ghetto, about 4000 stayed in Theresienstadt, and most survived the war. Of the nearly 50,000 deported to Auschwitz, Baeck was one of the few who survived. One might wonder what thoughts this man had for the remainder of his life about his decision not to warn his fellow prisoners.

Some of the survivors of the holocaust have written about themselves, their experiences, and their feelings. They all seem to share an overwhelming sense of guilt at having survived, when so many of their friends and families did not. This guilt seems inevitable and sad. Many have attributed some of their guilt to what they did in an effort to survive: their daily fight for food, shelter, and better work gangs, their stealing from their fellows and even denouncing others to obtain rations or favors. They rather uniformly describe themselves as grimly fighting to escape a fate which was claiming others, and which they recognized clearly. It appears from their testimony that the survivors of the holocaust came from the group which saw clearly that they were doomed to die, and fought endlessly to escape that fate. The majority of this group died, too, but some survived. In the group which either denied the reality of what was happening, or which, having recognized their doom, chose not to resist, survival was, apparently, almost nil. It must also be admitted that the will to resist could not have been a constant thing, and must have fluctuated and been affected by many chance and intentional factors.

HONESTY BETWEEN PHYSICIAN AND PATIENT

It seems to me that this lesson from the holocaust, and from their epicenter, the Polish killing camps, if I am interpreting it correctly, has a great deal to say to us about how we deal with people facing death from disease. If we deny them the relevant information about diagnosis, prognosis, and available remedies, we deprive them of even the choice of whether to fight for their lives. If, from their own denial, or unwillingness to fight, they decline to fight for themselves, it is another matter, but I deeply believe we are obliged, in honor and good faith, to acquaint them, and not just a family member, with the relevant facts about their situation.

In addition, patients who know that physicians will be honest with them about something as important as diagnosis and outlook may expect physicians to be honest about other details as well. In contrast, patients whose physicians lie to them usually are found out because patients are at least as smart as physicians, and can quickly pick up obvious lies. It is an imprudent patient indeed who, after being lied to, will believe other elements of what the doctor chooses or refuses to tell him. By being truthful, I do not mean that I advocate the rather sorry practice that some physicians have of telling a patient how long he has to live. I regard this as an effort on the part of the physician to pretend to a mastery that he doesn't possess, to pretend to a certainty of the future that would make a fortune teller blush. I have often heard patients say, "Well, the doctor gave me 6 months to live," and shared their amusement as we discussed this proffered gift several years later. This sort of imperial soothsaying does not dignify either the practice of medicine or the physician who does it. Nonetheless, patients and their families often ask how long they have to live, and it has seemed to many that this question concerns itself more with whether the physician is going to stick it out however long it takes than with knowing exactly the date on which the patient is expected to expire. Therefore, a reasonable response is "I don't know how long you are going to live, but I do know that we will go through it together, with whatever it takes, and for as long as it takes."

ANGER AND DEATH

One of the sad things that often happens while we are caring for a dying patient is that the frustration of the experience and the difficulty of dealing with the feelings that it engenders may lead us all to anger. If depression is perhaps the most common of the unpleasant feelings, anxiety is probably the least tolerable, and most of us substitute anger for anxiety. If we are anxious because of a patient's illness, and our inability to control it, it may be easier for us to be angry with the patient, to be angry with a family member who may have called once too often, or to be angry with another physician who has been involved in the patient's care. It is important to recognize that much of this anger very likely represents our expression of a general feeling of frustration rather than an appropriate reaction to someone's misdeeds. It is also worth remembering that both the physician involved in the care of a dying patient and the patient himself need all the support they can get. This support can most appropriately come from the family, but also in great measure, when the patient is hospitalized, from the nursing staff, from social workers, from ward attendants, and in a curious and delightful way, from other patients themselves. I have often thought that a good deal more therapy goes on in my waiting room than I am aware of, and at times, a good deal more than goes on in my treatment rooms.

ACCEPTANCE AND DEATH

Religious conviction is a great source of strength for those who believe. The threat of death represents a real test of the depth of belief and of the support it brings. Only yesterday I again saw the strength which profound belief in God brought to a young physician very close to death, but I have also recently seen deep disbelief appear in a dying woman, whose last words were "don't pray over me."

For many who face death the clergy are traditional, and occasionally helpful, members of the health care team. For those to whom religion is a source of strength, the clergy can be of great help in mobilizing this strength and in sustaining contact with the living. Many clerics are sources of strength themselves, and their humanity may make this help as available to those without specific religious feelings as to members of their own church. Like all of us, the clergy often have problems about death, problems which need to be worked through before they can become more comfortable with a dying person or his family. Like all of us the clergy have ways to achieve distance, to defend themselves against too much feeling. Where a physician may retreat behind a supposed life-sustaining machine, a clergyman may retreat behind prayer to prevent more personal involvement. Awareness of his own feelings and weaknesses is as important to the priest or rabbi as it is to a physician or nurse, and as uncommon.

What a human needs as he faces death is no different from what he needs in life, and love best expresses what he needs to receive and to give. Those of us in the helping/caring professions need the same in no less a sense, and profoundly need to be able to give love at the same time that we use our scientific and technical expertise. For all of us, whether with or without religion, the future involves accepting a common mortality. We all seem to seek "meaning" in life and in death, and in our personal and professional relationships. Peter deVries (1961), in his masterpiece *The Blood of the Lamb,* described this dilemma better than I can.

I believe that man must learn to live without those consolations called religious, which his own intelligence must by now have told him belong to the childhood of the race. Philosophy can really give us nothing permanent to believe, either: it is too rich in answers, each canceling out the rest. The quest for meaning is foredoomed. Human life "means" nothing. But that is not to say it is not worth living. What does a Debussy Arabesque "mean," or a rainbow, or a rose? A man delights in all these, knowing himself to be no more—a wisp of music and a haze of dreams dissolving against the sun. Man has only his two feet to stand on, his own human trinity to see him through: Reason, Courage and Grace. And the first plus the second equals the third [p. 241].

REFERENCES

Boehm, E. (ed.) *We Survived.* New Haven: Yale, 1949.
deVries, Peter. *The Blood of the Lamb.* Boston: Little, Brown, 1961.
Hackett, T., and Weisman, A. Denial as a factor in patients with heart

disease and cancer. In *Care of patients with fatal illness, Annals of the New York Academy of Sciences,* 1969, **164**, 802.

Housman, A. E. *More poems.* New York: Knopf, 1936.

Needleman, J. The perception of mortality. In *Care of patients with fatal illness, Annals of the New York Academy of Sciences,* 1969, **164**, 733.

Seneca. *Letters from a Stoic.* R. Campbell (ed. and trans.). Harmondsworth, Maryland: Penguin, 1969.

6

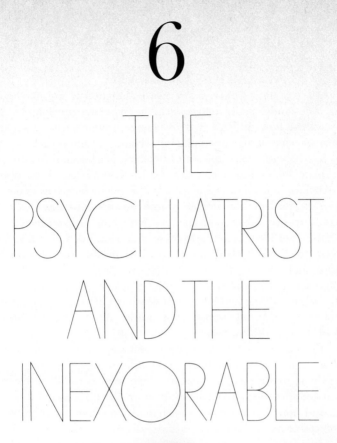

THE PSYCHIATRIST AND THE INEXORABLE

AVERY D. WEISMAN

A RECOGNITION AND REALIZATION OF DEATH

s a philosopher, I am aware that people are uncomfortable and usually bored with theory. As a psychiatrist, I know how difficult it is to change anyone's character, or even to alleviate what is most complained about. As simply another human being, I sense with every cell and fiber how fearful and dreadful it is to contemplate the certainty of one's death. Nevertheless, I am obliged to formulate how best we can cope with and reconcile ourselves to the inexorability of death. I do not propose simple answers posing as universal psychological truths. I can offer neither egregious encouragement to the fainthearted nor fatuous myths to those who regard denial as a way of life. My own proclivity is that fear of death is at the root of most human problems, and is woven into the solutions we propose. In some cases, turmoil and conflict are modulated into an acceptable ambiguity. Consequently, fears of dying and the fact of death can be ameliorated through a kind of transcendental despair, not unlike the tranquility supposedly found in the eye of a hurricane.

In the second half of this century, we have witnessed a strange resurgence of interest in topics related to death and dying. Although centered on the dying experience, discussions range from care of the bereaved to cultural considerations about funerals, from the high cost of dying to the nature and prevention of suicide. Currently, the number of publications, conferences, seminars, and courses about death far exceed anyone's capacity to assimilate everything that is being said or written. Much of this interest may be merely fashionable, and will soon recede. Even so, how can we explain this renewed interest, if not preoccupation, with the primary dread, death in the midst of life?

People have always been deeply concerned about death, so the resurgence of interest reflects no more than a new version of a very old enigma. Even a passing familiarity with classical and medieval times shows how other cultures dealt with death. Primitive people devised myths to explain how and why death entered the world. Of the Three Sisters or Fates, Atropos snipped the thread, reminding mankind that it has no control over the length of life.

Seneca wrote elegies in his essays about death, and then took his own life. Faust, according to the legend, fought against death, and lived to regret it. Myths about the Wandering Jew or the Flying Dutchman represent the futility and punishment inherent in the prospect of living endlessly. Destiny cannot be cheated. It is beyond quibble, quarrel, entreaty, and deception. Nevertheless, while we dread dying, we fear old age. Death is both sacred and sinister, embodying elements of evil or assurances of relief and release from suffering and injustice.

According to the now-popular opinion, we have stripped away the denial surrounding death. It is purported no longer to be a taboo topic because we talk more openly about death, implying that because of new-found candor we confront our own dying with equanimity. I am not con-vinced that resurgent interest in death-related topics is without its own anxiety. The process of making death more acceptable and less dreadful has generated many masterpieces in art and literature through the ages. Imbued as this generation is with the importance of "communication," "relationships," "real feelings," and "true selfhood," it is still reasonable to postulate that oversubscribed conferences and a plethora of publications may simply exemplify contemporary forms of denying death's personal reality.

I do not deplore openness, but like other professionals I am concerned about death becoming a chic subject. The hidden factors of death and dying as a central human experience may be in danger of again being obscured by counterfeit enthusiasm. It is a little like a dreamer who wants to talk about an intriguing dream, but is reluctant to analyze the elements that go into the dream. People seem to want answers, but prefer oversim-plified diagrams to the arduous task of asking researchable questions.

We are not so empirical that we do not dress up older ideas, as if they were innovations. Truth is only what we believe today, fortified by a faith that it will be true tomorrow. In short, every action has an equal potential for abuse of action. There is no idea so sublime, certain, or self-evident that it cannot be distorted and even become a form of insanity. Preoccupa-tion with "management of dying" is a noble and necessary quality of life, but it can also be a subtle tactic for exploitation of anxieties.

Stripped to essentials, the thrust of modern thought is existential. We have no authority to explain death: any theory about death is simply another version of how we cope and fail to cope with persistent problems of living. One major problem of this kind is the conflict between alienation and individuality, represented most often in the confusion between ideolo-gy and identity.

A link between alienation and individuality is to be found in the inexorability of death. We have no court of appeal, and it seems likely that all of us who struggle to make sense out of the mystery that finds us here can and will perish without a trace. Death is a property we hold in com-mon, but most of us would rather relinquish our claim. Death is whatever we choose it to be. It seems unfair, and yet so correct.

Death and life are inseparable companions, frequently in dispute, never very far apart, because each depends upon the other. Nevertheless, even thanatologists ask "What does it mean to die?" "Can I die?" "Will I die?" "Must I die?" "What is it like to die?" Their questions are no more sophisticated than those of a curious child. But their answers have a great-er ring of reality than that of a dogmatic adult. In the first place, our task is not to explain death, birth, maturity, or how we got here. As in antiquity, we are always changing and remaining the same. More specifically, to live is to strive toward a death we can live with. In the second place, our task is to reconcile ourselves with the inexorable, *death-as-it-is-lived,* uniting the satisfactions and conflicts of life with the consummations and frustrations of death.

By becoming and simultaneously ceasing to be, we change and remain the same, always undergoing little deaths and quiet transformations. The hackneyed split between an inner subjective reality and an obscure, obdurate aggregate called external reality is stagnant, static, and mistaken. Instead, by putting our unique stamp of recognition upon things we meet and are mindful about, we come to realize that death, too, is ours.

Realization has two meanings: perceiving something already there, and making something real that merely existed before (Weisman, 1974). In both senses, realization is preferable to the neutrality and vagueness of the term *reality.* It signifies personal participation, not passivity. We become conscious of something, and take action upon it according to our own dispositions. The distinction between reality and realization is not academic. Reality means that we simply await the inevitable, which is death. Realization is a directive, ordering us to be ever mindful of our mortality, because we just might have something to say or do about it. From this viewpoint, the old question about whether a tree falling in an uninhabited forest makes a sound is easily answered—I don't know, because I wasn't there.

Realization has still another meaning, signifying something beyond the immediate. A sound is just a sound until we realize it to be a word, then a word within a broader context of meaning, called language. From that point on, words become a call for action, designating something to be acted upon. Recognition and realization of death—my death and your death—depend upon using whatever resources we have, including that of language, to overcome obstacles and make effective use of our limited life spans. Alienation, annihilation, and constant endangerment are three major hazards that we risk in confronting death. Whatever resurgent interest in death is valid, therefore, is a result of the times in which we live. The human world has colored neutral events, and our values change. Different types of realization force us to recognize how much we are surrounded by calamity and potential catastrophe. We have few resources beyond ourselves. Words can join us briefly, but language can also be a barrier.

Plagues of the past have given way to other global reminders of our fragility and transience. Impersonal and highly efficient technologies can wipe us out, demonstrating once again that the "Angel of Death" always hovers nearby. Traditional authorities not only are ineffectual but can conspire to bring about rapid extinction. Precepts, policies, and principles, we see very clearly, are often exercises in self-serving rhetoric.

In the struggle to survive with a modicum of significance, we have only our own reality and resources. Realization goes beyond the present by insisting that we can participate in creating the words and worlds we live and die with. As youth discovered during the sixties, the search for realization easily slips into occultism, regressive panaceas, religious nirvanas, and pharmacologies that exchange one reality for another. This generation did not discover death. The reverse is closer to the truth. It is more difficult to hide from death today; perhaps that contributes to the feeling that we no longer "deny" death. In any event, to "face reality," using that quaint old phrase, we are required to face ourselves, set into a mirror reflecting how life-styles might become death-styles. We have our own life to live and our own death to die.

Consumerism and computerism have also helped us to become aware of personal death in contemporary society. We cannot simply be a bare fact, a statistic, an abstraction, a nullity. On the surface, consumerism seems very far from death. But it insists that we cannot trust established authorities. Ideas as well as products are suspect. Familiar and convenient objects, institutions as well as appliances, are sources of endangerment.

Computerism has vastly simplified many problems of a complex world, but it also threatens us with annihilation and anonymity. The computer helps the demographer in classifying causes of death, but does nothing to relieve fears. Ubiquitous fears about death concern not just the brooding fact of death but the loss of options to help create a reality suitable for survival until the very end.

From our growing awareness that institutions and inventions which often promise the most can be trusted least has come a resurgent apprehension about being helpless. Trust itself has become a potential instrument of duplicity. Professionals who work with death recognize that when we start talking about hope, usually no hope is left. Recognition of death is difficult to hide from, but realization of our own death is even more difficult to accept. We reach for almost any sophistry to relieve distress, especially that of bold and pretentious talk. Nevertheless, the presence of death is unmistakably a part of being alive, and even being fully alive. But unless we achieve mutual respect for our individuality, death will remain as an abstract symbol, dehumanizing mankind.

PSYCHODYNAMIC CONTRIBUTIONS TO A CONCEPT OF DEATH

Although psychiatrists will never see more than a tiny fraction of people facing death, it is startling, but scarcely surprising, that psychodynamic theory has given so little attention to death-related situations. In comparatively recent times, of course, psychodynamic psychiatrists have investigated the effects of severe psychic trauma, of serious losses, of bereavement and widowhood, and so forth. As a rule, however, psychiatrists have tended to sit aside, presiding over patients who consult them because of individual despair without alluding to or detecting the omnipresence of death anxiety.

Schur's contemporary study of Freud's thoughts about death and extinction underscores this anomaly (Schur, 1972). Suffering as he did from incurable cancer, Freud wrote much that would be useful for analysts. However, the clues that Freud offered have virtually been ignored. Psychoanalysts have preferred to revise the inexorability of death into a more acceptable form, which can then be "analyzed" as a symptom of something else, and whisked away. Like other people, psychiatrists are afraid of death.

A treatise about psychoanalytic thanatology has yet to be written. Nevertheless, it is possible to mention a few psychodynamic concepts and problems which have considerable pertinence for better understanding of death-related topics—anxiety, depression, suicide, guilt, destructiveness, mourning, suffering, masochism, despair, and so forth. Not the least problem is the nature of defenses, coping strategies, ego ideals, and libidinal fields. Transference and countertransference, infantilism, maturation, and senescence also deserve more reflection and reassessment on these terms.

I can only dip into the vast reservoir of psychodynamic concepts to show their implications. For example, the concept of a *dynamic unconscious* is the engine that makes psychoanalysis go. It is the equivalent of classical necessity (anánkè) in being an immutable force directing individual destiny. Psychoanalysts do not discover the effects of the dynamic unconscious. Rather, it is persuasively conveyed in most of what we do, think, or feel. We do not simply live with irrationality and impulsivity; we are lived by energies within us. Nevertheless, Freud's modest adumbrations about a "death instinct" have largely been disclaimed, and, with one noteworthy exception (Ricoeur, 1970), not carefully explored.

Narcissism is another central concept that fuels psychoanalysis. It refers, of course, to our body image, but more comprehensively, to our ego ideal, the image of perfection and perfectability. Narcissism holds us together, despite the demands and injuries inflicted by nature and people. Its abiding characteristic is that everything must yield to our reality. Regardless of our shortcomings and shabby behavior, narcissism keeps us from feeling too vulnerable. Nevertheless, it is appropriate to recall the original myth of Narcissus. He became so infatuated with his own beauty that he ultimately killed himself. Thus, in narcissism, excessive Eros can culminate in death (Thanatos).

Transference can serve similar aims. In a therapeutic situation, the patient may make severe demands upon the therapist. These demands are such that the therapist is asked to surrender part of his or her own autonomy and reality, to bolster the narcissism and diminish the deprivations that a patient has endured. Frequently, these deprivations derive from earlier losses and deaths of significant others.

Repetition compulsion is an awkward concept for analysts in that it combines Freud's views about instinct with a general pattern for mastery of persistent problems. Clinically, repetition compulsion can be recognized when patients find themselves undergoing certain painful experiences over and over, often with their own consent, as if repetitious activity alone will alleviate anxiety. And the most pervasive anxiety is that of death.

Conflicts are dissonances created by wishes and fears, appetites and aversions. The range of conflict, coupled with guilt, anger, and ambivalence, extends over the spectrum of human behavior. *Defenses* are habitual ways of dealing with conflict, especially when a problem is unspecified. *Coping strategies* are more public forms of behavior in which a tangible problem presents a threat or fright. These and other concepts offer much to thanatology. Application and reflection upon such ideas would help clarify problems met in dealing with dying patients. But concepts are only instruments needing someone to put them to use. Critics never tire of pointing out the therapeutic failures of psychodynamic psychiatry. This observation begs the question, because success or failure is defined in many ways. It is certain, however, that dynamic psychiatrists have been remiss in appreciating the pathogenic influence of death and dying upon what their patients complain about. Concepts such as the repetition compulsion correspond in some respects to what Kierkegaard, for one, lengthily described (Bretall, 1946). Overzealous expectations lead to disillusionment. Until psychiatrists understand more about coping and vulnerability in different forms of death anxiety, the results of psychotherapy are naturally going to disappoint many.

Modern psychoanalysts are sometimes embarassed by the obvious errors and oversights of their predecessors. The next generation may also be puzzled by the slight attention that analysts now give to the universality of death in their work. Professional rationalizations and occupational denials may be strategic avoidances of anxiety about death. Courses in thanatology are now demanded by college students, but there is hardly a psychoanalytic institute that offers such studies in its curriculum.

COMPASSION AND
CONSTERNATION ABOUT DEATH

One of the principal tasks of a psychiatrist is to accept the inexorability of death. This is probably also true of others professionally engaged in the care of patients—psychologists, social workers, the clergy, nurses, and others. By no means is this all that anyone so designated should know or even do in the course of professional duties. But confrontation with the facts of death exacts a heavy emotional price which partially can be met with an assiduous personal acquaintance and association with the phenomenon of dying. Personal realization, in the sense already described, is mandatory.

If death anxiety is always present, but only changes in degree, then we can expect it to modify our sense of reality. Consternation and compassion for the human predicament must include us all. Fear of dying is not like the fear of death. Fear of dying consists of different types of vulnerability—*helplessness*, to be without options; *hopelessness*, to be alienated from our distinctive reality; *guilt*, to have fallen from the expectations of our ego ideal; *truculence*, to be in danger and to be angry about our plight; and so forth. Severe sickness always compromises our autonomy, threatening us with weakness, as well as with unfamiliar perceptions. In order to cope with the psychosocial concomitants of chronic and progressive illness, we respond with strategies based upon a mixture of denial and acceptance—avoiding, postponing, minimizing, dispersing, redefining, reversing, rationalizing.

Evolutionary theory maintains that, for the species, only the fittest survive, while others die and become extinct. Despite constitutional myopia, however, we must also strive for an even shorter view, not yielding to fatalistic acquiescence that those who are very sick must die here and now as a "Law of Nature." One of the paradoxes of thanatology is that familiarity with death promotes a deeper appreciation of what it can mean to be alive. Consternation and compassion about individual illness, especially fatal illness, encourages a somewhat antievolutionary viewpoint: survival of the sickest as long and as well as possible. The problem is to find a death we can live with, to cope with the ongoing process by calling upon successful strategies from the past while correcting for differences in the present. The ultimate test of coping effectively with our deaths, yours and mine, is a type of transcendental despair, a process of creative acceptance of limitations and possibilities, without relying on linguistic or theoretical legerdemain.

It is very easy to offer palliative platitudes, to confer with colleagues, to interpose depersonalizing procedures, and to do practically anything but realize our own mortality, especially as reflected in someone else's demise. Even at peak moments of experience, we do not succumb and wait for evolution to alter acceptance of extinction. In the here-and-now, the salient question is not who is fittest to survive, but who is in danger of dying?

Physicians cannot safely predict who will die at what moment, even among incurable patients. By the time that a clinician can determine with certainty that this patient, not another, will soon die, it is already too late for psychosocial intervention. What we already have learned about the psychology of death has largely come from study of people who are comparatively healthy, or at least only in the preterminal stage of life (Kastenbaum, 1972; Shneidman, 1973).

Because death is an inescapable allotment, psychosocial interventions are appropriate at almost any time, even when death is indeed remote. But as a practical consideration, specific interventions can take place advantageously whenever chronic and very serious illness threatens to lapse into an intractable stage. There are many death-related situations which are still far enough from biological death but near enough to evoke consternation, concern, and compassion, lest the patient slip further towards death. Under these circumstances, it is proper to consider the following elements of preterminal intervention as steps towards inexorable, if not incipient, death: (1) informed consent (2) safe conduct (3) significant survival (4) anticipatory grief (5) timeliness and (6) appropriate death.

Informed Consent

The phrase has a contemporary ring, but by no means is a recent ethical, legal, or psychological problem. At present, hospital associations and government agencies have provided guarantees and guidelines to protect patients and physicians against unwarranted, uninformed, violations and transgressions. Risks are weighed against benefits; side effects and consequences, experimental and expected, have become part of the physician-patient contract.

Informed consent does not end with a bill of rights (Kessenick, 1973). Indeed, legal considerations are only one aspect of the rapport presumed to exist between doctor and patient. At best, laws simply circumscribe and define the limits of transgression, and do not automatically restore rights forfeited to technology and overinstitutionalization of medical care. As an ethical problem, informed consent recognizes that doctors and patients should be allies, not adversaries, who must be very cautious before agreeing to any procedure.

In its psychological dimension, informed consent is an act of freedom within one's sense of responsibility. Were it not for the fear of dying, with all its component characteristics, informed consent would merely be an expression of mutual respect. However, sickness is the opposite of responsibility (Weisman, 1965). Part of the predicament of illness is that a very sick patient fears being victimized. The inroads of disease are less to be dreaded than the indifference of strangers, however competent in their skills. Informed consent is an obligation which guarantees the prerogative to choose or refuse. No one can be absolutely sure about any treatment, but informed collaboration does not require much more than prudence. It does insist that among the risks of being very sick, fears about alienation, abandonment, and anonymity can be exceedingly strong. Few patients demand omniscience from their doctor, but trustworthiness is a pivotal consideration, especially when therapeutic resources are limited, and patients are vulnerable. Rights are of little use to people with few options; vulnerability to wrongs requires the pledge of compassionate allies, physicians among many others.

Safe Conduct

There are several rights that any patient should expect from a doctor— knowledge, skill, and compassion. Medical care itself has three widely recognized aims—diagnosis, treatment, and relief. A fourth aim is also a right: safe conduct. For the terminal patient, safe conduct may be all that remains to help neutralize his or her consternation.

Safe conduct means two things: to behave cautiously and prudently, and to guide another through peril and the unknown. It does not mean to play it safe in a constrained manner, caring simply for one's own safety. Safe conduct is part of informed collaboration, extended to the point of incipient death. For many doctors, safe conduct consists of giving more drugs, and delegating authority to others. Very sick patients need more than this, however, especially since their options are usually limited to simple activities near the bedside. A psychiatrist, or someone else skilled in human interaction, can behave compassionately, and prevent dehumanization of patients as the lifeline comes to an end. If the therapist cannot collaborate and share the uncertain certainty, it is far better to recognize intractable consternation and quietly transfer responsibility to another.

Significant Survival

For most of the world's population, mere survival is difficult. But given the good fortune to be free from intense suffering and to have a decent degree of emotional and economic solvency, it is not enough merely to survive. Individuality, as opposed to alienation and annihilation, depends upon survival for a purpose.

Survival for a purpose is significant survival when we realize a value in what we are and do. A sense of self-esteem is necessary for a congenial reality, i.e., a world in which we are willing to live. Because living and dying are always in a precarious equilibrium, threatened at every moment by forces and caprices beyond foresight and control, the psychosocial therapist (I know no better general term) who offers safe conduct is also obliged to find an Archimedean pivot enabling a dying patient to find significance in what is, after all, part of his or her living, the penultimate portion. Besides relief of suffering, the therapist looks for whatever an individual has found significant during earlier and healthier days. To be sure, much of this is beyond recall, but significance is a sense of well-being and self-esteem, treasured in reminiscence as much as in reality.

In the succession of days and years, values and activities, motivations and outcomes once charged with excitement and enthusiasm tend to abate, to be relinquished, sometimes ruefully, but often with relief. Ends and means usually fuse, and we come to accept limitations in time, space, and opportunity. Safe conduct is measured by the extent of significant survival that informed collaboration imparts.

Significant survival accepts oscillations between sickness and responsibility without loss of self-esteem. There is risk, however, that in caring for the very aged or terminally ill we may tilt the balance toward denial, rather than acceptance. This can lead to an unwitting duplicity in which we talk vainly about "hope," when we mean courage, about "reassurance," when we mean regret. Frequently, it is the doctor who loses hope and becomes vulnerable, exchanging the devalued coin of "encouragement" to cover his or her therapeutic bankruptcy.

Anticipatory Grief

To rehearse death, at least in the privacy of one's own mind, is a way of anticipating it. To anticipate a loss is the first phase of bereavement. While absolute pessimism about a patient has no more to recommend it than unqualified optimism, the question of whether terminal patients prefer not to be kept in ignorance is moot, if not irrelevant. With some exceptions, most dying patients do not need to be "told the truth," because they are already aware of being very sick. However, it is simply practical for doctors to be compassionately candid. Not only does this make their task easier but it encourages both the patient and family to initiate bereavement, without waiting for death to take them seemingly by surprise.

Anticipatory grief is a phase of coping with inevitable death, to be followed by other forms of mourning and resolution. Bereavement, of which grief is a part, comprises a series of adjustments in which people realize and reaffirm relationships. Although bereavements differ, absence of grief is apt to signify a disturbed relationship, or one in which the relationship has little functional meaning to survivors. To be saddened and undergo bereavement means that someone cares, recognizes the transience and transcendence of existence, and can personify inexorability.

Timeliness

In a society that prizes longevity and productivity, it is curious that workers are now being required to retire at younger ages. Productivity ceases, and enforced retirement imposes a sense of both obsolescence and guilt upon people through no fault of their own. As a result, some exworkers feel not only that it is time to retire but that it is even time to die as a significant individual.

There are many untimely deaths—premature, unexpected, and calamitous (Weisman, 1973). While not acknowledged so openly, there are also many hypermature deaths. However, timeliness of death is not like condemning someone to the limbo of obsolescence, nor is it simply a demographic probability. It is a highly personalized realization of completeness, in which actual survival corresponds to expected survival. The allotment of life that the ancients called *Moira* is still relevant, steeped though we are in the philosophy of survival for its own sake.

Perhaps it is the very notion of success in our culture that is antagonistic to the timeliness of death. Were people given a choice of when and how they would die, many would, of course, hesitate, stall, and compromise, denying their vulnerability as much as their mortality. But other people consent to die, not as a sign of depression or despair, but as an acceptable realization. Arguments about euthanasia abound today, and it has always been easy to say that someone else, about whom we care very little, has lived long enough. However, if we truly believe that each person's death is his or her own, then to accept death as our decision is a reasonable consequence.

These thoughts should not be construed as an advocation of unilateral, active euthanasia. Many aged and infirm people assert that they are living on "borrowed" time. But borrowed from whom? We can be loyal to our pledge of safe conduct and still question the quality of someone's remaining life.

It would be foolish to pretend that dying people usually welcome death, but equally obtuse to ignore patients who feel prepared to die, although with a mixture of anxiety and serenity (Feifel et al., 1973). Anticipatory grief does come to an end for the individual as well as the survivor. Stewart Alsop (1973) observed that a dying person needs to die, as a sleepy person needs to sleep. In medieval times, the craft of dying consisted of creating a situation in which death became more significant, socially acceptable, and less terrifying. In these secular times, the same aims can be reached without rituals, provided that we are not always expected to fear death with the same intensity.

Appropriate Death

An appropriate death is one we might choose, had we a choice. It is not necessarily an ideal death, whatever that might mean. As Becker (1973) pointed out, our heroes are those who defy death, and vanquish it, thereby enabling those of us who are not heroes to deny death.

Birth and death are really the most banal events imaginable. Everyone is born and therefore dies. The silent totality is not a very exclusive society. It is what can be interposed between birth and death that makes one life distinctive and another futile. However, the facts of life and death do not prevent us from seeking to reduce infant mortality, eliminate pollution, treat disease, and generally improve the quality of life. We can also include searching for an appropriate death.

Just what is an appropriate death? It means an absence of suffering, preservation of important relationships, an interval for anticipatory grief, relief of remaining conflicts, belief in timeliness, exercise of feasible options and activities, and consistency with physical limitations, all within the scope of one's ego ideal. Resolution of qualms and equivocations about the inexorability of death ensures that a dying person, through the final version of an informed consent, will die with dignity, perhaps with greater self-esteem than was possible during life. The dying person can realize extinction without false promises, but with safe conduct, renouncing autonomy without feeling helpless. Appropriate death is not a visionary consummation, but one in which the reward is to confront our mortality as if we had created it.

PSYCHIATRIC INTERCESSIONS

Caring for the dying is a special instance of safe conduct for patients beyond cure, just as informed consent is for patients who need treatment, but have few options. In this book, generally devoted to the meaning of death, I have chosen to discuss guiding principles without detailed clinical instructions or case illustrations which are found elsewhere (Weisman, 1972). As a prerequisite for asking patients to confront mortality, I have advised professionals first to confront their own. This is not a matter of theory versus practice, but a series of ongoing maturational pauses, progressing from principles to practice, then back again. We move ahead with small leaps and quiet insights. Without a grasp of theory to guide our efforts, we risk floundering amidst myths, preconceptions, value judg-

ments, and anecdotes. Without clinical contacts, we risk interposing notions that have little to do with dying as a human experience.

Several tactics can be recommended, but most can be reduced to the
realization that our image of death is constructed on living experiences of
compassion and consternation. The psychosocial dimensions of care need
informed collaboration between allies, one of which is the patient, because
there is a common threat to autonomy and individuality in contending
with death. Finally, we face a common fright together, lest we undergo
alienation, annihilation, and endangerment—an existential plight that
prevents us from fully realizing each other.

"What can a psychiatrist do?" The question can be turned around:
"What can death do for the psychiatrist?" He or she is only incidentally a
physician. Unlike other doctors, psychiatry is a field in which death seldom occurs. On the other hand, psychiatry studies the human condition
within the context of illness. Consequently, to study the human condition
without including death is a lopsided enterprise. Moreover, what is real for
a psychiatrist can be made very real for others in coming to terms with
death. Regardless of their professional, paraprofessional, or semiprofes-
sional status, thanatologists can both reach and teach others by example,
precept, supervision, and open, shared concern (Weisman, 1972).

The role of a thanatologist is not determined by psychiatric training.
Psychiatry is simply one advantageous avenue; there are others. But if a
psychiatrist sets out to become a thanatologist, it is essential to modify the
excessive anonymity and reliance upon words that conventional training
imposes. One should not insist upon talking about death incessantly, as a
kind of litany or counterphobic leap into the unknown. On the other
hand, a psychiatrist should not withdraw from openly and dispassionately
permitting patients to talk about their plight. As an informed participant,
tact and mutual respect should prevail. Each session is individualized as
an opportunity to deal with a host of mutual responses—denial, depression, resentment, apathy, defensiveness, despair, and so forth. Like the
bearer of bad tidings, a psychiatrist may become a target for all the frustration that a dying patient feels.

Compassion is not the same as offering consolation, if the latter means
simply to voice reassuring comments. Knowing something about physical
illness and the expected effects of medication may be even more helpful.
Denial is certainly not to be encouraged, but in some instances, denial
may be impenetrable. Nothing is to be gained from confrontation for its
own sake. In fact, realization of death is an instrument not unlike insight
during psychotherapy. It is not achieved in a flash of illumination, nor
darkly intimated. Effective insight comes from the patient, not the therapist. Intelligent appraisal of one's situation is a less ambiguous aim than
that of insight.

The physician's goal is to treat the cause of disease, and if he or she fails, to know the cause of death. The psychiatrist's goal is to modify the social and emotional context of fatal illness, and by succeeding, appropriate death itself becomes a cause. Other goals are to neutralize dread without ponderous, apathetic, and philosophical pronouncements. Those who are afraid of working in vain with patients who are destined to die anyway should get out of the field; vanity has no place. There is no reason to keep secrets from patients, but we may ask patients what to tell others. We can answer questions, provided that we are not afraid to admit ignorance or uncertainty. One cannot predict the significant concerns of every patient. Schematic stages—denial, anger, bargaining, depression, acceptance—are at best approximations, and at worst, obstacles to individualization. Properly realized, a good death, like a good life, has elements of informed consent, anticipatory grief, safe conduct, timeliness, and significant survival.

No psychiatrist should underestimate his or her vulnerability and tendency to deny. Sharing concerns with others, even role playing the final scene in the company of colleagues, can be instructive and beneficial. Later, psychological autopsies collate the information and insights gained from the encounter.

A final word about intercessions with the dying. Constant self-monitoring means that we ask questions, but we should also know the value of silence. Welcome awareness of dread and despair, because this helps transcend anxiety and prevent unwarranted feelings of inadequacy and guilt.

Death always arrives at the allotted time. Days and nights follow each other with relentless and inexorable impartiality. To find significance in death we must find significance in our own transience. In a very brief time, we shall all be nothing—a mossy gravestone somewhere, a slot in a columbarium, a few ashes in the sea. The rhythms of nature and the uncertainty of being alive bear witness to how we can mourn, forget, and be immersed in mankind's anonymous continuity, like waves breaking against the rocks, challenging time and nothingness.

REFERENCES

Alsop, S. *Stay of execution: A sort of memoir.* Philadelphia: Lippincott, 1973.

Becker, E. *The denial of death.* New York: Free Press, 1973.

Bretall, R. (Ed.) *A Kierkegaard anthology.* Princeton: Princeton University Press, 1946.

Feifel, H., Freilich, J., and Hermann, L. J. Death fear in dying heart and cancer patients. *Journal of Psychosomatic Research.*, 1973, **17**, 161–166.

Kastenbaum, R., and Aisenberg, R. *The psychology of death.* New York: Springer, 1972.

Kessenick, L., and Mankin, P. Medical malpractice: The right to be informed. *University of San Francisco Law Review,* Winter, 1973, **8,** 262–281.

Ricoeur, P. *Freud: Living and dying.* New York: International Universities Press, 1972.

Shneidman, E. *Deaths of man.* New York: Quadrangle/New York Times Book Co., 1973.

Weisman, A. D. *The existential core of psychoanalysis: Reality sense and responsibility.* Boston: Little, Brown, 1965.

Weisman, A. D. *On dying and denying: The practical significance of mortality.* New York: Behavioral Publications, 1972. (a)

Weisman, A. D. Psychosocial considerations in terminal care. In B. Schoenberg, A. Carr, D. Peretz, and A. Kutscher (Eds.), *Psychosocial aspects of terminal care.* New York: Columbia, 1972. (b)

Weisman, A. D. Coping with untimely death. *Psychiatry,* November, 1973, **36,** 366–378.

Weisman, A. D. *The realization of death: A guide for the psychological autopsy.* New York: Jason Aronson, 1974.

7

NURSES AND THE HUMAN EXPERIENCE OF DYING

JEANNE QUINT BENOLIEL

Dying is a lonely passage in that no one can "live through" the experience of terminal illness for another. Yet dying is also a social passage. What happens to anyone defined as dying is affected by the actions and choices of the other people who comprise his or her social world. In modern urbanized societies, the process of dying has shifted from the moral to the technical sphere of control, and the care of dying persons has increasingly become an institutionalized and depersonalized phenomenon (Cassell, 1974). Yet within this bureaucratic system not all dying patients experience depersonalization as they undergo the journey toward death. Because nursing as a service functions in the interface between consumers and the technical aspects of medical care, nurses often play singularly important and unrecognized roles in assisting patients and families to cope with the exigencies of death and dying.

The different ways in which nurses contribute to the lives of patients and families during terminal illness can best be understood by examining some changes that have altered both the practice of nursing and the social contexts in which death and dying occur. In the last half of the twentieth century dying has increased in complexity as a social problem, and caregiving services have become difficult for at least two important reasons. The society contains increasing numbers of elderly and physically disabled people who are undergoing prolonged dying, many of them isolated in special institutions organized and funded to provide essentially custodial services. The expansion of life-prolonging technology has increased the complexity of services delivered in hospitals through the creation of special purpose intensive care settings and a proliferation of highly specialized modalities of medical treatment. Both changes have clearly affected the work performed by nurses. The populations in need of nursing services have increased in number and have changed in character. The specialized skills required of nurses have been expanded under the influence of science, technology, and changing social conditions.

CHANGED NATURE OF NURSING PRACTICE

Nursing has long been identified as an occupation that offers personalized services and physical ministrations to sick people, including those who are dying. In days gone by direct physical care given by nurses often played a

Note: This chapter is based, in part, on research supported by Public Health Service Research Grant NU-00047 from the Division of Nursing, Bureau of State Services-Community Health, and conducted at the University of California, San Francisco.

124

major part in effecting recovery from pneumonia and other serious infectious diseases. The advent of antibiotics and complicated recovery-oriented medical therapies changed the character of nursing practice and created new clinical problems in which decisions about termination and prolongation of life have become occupational issues of serious concern.

Direct Care and Personal Satisfaction

Prior to World War II, nursing care of critically ill patients was often provided by special duty nurses working in either hospital or home or by student nurses on special assignments. With shifts extending 8 to 12 hours or more, the delivery of direct care in each case brought patient and nurse into prolonged daily contact, thereby creating circumstances conducive to involvement with personal as well as professional issues in the relationship. Technical activities and nursing procedures were relatively simple yet often added greatly to the patient's comfort and the nurse's sense of personal accomplishment. Direct physical contact was a source of satisfaction for both parties, and even when the patient did not survive, the nurse had the opportunity to experience directly the feeling of having made a singular contribution to the patient's comfort and well-being.

In many ways the curative effectiveness of new medical treatment removed from nurses the personal satisfactions associated with concrete acts of physical assistance. For instance, the sense of personal reward achieved through giving a tepid sponge bath that lowered a patient's fever originates in strong subjective feelings that these nursing actions did indeed make a difference in the patient's recovery from his illness. In contrast, the administration of penicillin by injection is an impersonal, instrumental act that offers limited opportunity to experience personal satisfaction in the recovery process. In a very real sense, the increased use of medical technology in patient care fosters a depersonalization of experience for the deliverer as well as the recipient of that care.

Specialization, Fragmentation, Depersonalization

Specialization in medicine has clearly added to the technical elements of nursing practice and, not surprisingly, has stimulated the growth of specialization in nursing. More importantly perhaps, specialization in medicine has transformed the context of patient care by increasing the numbers and types of paramedical personnel involved. No longer are services to sick people given by small teams of doctors and nurses working side by side in close communication. In the 1970s services to sick people are provided by large teams composed of many different specialists, and nursing occupies a middle position in the delivery system such that clinical nursing management of patient care has become an involved and often intricate social and interpersonal process.

Whereas direct physical care was once the major component of nursing practice, it is no longer sufficient in large, multipurpose health-care systems in which services to consumers are provided by many different types of workers. Indeed, communication among these various participants has become a key element in the nursing management of services for patients with critical, life-threatening diseases and injuries. Whenever the threat of death is present, clinical nursing management becomes an especially delicate matter because the problematic nature of team relationships is compounded by the conflicting demands of care and cure and the tensions associated with death and dying (Quint, 1967a).

There can be little doubt that the United States has evolved a cultural system for depersonalizing, specializing, and fragmenting the experience of human death (Kastenbaum and Aisenberg, 1972). Dying patients and their families find themselves in a complex medical system that attaches high priority to lifesaving procedures and technical activity and is poorly organized to offer personalized services. Yet not all patients facing death experience depersonalization in their encounters with the system, nor are their meetings with health-care personnel of necessity impersonal, detached, and devoid of personal meaning.

Visibility, Social Rewards, Public Recognition

Physicians play an important part in the lives of these patients, and public recognition of the doctor-patient relationship as central to personalized care is reflected in the amount of publication devoted to the topic. Far less attention has been focused on the contributions made by nurses to the welfare and well-being of patients during terminal illness, and this lack of public accolade may well be tied to the sex-linked and interstitial nature of the tasks performed by nurses. As Adams (1972), has noted, the low visibility of work performed mainly by women is associated with its nonspecialized character and coordinating function. The paucity of public recognition accorded to nursing's activities in patient care undoubtedly reflects the low social value attached to occupations defined as traditionally female.

In part then, society's failure to recognize nursing's contributions to terminal care rests in a cultural definition of nursing as a second-class occupation. The work performed by nurses tends to be taken for granted, and the value of their actions is obscured behind the cure-oriented goals of medical practice. Equally important, however, society's failure to identify openly the significant activities performed by nurses during terminal illness effectively shields the public from open awareness about the realities of dying. Few human beings, if any, want to be reminded of the suffering and indignities that are part of the process of dying.

The movement of human death from a public and accepted reality of life to a covert and tabooed position outside the mainstream of ongoing human experience has produced a society of people ill-prepared to cope with the problems and changes imposed by terminal disease. As control over the events of terminal illness—the ritual ceremonies of dying—passed from the dying person to the family and eventually to the doctor and the hospital team (Ariès, 1974), training for the social roles expected at the bedside of the dying became a major task for nurses and other direct-care providers. Adding yet another dimension to the formidable task, expanded medical technology and increased public demand for a broad spectrum of health-care services together created new situations in which death and dying exist as clinical nursing problems of central importance.

TYPES OF DEATH-RELATED, NURSE-CONSUMER CONTACTS

Death, near-death, or fear of death is a characteristic of many situations in which nursing personnel provide services to patients, yet in not all cases is the consumer of services explicitly defined as a "dying patient." Indeed, much of the time consumers of nursing services are viewed as recovery bound regardless of the seriousness of their physical states. For analytic purposes there are at least five kinds of situations in which nurses are in contact with patients who are facing death, and in each case, the death-related problems of practice are somewhat different.

Intensive Care

Expansion of medical technology in the 1950s and 1960s created new hospital settings designed specifically for the intensive treatment of critically ill patients. These intensive treatment wards share a common goal of recovery through application of new modalities of medical treatment, including recent advances in life-prolonging technology. Some wards provide services to patients with generalized medical or surgical problems. Others offer specialized therapies to patients with particular medical problems, such as extensive burns, acute coronary occlusion, massive trauma, or life-threatening complications associated with premature birth.

Organized around the work ethic of cure, these units are designed for rapid action in sudden emergency. Because the patients are in serious to critical condition, careful and frequent observation is an important nursing activity, performed increasingly with the assistance of specialized monitoring equipment that requires additional training and special expertise. Treatments and medications are given at frequent intervals, and technical equipment and new procedures are the order of the day. Although high in prestige on the cure-care continuum of services, the work is also time-consuming and energy-depleting.

Although many patients in these settings are in life-threatening circumstances, they are not necessarily labeled as "dying." Rather, the context is one in which uncertainty about prognosis is likely to be a common, though unspoken, norm. Usually these units are spatially arranged to maximize the goal of constant vigilance, often sacrificing the privacy of the patients in the process. To achieve the goal of recovery, nurses are expected to maintain a state of constant readiness for lifesaving action should such action be necessary. It should come as no surprise that constant vigilance creates a work atmosphere in which underlying tension is high, and personal concern about negligent performance is not uncommon. Hay and Oken (1972) likened the nurse's situation in intensive care to that of soldiers serving in an élite combat team.

Not only are intensive treatment expectations conducive to strain but the daily work itself brings nurses into contact with formidable stress-producing problems that reproduce themselves again and again as new sets of patients pass through. Despite the lifesaving ideology, nurses in intensive care settings face and live with repeated exposure to death and dying, regular contacts with unsightly and comatose patients, distraught families waiting outside the door, limited work space and intricate machinery, and communication problems involving physicians, staff, and families. Many deaths at once and the deaths of young people are experiences that intensive care nurses find difficult to tolerate. A head nurse on one surgical ICU made the following statement about her situation:

> Right now the staff is feeling very low, and there are several contributing factors. During the autumn there were several deaths all of young people, and this really got to the staff. One patient was a woman student from a nearby campus. Her illness began with vague symptoms, going downhill, but nothing could stop the progress. At autopsy they still could not find the cause. The girls worked very hard in giving care to this patient, and it is because they identified with her. A woman anesthetist, a resident assigned to the ward, identified so strongly that when the girl's condition got bad, she could not stay home but had to come back to the ICU to spend the night.

Whether en route to death or recovery, patients in these settings are heavily dependent on the nurses for both lifesaving activities and the comfort provided by personalized care. Sobel (1969) reported that the nurses working on a coronary care unit made a singular contribution to the emotional well-being of these patients when they communicated with them on a human-to-human level of understanding. Yet human-to-human contact increases the nurse's underlying concerns (including fear of death) and adds to the strain of trying to perform well in a context of conflicting demands.

Some nurses respond to intensive care work by depersonalizing their contacts with patients, families, and physicians. Others remove themselves to forms of nursing work less draining of personal resources. My contacts with nurses who cannot tolerate continuous assignment to intensive care wards suggest that they leave because they feel caught between the task of "lifesaving at all costs" and a personal wish to help the patient have a humane and dignified death. I have come to believe that intensive care nursing creates dehumanizing conditions for the staff in that they must continuously cope with conflicting expectations and demands, frequent life-death decisions, information overload, and patients who look to them for both cure and care (Benoliel, 1975a).

Emergency Care

Another context in which nurses encounter life-threatening problems of practice is the emergency room, a setting designed and organized for the rapid treatment of accidental injury and sudden critical illness. Typically located as subunits of large county or city hospitals, emergency wards provide lifesaving services to injured people from all segments of society. The problems brought for treatment range from simple cuts and bruises in a single individual to massive and extensive injuries involving multiple numbers of people and requiring rapid mobilization of additional personnel and emergency resources. Some units have as an adjunct mobile units that can travel to the scene of an accident to deliver emergency care with rapidity not unlike the services provided by military emergency teams in the treatment of battle casualties. Sometimes nurses are part of the mobile team, but more commonly nurses remain at the central emergency room with the mobile lifesaving care being delivered by physicians' assistants specially trained for this activity.[2]

---

[2] In Seattle, Washington, the Medic I program was first developed with firefighters selected and trained to offer first aid and cardiopulmonary resuscitation as needed. The actual delivery of emergency mobile services was done by these selected individuals who also had two-way radio communication with the physician in charge of emergency for help in evaluation of difficult cases.

Nurses who work in emergency rooms located in the inner cities of large metropolitan areas are exposed to the reality of unexpected and sudden death almost on a daily basis. More than that, they are exposed to death and near-death in its messier forms; i.e., the work often requires them to give aid to victims of suicide, homicide, fire, hit-and-run, and other forms of violence and destruction.

When patients are admitted in critical condition, emergency room work requires rapid evaluation of the type and seriousness of the patient's physical state followed by rapid decisions and actions appropriate to the situation. Often these decisions must be made in a context of incomplete data and uncertainty, and choice of action may mean the difference between a life lost and a life saved. When more than one emergency presents itself or when multiple emergencies appear simultaneously, decisions must also be made as to which patients are to be given priority. Although ideologically the staff would probably identify "critical physical state" as the major criterion used in making these choices, evidence from research suggests that these decisions are also influenced by social factors. According to one investigation, staff evaluations of the perceived social worth of clientele coming for emergency care strongly affected the treatment they received; for instance, Roth (1972) reported that patients labeled as drunks were more consistently treated as undeserving than were any other category of patient.

Since the work is organized to implement immediate lifesaving goals, emergency room staffs are not surprisingly heavily invested in the tasks of diagnosis and treatment of physical problems and the challenge of rapid choice. The short-term nature of these services results in relatively brief contacts between nursing personnel and the patients and their families. The intense character of emergency work in combination with the brevity of time involved fosters depersonalization in the contacts that take place between nurses and the people who come for assistance.

Following a period of participant observation on one emergency ward, Hess (1970) observed that staff behaviors that appeared "callous" at first came to be understood as a necessary "coping mechanism" for dealing with the difficult choices and decisions that had to be made on a regular basis. As a nurse not directly engaged in the delivery of lifesaving services, she was able to identify major psychosocial problems that some patients and families were facing and to provide them temporary assistance mainly through listening and referral to others in the clinic. Like many such places, the emergency ward observed by Hess was not structurally organized to offer crisis-intervention services on a regular basis nor to provide follow-up care to bereaved families and others affected by the aftermath of sudden psychosocial crises of major proportions. A few places have developed crisis teams containing clinical nurse specialists in psychiatric care to assist the regular staffs in coping with the psychological and social problems associated with emergency work (Jensen, 1973).

Recovery Care

A third contact occurs in settings in which ordinary medical treatments and diagnostic procedures are used to assist patients in recovering from minor and noncritical illnesses, injuries, and surgical operations. Nurses who work in doctors' offices, in outpatient clinics, and on general hospital wards encounter many patients whose conditions are of this type. Notwithstanding the noncritical nature of their illnesses, many of the patients have fears about death or dying regardless of whether these concerns are verbalized or not. Sensitive nurses are aware of these tensions, but the availability of a sensitive nurse at the right moment for a frightened patient occurs as much by chance as by plan.

The work in these settings is oriented mainly toward cure, and death-related problems are relatively infrequent as nursing tasks (Menzies, 1960). On occasion a patient moves into a critical state requiring intensive or emergency treatment on a temporary basis. The most difficult problem causing deep concern among the nursing staff is the unexpected death of a patient who was fully expected to recover. Unexpected death triggers in nurses (and physicians also) many questions about personal negligence regardless of whether negligence is at all a reality. Such deaths also lead to unusual channels of communication and stressful interactions as all persons involved strive to cope with a social event for which their established protocols (both personal and occupational) do not provide direction (Spitzer and Folta, 1964). The extent to which nurses can be helpful to other people under the circumstances of unanticipated death depends in great measure on the maturity they have developed through personal life experience and the knowledge they have accumulated about human behaviors in response to sudden loss and major change.

Chronic Care

A fourth type of nurse-consumer contact occurs with people who have chronic and life-threatening diseases at various stages of incapacitation, with different requirements for assistance depending on the physical and psychosocial problems that need to be solved. People whose lives have been altered by such diagnoses as diabetes mellitus, multiple sclerosis, emphysema, stroke, congestive heart failure, or cancer need different kinds of helping services depending on whether the disease is new and responsive to active medical treatment, whether secondary complications have appeared, or whether the terminal stage of illness is approaching.

One of the commonalities of persons who are adapting to the experience of chronic illness is the process of grieving, and nursing personnel are frequently in contact with patients and families at critical moments when support and communication are helpful to this process. During early stages of chronic illness, nurses are often involved in helping patients and families to educate themselves to live with the changes imposed by the disease and its treatments. Some patients with long-term problems are also subject to acute episodes of illness that may require hospitalization and application of recovery-oriented, intensive treatment regimens. Other patients may require long-term, rehabilitative and direct-care services to assist with the disabling impairments produced by progressive disease. My point is that chronic care consists of a broad range of nursing services that include lifesaving assistance, direct physical care, teaching-socialization, emotional support, and many others.

Although people can live for years with life-threatening diseases and disabling conditions, the process of dying probably begins for the person himself at that point in time when dependency on other people becomes mandatory rather than optional due to extensive physical regression and progressive limitation in activity. The form of physical restriction imposed by chronic illness varies depending on the part of the body most heavily involved. A young person paralyzed by cervical cord injury finds himself totally incapacitated as a social being and completely dependent on others for assistance with even the most intimate of personal tasks. An elderly person with advanced obstructive pulmonary disease finds his movements progressively diminished by an inability to breathe, a physical state that eventually forces him into total invalidism. Whether the change comes suddenly or gradually, the person with chronic illness or disability finds his social world either diminished or destroyed by the onslaught of physical deterioration over which he has little or no control.

In many ways, chronic disease brings *social death* for many long before the physical process of dying actually begins. As time goes by, the person undergoing the process of prolonged dying is forced by circumstances to relinquish personal control over many ordinary decisions about daily living. Whether at home with the family or in an institution, the person with fatal illness is at the mercy of other people. The extent to which control can be maintained over the circumstances of his forthcoming death is ultimately influenced by the choices and decisions of those persons who comprise his social milieu.

NURSING FUNCTIONS IN TERMINAL ILLNESS

Terminal Care

Terminal care consists of two classes of activity: physical and psychological assistance provided during that period of time the patient is defined as in the final stages of living, and necessary legal tasks performed at the time of death and immediately after. The terminal stage begins when there is recognition that curative medical treatments have little, if anything, to offer the patient, and palliative and supportive assistance is all that remains. The actual duration of the terminal stage varies a good deal, however, and the problems encountered by patient, family, and staff alike are closely linked to the amount of time existing between the point of definition of dying and the actual event of death.

From the perspective of nurses, different forms of emotional impact and different needs for nursing assistance are created by the length of time required for dying and the type of disease or injury involved. Massive head injuries, for instance, produce rapid dying, compounded by the psychological shock for survivors of viewing the traumatic aftermath of accidental injury. In contrast, brain tumors can mean living for relatively long periods of time before death finally comes, but not uncommonly in a state of disruption as the tumor extends and leads to aberrant patterns of behavior. As another example, a patient with brain damage can enter a comatose state that lingers indefinitely and may create problems relating to the initiation or the removal of life-prolonging procedures. Each pattern of dying produces its own set of special stresses and strains, and all make demands of some sort on the nursing staff providing care.

Whenever a patient is explicitly defined as dying, the burden of care shifts from the medical to the nursing staff even though the physician still carries responsibility for medical management of the patient's disease or injury. Like other patients in serious physical condition, the dying patient needs to be fed, bathed, and assisted with personal matters he or she cannot manage alone. Medications and treatments need to be given, and special assistance is required when the patient's physical state becomes one of extreme debilitation and weakness.

The provision of these personal services is difficult at best because work with the dying patient does not afford the same satisfaction as that with patients who recover. To compound the problem, the delivery of nursing services is often complicated by the continuation of recovery-oriented treatments and/or the withholding of prognostic information from the patient. The tendency for family and health-care personnel to withhold from the dying person information about his disease, its treatment, and related matters is often justified on the basis of "protection of the other" or "not taking away the other's hope." Yet whenever the doctor and family decide that the patient is not to be told the truth about his condition, the provision of direct assistance to the patient becomes tension-producing and awkward for nurses, because the constraints imposed are not realistic to the situation. Such directives encourage many nurses to utilize distancing behaviors in their contacts with patients. The resulting atmosphere of depersonalized care giving adds further to the socially isolating experience of dying and limits opportunity for the patient to bring closure by means of interaction with significant others.

The provision of terminal care is relatively simple if the time for dying is short, the patient is nondemanding and quiet, and the family is cooperative. The observation period just prior to death and the care of the body afterward are also relatively simple if agreement has been reached to allow the patient to die without heroic intervention, and the body of the dying person is not grossly distasteful to smell, touch, and sight. Necessary legal and administrative tasks required at the time of death are easiest to complete when family members as well as staff are prepared for the event of death and are not taken by surprise when it arrives.

Problems appear, however, whenever the circumstances of dying are conducive to stress and strain. Terminal care becomes complicated and often difficult when the course of dying is prolonged, when pain is difficult to manage, when the staff become personally involved with the patient or family, or when the use of life-prolonging activity continues indefinitely and indiscriminately. Scenes are likely when family members are not prepared for death. The work itself can be thrown out of phase when doctors and nurses are faced with the shock of unanticipated death. Indeed, the most difficult problem for health-care professionals following the unexpected death of a patient centers in the question that each person asks himself—"Was I negligent in any way?"

As a work assignment, terminal nursing care includes difficult decisions and serious responsibilities. Nurses make many judgments about continuing and discontinuing treatments, offering explanations to patients and families, communicating with physicians, and taking steps to relieve discomfort and pain. Far more than is true for physicians, nurses are in positions to influence the social milieu of dying and to set priorities based on the patient's stated wishes.

In many ways, terminal care is a curious mixture of the traditional tasks of nursing and opportunities to assist the dying person in maintaining personal contact with the social world he is about to leave. The terminal period of dying is a status passage of considerable importance not only to the person who faces death but also to the survivors, for whom the period serves as a major transition. The activities that nurses perform on a day-to-day basis not only are important for the physical well-being of the patient, but also contribute in important ways to the patient's relationship with his social network as life draws to a close.

Priorities in Nursing Services

In a very real sense, all health-care practitioners must find a balance between the cure goal of practice and the care goal. Whereas the former deals principally with the objective aspects of the case and the application of science and technology to diagnosis and treatment of disease, the latter is concerned with the subjective meanings of the experience of illness and the welfare and well-being of the person. Operationally, cure involves "doing things to" people. Rooted in human compassion and respect for the vulnerable members of society, care is manifest through actions of "doing things with" people.

The dilemmas of nursing practice are fundamentally ethical ones. Choices about when and when not to intervene in the lives (and bodies) of patients have increased in complexity with the addition of life-prolonging procedures and new techniques of treatment. My bias, and the bias of many nurses, requires that the patient be involved in the choices and decisions about his or her illness, its treatment, and the circumstances surrounding the final days of living (Benoliel, 1976). Yet nursing as a service to patients cannot be offered in isolation from the overall social environment in which nurse and patient interact. Hence the functions of nursing in terminal illness must also encompass the coordination of activities by many different people whose decisions make a difference in the day-to-day living of the person who is dying (Summers, 1974).

Nursing is fundamentally an interpersonal relationship with two important functions in terminal illness (Benoliel, 1975b). Nursing provides continuity of experience for the person who is dying. Nursing offers personal care and direct assistance when the individual is unable to provide these on his own.

The provision of assistance to the patient facing death is designed to achieve four general purposes: to facilitate normalization of living according to the patient's preferences throughout the process of dying; to maximize opportunities for the patient to participate in decisions affecting living and dying; to foster and encourage open communication between the dying person and those who are important in his or her life; and to help the patient find an "appropriate death" (Weisman, 1972). Achievement of these purposes requires that nurses be concerned with the complex interrelationships among the personal, the interpersonal, and the social experiences that together comprise the process of dying. Achievement of these purposes also depends on access to a broad spectrum of nonmedical services including home health care, visiting nurse services, transportation assistance, child-care services, financial help, legal services, and many others depending on the particular needs of the particular situation.

Continuity of Experience

The provision of continuity of experience for patients who are dying comes about when nurses are willing to assume roles that help patients, either directly or indirectly, to find direction for the journey they are taking. The role of guide is especially important in helping the patient to become informed about what is happening and to understand the alternatives available to him or her at any given point in time.

> ### Case example
>
> Mrs. K. came to see me because she was progressively losing her capacity to function and believed she was approaching the terminal stage after seven years of her battle with cancer. She knew that her tumor had metastasized to the liver and forthrightly described herself as having a limited amount of time, perhaps two to four months more. She realized her energy was rapidly diminishing and found herself wakening suddenly in the middle of the night terrified by the realization that her universe was about to end. She was concerned about burdening her husband with these experiences yet also wanted to share them with him. She had the feeling that her time was changing, even though the doctors protested otherwise. She also wanted to die at home. I asked whether she had discussed her wishes to die at home with her physicians, and she said that she had not. I then indicated that I thought she must begin to discuss her desires with them if being at home was what she truly wanted. We also talked briefly at that visit about nursing needs and requirements for assistance as time went by.

A related role of singular significance is that of intermediary and sometimes negotiator for the patient with the physician(s), with members of the family, and/or with other health-care personnel.

> ### Case example
>
> Mrs. T. whom I had met the previous week in oncology clinic was admitted to the hospital with intense pain and a suspected bowel obstruction. The doctor called me to discuss her situation and to request my help in obtaining her perspective on what was happening. Mrs. T. knew that she had far advanced cancer and that continued chemotherapy was of little value to her. The nurse in the clinic said that Mrs. T. seemed very angry about information not having been

made clear to her. When visiting her, I asked directly what was taking place. She immediately began to talk about the possibility of surgery and her wishes to have no more surgery. She added that if surgery meant only a couple of months, she really was not inclined to consent to it. She recalled that recovery from her last surgery had been very prolonged, and she did not want another such experience. Later in the day I met with the medical team for a pooling of information, and out of that meeting came a decision that surgery was not essential but better pain management at home would be helpful. She went home the following day, to return one month later to die—without the necessity of surgery and with her husband beside her.

Implementation of the role of negotiator means a willingness to break through any conspiracies of silence that impose constraints on the well-being of the patient. It also depends on a tempered sensitivity to the importance of time and timing in social interventions when all participants are affected by underlying currents of emotional tension and strain.

Acceptance of responsibility for continuity of experience means the development of a system whereby access to necessary people and resources is available to patients on an ongoing and regular basis. Acceptance of responsibility for continuity of experience means helping families to come to terms with the reality of what is happening by making available to them support, guidance, information, and assistance in locating community resources appropriate to their needs of the moment.

Case example

Mr. K. called me in a very upset state. He had taken his wife in for her regular treatment, and the doctor had called him aside to say that Mrs. K. was going downhill very fast (news the doctor did not share with Mrs. K. because he thought she could not take it) and that the doctor would find an excuse for hospitalizing her if the going got tough at home. I asked Mr. K. what he thought of the doctor's suggestion, and he said he did not like it. He wanted to have Mrs. K. stay at home as long as she wanted, but he also had lots of concerns about how to handle the situation if she had lots of pain or a medical type emergency took place. We then discussed the need for finding nurses to provide care at home and resources to contact for making these arrangements. I also suggested that he ask the doctor directly to explain what kind of medical emergency—if any—might be likely to take place during the period of her dying. As an outcome of this discussion, arrangements were made for nurses in the home, and Mr. K. did obtain information that gave him a sense of security of what to expect and do in the immediate future.

Acceptance of responsibility for the patient's right to have a death appropriate to his needs and wants means a willingness to help patient and family make known their wishes about the use or nonuse of life-prolonging procedures and treatments and their choice of setting for the final event of death. The opportunity to die without heroic intervention comes about when all who share in the process of dying can reach a point together of allowing death to come in a context of quiet waiting. Families, however, often need several kinds of assistance to enable them to cope constructively with the various stresses and strains that the process of dying carries with it.

Continuity of experience for the patient depends on open channels of communication among the many different people involved—patient, family, and staff. The achievement of open communication is far from easy in large, cure-oriented medical centers and hospitals, but it can be facilitated when both the spirit and the process of teamwork can be introduced. Consensus about goals and directions among all concerned depends on opportunities for exchange of ideas and information in an environment of mutual respect and support, such as the model of personalized care provided by St. Christopher's Hospice.

Recently in the United States efforts have been made by nurses and others to establish workable support systems in hospitals and other institutions offering services to dying patients, but these efforts to date have not been very effective. Despite increased attention in nursing education to the psychosocial needs of dying patients and the development of a corps of clinical nursing specialists who have learned to interact constructively with dying patients and their families, the structural conditions of health-care work—especially in hospitals—work against the delivery of personalized services by even the most committed of individuals. The problem is not so much that there is lack of interest among nurses for bettering the services offered to dying patients. The problem fundamentally rests in a societal value system that institutionalizes recovery-oriented practices, methods, and instrumental activities at the expense of human-to-human contacts.

Some Dimensions of Care

The second nursing function in terminal illness becomes increasingly important as the person who is dying moves into the stage of total dependence. Direct physical assistance that provides relief from some of the sufferings of illness is a singularly important nursing activity and is central to the functions of nurses in their work at St. Christopher's (Ingles, 1972). The act of personal assistance is enhanced in personal value when the patient participates actively in decisions about the form of that assistance.

In fact, collaboration in decision making about the implementation of personal care permits the patient to maintain some semblance of control over the management of his or her life and provides nurses with opportunities to individualize the care that they offer. The effectiveness of using an individualized approach for pain management in terminal illness as reported by Bader (1972) highlights the human as well as the therapeutic value of involving the patient in the decision-making process. The article also suggests that teamwork involving physicians and nurses may well be enhanced when they work together in solving troublesome clinical problems.

The nurse's manner of administering physical assistance is critically important to the physically incapacitated person because it conveys a sense of respect (or disrespect) toward him or her as a human being. The nurse's approach is especially important when energies are taken up with responses to such unpleasant experiences as nausea, vomiting, breathing difficulties, or chronic pain (Quint, 1967b). The dying person wants and needs a caregiver who is calm, confident, matter-of-fact, and unhurried in manner. Such an approach serves as a source of comfort above and beyond the actual assistance that is given by a treatment or procedure. It carries a message of respect and care that is not easily appreciated by people who have never been ill or totally dependent on others for help. It is also difficult to provide day after day because it makes tremendous demands on the nurse's capacities and resources and is psychologically draining because of these demands.

Good physical care is a form of psychological support. But nurses have other opportunities to provide care directly to patients during the time when life is declining. Because nurses have the privilege of being present when many other health-care professionals are not, nurses have unusual opportunities to share the human experience of dying and to interact with the dying person in terms of his needs of the moment. Thereby nurses are often present to offer the comfort of listening when the patient wants to talk about his or her past and future, to share the fleeting moments of joy when small events in living become terribly important, and to sit quietly when sorrow and sadness permeate his or her being. Events such as these do not normally become part of the patient's hospital record, nor are they necessarily shared by the nurse with other people. Yet they make the process of dying an experience in living, and they are as important to the person as the traditional tasks ascribed to nurses.

THE PARADOXICAL POSITION OF NURSING

It would be a mistake to end this discussion without openly admitting that involvement in another person's dying is far from easy. At the same time such involvement offers profound opportunities for sharing the experience of living at a depth of personal investment not generally found in human relationships. Ultimately no one can protect another human being from the loneliness inherent in the personal experience of dying, but nurses can and do provide for many people a thread of continuity and care as they live through their final days. Paradoxically, nursing's promise and nursing's problem rest in the power and the pain of human presence at moments of crisis and the unique opportunity the nurse's position provides to be present when patients are dying.

REFERENCES

Adams, M. "The Compassion Trap," in V. Gornick and B. K. Moran (eds.), *Woman in sexist society.* New York: Signet Books, 1972. pp. 555–575.

Ariès, P. *Western attitudes toward death.* Baltimore: Johns Hopkins, 1974, pp. 85–107. According to Ariès, this change in control took place as part of an overall shift in moral duty. Ritualized ceremonies acknowledging death as transition were replaced by a social obligation to avoid any and all causes of sadness and to support the public happiness by constraining demonstrations of grief and despair.

Bader, M. A. Personalizing the management of pain for the terminally ill patient. *The Journal of Thanatology,* 1972, 2(3–4), 757–766.

Benoliel, J. Q. Causes and consequences of dehumanization—A commentary. In J. Howard and A. Strauss (Eds.), *Humanizing health care.* New York: Wiley, 1975a, pp. 175–183.

Benoliel, J. Q. "The Terminally Ill Child," Gladys Scipien *et al.* (eds.), *Comprehensive Pediatric Nursing,* McGraw-Hill, New York, 1975b, pp. 281–295. The functions of nursing in terminal illness are herein identified and described somewhat differently as supporting, teaching, coordinating, and caring.

Benoliel, J. Q. "Overview: Care, cure and the challenge of choice." A. Earle et al. (eds.), *The Nurse as Caretaker for the Dying Patient,* New York: Columbia University Press, 1976, pp. 6–18.

Cassell, E. J. Dying in a technological society. *The Hastings Center Studies,* 1974, 2(2), 30–36.

Hay, D., and Oken, D. The psychological stresses of intensive care unit nursing. *Psychosomatic Medicine,* 1972, **34,** 109–118.

Hess, G. Health care needs inherent in emergency services—Can they be met? *Nursing Clinics of North America,* 1970, 5(2), 243–249.

Hoffman, I., and Futterman, E. H. Coping with waiting: Psychiatric intervention and study in the waiting room of a pediatric oncology clinic. *Comprehensive Psychiatry,* 1971, **12**(1), 67–81. Describes the special problems of mastery when the person facing death is a child.

Ingles, T. "St. Christopher's Hospice," *Nursing Outlook,* 1974, **22**(12), 759–763. Describes in some detail the intertwining of professional services and personal care that together create an atmosphere in which each patient can live out his/her final days with full attention given to the problems of pain, discomfort, loneliness, and grief which can interfere with the more general problem of bringing closure to life in a dignified way.

Jensen, D. Crisis resolved: Impact through planned change. *Nursing Clinics of North America,* 1973, **8**(4), 735–742. Describes the development of one crisis team composed mainly of psychiatric nurses working in collaboration with the emergency room staff and other mental health specialists.

Kastenbaum, R., and Aisenberg, R. *The Psychology of Death.* Springer Publishing Company, New York: 1972, pp. 205–208.

Menzies, I. E. P. A case-study in the functioning of social systems as a defense against anxiety: A report of a study of the nursing service of a general hospital. *Human Relations,* 1960, **13**, 95–121. In reality many of these general recovery-oriented settings have both types of patients—those facing death and those who are not. Because the primary orientation of the work is towards the goal of cure, patients are generally defined as recovery bound, and nurses are not especially oriented toward the death-related concerns of patients and families. Menzies concluded that the nursing service department developed a particular kind of social system to protect the individual nurses from the anxiety-producing aspects of patient care.

Quint, J. C. When patients die: Some nursing problems. *The Canadian Nurse,* 1967a, **63**(12), 33–36.

Quint, J. C. "The Dying Patient: A Difficult Nursing Problem," *Nursing Clinics of North America,* **2**(4), 763–773, 1967b. Contains a more complete description of the nurse's difficulties in work that involves dying patients.

Roth, J. A. Some contingencies of the moral evaluation and control of clientele: The case of the hospital emergency service. *American Journal of Sociology,* 1972, **77**(5), 839.

Sobel, D. E. Personalization on the coronary care unit. *American Journal of Nursing,* 1969, **69**(7), 1439–1442.

Spitzer, S. P., and Folta, J. R. Death in the hospital: A problem for study. *Nursing Forum,* 1964, **3**(4), 85–92. Noted that interactions among hospital personnel increased and unusual communication channels developed in response to unexpected death—behavioral patterns quite in contrast to those observed when expected death took place.

Summers, D. H. The role of the nurse. Paper presented at a symposium,

Living, Dying and Those Who Care, sponsored by the Foundation of Thanatology in New York City on November 2, 1974.

Weisman, A. D. *On dying and denying.* Behavioral Publications, Inc., New York, 1972, p. 6. Describes an appropriate death as "a death that someone might choose for himself—had he a choice."

8

IMPACT OF DEATH ON THE HEALTH-CARE PROFESSIONAL

CHARLES A. GARFIELD

Most would readily agree that from an experiential point of view that we, the living, know little of death or the process of dying. Yet, as health-care professionals who work with the terminally ill, we often collude in the belief that we are experts in the psychosocial issues surrounding life-threatening illness. This somewhat illusory expertise often translates in practice into an attempt at hyperefficiency in biomedical duties, the use of heavy sedation to reduce severe pain but also to diminish the likelihood of having to relate to emotional needs expressed by the patient, and diminished contact with and withdrawal from the patient using the rationale "we've done all we can do." The basic and often unacknowledged premise is that dying is a biological process demanding biomedical intervention. As death approaches and treatment toward improved health is no longer a possibility, staff may initially adopt a more rigid, inaccessible posture especially with more assertive patients who express their emotional needs. The dying patient is clearly not a neutral element in the psychosocial field of the health-care professional. At times, the extreme anxiety of physician or nurse becomes the major issue in the relationship between staff member and patient. Dying is not solely a biological or even psychobiological set of events and experiences. The social or interpersonal concomitants of the dying process, which impact powerfully on patient and health-care professional alike, expose the fact that we are dealing with a sociopsychobiological process with extensions to the religious realm. However, we rarely consider the impact on the professional of intensive or extensive contact with the dying. What follows is a personal case history of my initial encounter with a dying patient. The data were journal notations written throughout the death trajectory and reexamined after 5 years of research and clinical work with dying individuals. These writings constitute as powerful an introspective exercise as I have ever done.

TO BE WITH ONE WHO IS DYING

All I could hear was my father singing "Sunrise, sunset, sunrise, sunset, swiftly go the years." Over and over this seemingly endless refrain pounded through my head as I left the hospital. Periodically, it mixed with the Tibetan mantrum "Om Mani Padme Hum," my fifth grade teacher singing "America the Beautiful," or Mick Jagger shrieking "I can't get no satisfaction." Larry had just died. This was the first time in my work with cancer patients that I was forced to confront the death of someone with whom I had shared many hours. I walked around the university campus the rest of that day wondering why no one else understood what had happened. It seemed outrageously bizarre that everyone else, in uniforms as diverse as professional-looking white coats and jeans à la Haight-Ashbury "street freakery," was not attending to the monumental event that had just occurred.

I had met Larry 2 months before, following a psychological consultant request from his physician. The request stated simply, "Patient having problems dealing with emotional aspects of malignancy." I imagine so! Since then I've received many similar requests and have always wondered how bizarre they seemed. For instance, what would be the reverse? "Patient having no problems dealing with emotional aspects of malignancy"? Then I might truly be concerned. It appears strange that anyone would even question the existence of strong feelings connected with so monumental a process as an advanced cancer. In work with both inpatients and outpatients I have rarely encountered an individual with cancer who did not at times manifest powerful and often painfully disorienting emotional reactions. What I have seen frequently are well-intentioned but overburdened medical and nursing personnel without the time or psychological expertise necessary to assess accurately the emotional status of their patients.

In some settings, when a psychiatric or psychological consultant is requested, a different drama unfolds. The mental health professional, encumbered by psychotherapeutic systems usually requiring extended therapeutic processes over time, may fail miserably with the patient who has a limited life span. With rapid changes in physiological status, body image, and mood resulting from both the disease and its treatment, interpersonal consistency tends to be the exception rather than the rule. To assess this as psychopathology is frequently nonsense, since it is often an appropriate response by the patient to an extreme stressor. To pretend that we, the professional staff, would not respond similarly, given the same diagnosis and contextual demands, is harmfully naïve. What appears true, despite the reality of our time pressures and biomedical duties, is that we ourselves are not psychologically comfortable around the dying and may resort to extreme psychological defensive postures, i.e., denial, intellectualization at case conferences, etc., to avoid meaningful relationships with our patients.

WHO HELPS WHOM?

I think my ability to work with people such as Larry is directly related to the degree to which I risk being emotionally accessible to them. This work continually forces me to confront fears about my own death and to realize that my primary data are secured by trusting the patient as an accurate source of information. The largest single impediment to providing effective emotional support to the dying is the powerful professional staff distinction between *us* and *them*. It is a deeply conditioned and tradition-bound assumption in the hospital context that *we* are the professionals and you are the patients, and *we* will help you out of our technological mastery and beneficence. This distinction is most unfortunate. With regard to emotional reactions to life-threatening illness, *we* are literally *they*. We use all our biomedical and psychological sophistication to facilitate healing, but then what? For myself, it is to imagine "my" experience, feelings, thoughts, and emotional needs as patient in the same demanding situation; to share even if mininimally the pain, confusion, and insight resulting from yet another human encounter with death. Whenever a professional colleague tells me, "I can't get emotionally involved," I think, "How unfortunate," and wonder to myself "How long has this horrid affliction persisted?" To identify emotionally with a person(s) under duress to the point of being dysfunctional is of little help to anyone. However, to deny any emotional connection is violence. I understood Larry's plight as well as I did because I could imagine my own response in the same situation. When I was confused about how best to help him, I'd immediately confer with Larry. My skills as a clinical psychologist are, of course, a tremendous asset, but the issues revolve more around human authenticity than professional expertise. I've learned since my work with Larry that a primary assumption in working with seriously ill cancer patients is that there are always emotional issues and that people trained to be sensitive to these issues can be an enormous help. Patients with "emotional difficulties related to malignancy" are the norm, certainly not the exception.

My initial reaction to Larry was one of surprise. Here was a man sitting stripped to the waist with a muscular body and appearing at least as strong as I. The difference was that Larry had a presumed diagnosis of childhood leukemia. We spoke for some time, and I learned that Larry was an ex-Marine, 20 years old, who had spent a great deal of time distancing himself emotionally and psychologically from his family. He had been somewhat of a rebel all his life and had joined the Marines on a bet. Two of Larry's major problem areas were (1) the fact that although he had been told that there was a 75 percent cure rate for his form of childhood leukemia, he was not feeling well; although he was receiving positive feedback from his physician and the nursing staff concerning his medical condition, he did not feel the improvement, and (2) his relationship to his family. Channels for communication on an intimate level had never been established. Larry's life experience thus far had been based on an extended adolescent rebellion. Now, however, he was sick, frightened, and needed his family desperately but was without the interpersonal skills and the insight needed to establish communication. The reverse was also true. There was no one in Larry's nuclear family who could openly and honestly relate to him.

We spoke about both of these issues, and I decided that I could do something very concrete concerning (1). I would consult with Larry's physician and find out if he had any ideas. First, I decided to check Larry's chart. Much to my dismay, I discovered that 2 weeks before Larry's diagnosis had been changed to acute adult leukemia, and that his prognosis was now very poor. Larry had not been informed of this change in diagnosis. He was still operating on the old assumption that there was a 75 percent chance of cure for his form of "childhood leukemia," and that he would be up-and-around in several weeks. This seemed outrageously unfair, and when I mentioned this to Larry's physician, he responded, "I just started this rotation. It's not my responsibility to tell him. It should have been done by his previous physician." I was unable to accept this response, and in further discussion with the physician I volunteered to tell Larry about the change in his diagnosis. Larry's new physician was a young, sensitive, and intelligent man who identified strongly with Larry. He realized that Larry should know about the change in diagnosis but was tremendously afraid to break the news for fear of devastating Larry (and himself!). When he saw the strong feelings I and Larry had concerning concealment of such information and recognized I was correct, he broke down, and I spent an hour in supportive psychotherapy with the physician before he was able to go in and talk to Larry. This was one of the most moving situations in which I have ever been involved.

Early in my work I learned the difficulty inherent in the physician's role. Culturally defined as a *healer*, he may be forced to resort to an extreme psychological defensive posture to deny the reality of many of the situations in which he works. That is, with regard to many forms of cancer, medical tools toward care are minimal, and the physician must face the fact that the patient will die. For a culturally defined healer, death is tantamount to failure, and the emotional consequences for the physician are often severe. Little has yet been written on the emotional impact of patient death on the physician, and yet this appears to be a vital area of inquiry.

THE FIRST BREAKTHROUGH

We went in to see Larry together, and for 10 minutes the physician did his best to break the news. Larry was painfully aware of the inconsistency of the situation; i.e., he had never before seen his physician and me together and knew something was wrong. His heart was pounding in the manner of people and animals responding to stark terror. After this brief visit his physician left hurriedly, and I remained to deal with the emotional aftermath. Larry experienced an enormous amount of emotional upheaval. He cried and raged about not having been told the truth and was furious at the Cosmos for this horrible turn of events. Finally, after much pain, he asked me to thank his doctor for attempting to carry out what must have been a very difficult task.

From then on the nature of our work changed. Larry was extremely intent on establishing meaningful contact with each member of his family and I suggested that we meet as a group. On the scheduled day, I arrived a few minutes late, looked in, and saw each family member standing in an opposite corner of the room as far from Larry's bed as possible. The general tone of the situation was conflictual, and I felt I had walked into the middle of an argument. I apologized, saying that I'd wait outside until their discussion was completed. Larry's mother hurriedly said, "I'd like to come out and speak with you." As soon as we left the room, she broke into tears saying that she did not know how to talk to Larry anymore. She had always felt close to him but didn't understand what was happening with his illness. She was very unsure of what to say to Larry for fear of upsetting him.

AVOIDING THE FACT OF DEATH

What had developed was the kind of conspiracy of silence that often engulfs and isolates the dying. Although the family knew what was going on medically and realized the gravity of the situation, and Larry similarly understood the severity of his condition, neither party was able to discuss this information openly for fear of upsetting the "emotional equilibrium" of the other. I decided to speak with the various members of the family, discussing their feelings about Larry, his deteriorating physical condition, and ways in which they thought they could assist him. I learned from Larry's mother that she wished to be close to her son and saw this as a long-desired opportunity to breach the communication gap that existed between Larry and the other family members.

Larry's father, with whom he had never shared anything more intimate than a slap on the back and a can of beer at a football game, revealed an enormous amount of previously unexpressed feeling about his son's plight. Although he wished to say much to his son, channels of communication on an emotional level had never been developed. Larry's father asked me to help him in "getting the two of us together." By his own admission, he cried for the first time in 30 years and explained that he couldn't let his son go to his death without some communication of love between them.

Larry's sister and brother followed closely the model of their parents. They were also interested in communicating with Larry about his illness and had a somewhat easier time doing so. By acting as a facilitator, friend, therapist, and participant, I was able to give the family permission to discuss all aspects of the situation freely and openly with Larry. It is important to remember that I had spent hours with Larry in advance of this meeting and knew very well what his feelings and preferences were with regard to such communication. Larry was extremely adamant about demanding as open a communicational context as possible. Within a short period of time, Larry's family was sitting on or near his bed, laughing, joking, crying, and sharing in a far more authentic manner, the essence of what was transpiring.

As with many dying adults, Larry was frightened and puzzled by those issues and feelings summarized by the phrase "How could I not be among you?" He wanted to explore the possibility of leaving something behind—a personally relevant extension of himself to those people for whom he cared. I helped him secure the tools for doing leather work, and Larry fashioned leather goods for his family: wallets for his father and brother and purses for his mother and sister. On each item he etched "with love always—from Larry." Sensing that part of him would survive, these items meant a great deal to Larry. Such self-extensive forms of expression have been important to many dying people and amount to personal symbols of (or "testimonials" to) one's incarnate existence.

MOMENTS BEYOND THE PAIN

My work with Larry continued to change form as we discussed many topics formerly inaccessible to consciousness. He asked whether I believed in a life-after-death, and if so, in what form. We spent hours discussing the purpose of his life (and mine); whether he (Larry) and I (Charlie) would ever meet again, in a recognizable form, in another time and place. We spoke of loving people, of relationships, of the pain inherent in confusing roles (such as patient, psychologist, or doctor) with people. It was no longer theoretical analysis or philosophical debate in the manner learned during my quarter century of "academic tutelage." Larry's limited life span gave the interchange an urgency and vitality absent elsewhere. We were two representatives of the somewhat odd and physically vulnerable species *Homo sapiens* struggling to understand why we were sitting (or lying) on an oblate spheroid whirling somewhere in the Milky Way. It was both frightening and exhilarating, and I'll not likely forget those shared "struggles." Perhaps the content didn't matter at all. Perhaps we were "only" defining our relationship while protecting each other from the void like children huddling together in the dark . . . perhaps . . . perhaps . . . perhaps.

THE PATIENT AS TEACHER

As his disease progressed, Larry grew weaker and his family, sensing the outcome, withdrew emotionally. This process, sometimes accurately called *anticipatory grief,* is a psychological reaction to impending death frequently experienced by family members and hospital staff. While helping to prepare the survivors psychologically, this reaction can easily be experienced by the patient as a painful abandonment. While I, too, was bracing myself for the worst, I remained with Larry, discussing those things that were uppermost in his mind. He suggested that I take notes so that I might subsequently use his "story" in teaching health-care professionals. When I agreed, Larry seemed to know that his painful drama might positively affect the experiences of other seriously ill people.

I saw Larry on Friday before returning home, and we talked about pain, both emotional and physical, loneliness, and the fact that he felt his family withdrawing. He also felt the staff withdrawing and was enormously saddened by the fact that both his physician and favorite nurses were now visiting much less frequently. He repeatedly thanked me for being "the one person who was not afraid to share this awful pain," and asked if there was any way he could repay me. I assured him that I had been repaid many times over, but Larry insisted on giving me something. I asked him to be my teacher and translate his experiences for me. "When you're alone, Larry, what thoughts and feelings do you have?" "Specifically, what is it that makes you afraid?" "Teach me how best to help you." In a situation that I have since encountered many times, Larry faded in and out of waking consciousness. In lucid moments, he was extremely clear in responding to my questions, but then would drift into a sleeplike state. He taught me much during that period, and I know I was a support to him as well.

I learned how vital it is to remember that we are dealing not with a professional issue, but a human one. As health-care professionals we are trained as healers, and it is clear that death is an unacceptable outcome for many of us. To imagine that trained healers—i.e., doctors, nurses, and other biomedical personnel who experience themselves as adversaries of illness and death—can respond effectively to the dying patient is often an erroneous expectation. It is more often the case that the professional's anxiety and sense of impotence drives him away, leaving the patient emotionally and psychologically isolated and often physically abandoned. I learned the importance of training both professionals and lay people to relate effectively to the dying person. If we are ever to transcend our barbaric isolation of the terminally ill, we need to stop relating to dying people as lepers. We must realize that at our current level of scientific expertise, death is not always the result of a biomedical mistake or a mysterious virus, but may be seen as a natural winding down of the human psychobiological totality.

THE GOOD-BYE

Shortly before I left that Friday, I sat watching Larry with his black and blue body, sunken eyes, and yellow skin. As he lay there with his intravenous "life supports," I thought of Auschwitz and Treblinka, my grandfather Aaron, and Vietnam. Suddenly, as if sensing my despair, Larry awoke, looked straight at me, and said, "I have something very important to say to the people who will read your book." I listened carefully, somewhat surprised by Larry's intensity. Finally, he said, "Dying alone is not easy."

There was a calm and clear tone to Larry's message that was uncanny, and he smiled peacefully, adding to my uneasiness. His words haunted me for days. The following Monday I hurried to visit him again. When I arrived at the nurses' station, I was told that Larry had died. I was sad, angry, relieved, confused. Finally I was left with the feeling that somehow I should have known that what Larry was really saying on Friday was good-bye. Yet it didn't feel like good-bye. There was a tranquil and accepting look on Larry's face so remarkably discontinuous with those tormented, pain-wracked experiences I had witnessed previously. There was a powerful sense that Larry had transcended the somatic entrapment that bound him for so long. I believe that what Larry was communicating to me that Friday was "Dying alone is not easy, but the job is done, and I've reached a place of peace. . . . I appreciate and love you for what you've shared with me, and if by chance we meet again . . .

9

DYING THEY LIVE: ST. CHRISTOPHER'S HOSPICE

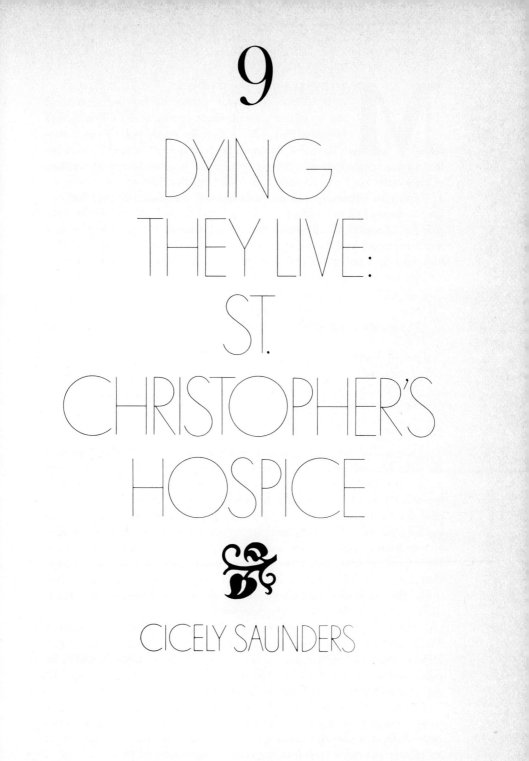

CICELY SAUNDERS

M
LIFE HAS A PATTERN
r. B. (Figure 9-1) was sitting by his bed in one of the small number of single rooms at St. Christopher's Hospice. Now 63, he had, for many years, been a firefighter in London. He had been admitted 2 weeks before with a fungating and offensive recurrence of a carcinoma of the floor of his mouth. He had had surgery 4½ years earlier, followed by radiotherapy and chemotherapy. His previous hospital had now decided that further treatment of this nature was inappropriate and had asked the Hospice for admission to alleviate his terminal distress. His pain was by now well controlled, and the odor, previously his greatest distress and humiliation, no longer noticeable. We greeted each other, and after he had reported that his previous symptoms were under control, we went on talking.

"What do you do with yourself all day?"
"I read a bit and watch television; my wife and daughter spend a lot of time visiting me."
"Do you get bored?"
"No. I am contented—all my life I've been as you might call it, succouring people, helping others; now I am on the receiving end."
"Do you find that hard?"
"No—I don't now—life has a pattern."

A few days later I joined him in a three-cornered conversation with his wife. She told me about the rest of the family and that her elderly mother was in a nursing home. Mrs. B. saw her often, and she told me that her mother and her roommate, both now in their eighties, were good and cheerful companions and that they were happy there. She went on to tell me how the second old lady had arrived about a year ago, severely incapacitated from a recent stroke, and so unhappy that she had asked first her own daughter and then Mrs. B. if they would bring her in some pills so that she could kill herself. "Now," said Mrs. B., "she has changed her mind; she can walk with a frame and can do crochet. She does not want to die now, her whole outlook has changed."

His wife reported to me later that, although it had been hard to bear, Mr. B. had not been overcome by his previous distress. Indeed she felt that all along he had been supporting her. Now the whole family joined in his relief and were able to relax. His freedom from pain had enlarged his capacity to use this part of his life's pattern to the full.

Mrs. B. is fortunate in that her mother is in a capable and compassionate nursing home where an old lady has been helped from a desperate wish to die to a cheerful readiness to live. A similar change of attitude in an elderly patient is shown in the conversation notes of Mrs. D., aged 82

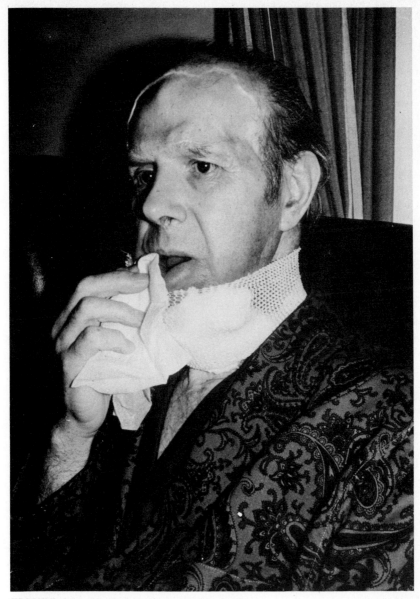

FIGURE 9-1 Mr. B. 2 weeks before his death.

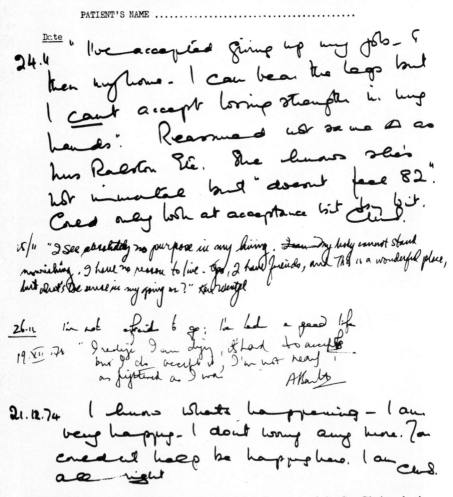

ST. CHRISTOPHER'S HOSPICE

THIS FORM IS FOR THE USE OF ALL NURSING STAFF FOR NOTING ANY
SIGNIFICANT COMMENTS MADE TO THEM BY THE PATIENT REGARDING
HIS/HER ILLNESS AND PROGRESS

PATIENT'S NAME ....

FIGURE 9-2 Conversation notes with Mrs. D. as used in St. Christopher's Hospice ward notes.

years, and a patient in St. Christopher's (Figure 9-2). Her physical condition was deteriorating throughout the time covered by this record yet her outlook was developing all the time. Once she reached acceptance she did not lose it again. A few days before her death (3 weeks after the last entry) she was overheard discussing the world to come with her friend, the long-stay patient in the next bed. "Wouldn't it be good if we both went together," she was heard to say, and the subsequent conversation made it plain that their expectation was to go to a place of excitement and interest. In fact, Mrs. D. died 36 hours after her friend, staying long enough to comfort the nurses and the many friends of that much-loved patient.

"Life has a pattern," said Mr. B., and no one meeting him could doubt that this pattern had been accepted or that the acceptance had enabled good to emerge from what was indeed a desperately hard situation. Those who meet and listen to such people as Mr. B. and Mrs. D. have seen repeatedly how much strength there is in accepted weakness and how often it is the person who is "on the receiving end" who is giving courage to those around him or her.

Patients who have intractable pain or other terminal distress from malignant disease and the elderly with deteriorating illnesses or diminishing powers are the two groups who are most often referred to in the literature demanding the legalization of some form of voluntary euthanasia. It is claimed that the only way in which they can die with peace and dignity is for them to be given, when they ask and with due formalities and safeguards, a lethal injection. It is taken for granted that many *will* ask, and the complex issues behind this suggestion are rarely explored. Little account is taken of the inconsistencies of the ill or of their vulnerability to the suggestions of others. Family discussions and divisions, doubts, and guilts are ignored, and no account is taken of the great difference between experiencing a situation and watching it from without. The suggestion that a declaration should be made earlier in life ignores this fact. It also takes little account of the shock reaction of the well on seeing the very ill and the frequency with which they project their own feelings upon the sick person.

It is also taken for granted that dying people will suffer inevitably increasing pain or other physical symptoms which cannot be relieved or which can be alleviated only at the cost of the impairment of their mental faculties. It is implied that the elderly will inevitably deteriorate to a stage of senile dementia, confused, incontinent, and a travesty of the persons they were. Sadly, these assumptions are all too often reinforced by stories of truly horrendous cases, where pain was not controlled and all drugs appeared to have lost their effect; where people were subjected, apparently with no choice, to more and more surgery or life-supporting measures which were at best inappropriate and at worst correctly described as forms of torture no one would have permitted an animal to undergo. Far too many elderly people end their days in pitiful and degrading isolation, with the reality around them so distressing that they retreat into confusion and do not even recognize those they love. It is no help to this discussion if we deny the distress which many people are suffering at this moment.

Such patients are not easily given appropriate care in a busy general ward. Often it is not the right place for them nor do their needs arouse the interest of many of the doctors who look after them. One reason for this is no doubt the fact that such patients are not seen often where most medical education takes place. Ann Cartwright's study, *Life Before Death* (Cartwright et al., 1973), gives the details of the last year in the lives of 785 people, a random selection from different areas in the United Kingdom. Only 2 percent of her sample died in teaching-hospital beds. Such wards are geared to active diagnosis and the treatment of acute conditions, and their implicit standards do not help students to learn how to help people who are dying. Many of the staff feel that treatment must mean active therapy designed for cure or rehabilitation and that ethically this can never be discontinued. We may add that it is implied that "satisfactory" patients should get better or at least die without fuss before those treating them have come to the end of their (largely irrelevant) resources. It is often thought that the strong analgesics which some patients need desperately for adequate relief are virtually unusable because of ill-understood risks of tolerance and dependence. Even when they are given, it is implied that they are somehow a disgrace. As one medical student told us, "In our hospital, the patients have to earn their morphine." If we add to this the implicit demands that patients should not ask awkward questions and that families should be unobtrusive and not disturb others with grief or anger, we see some of the reasons for the sad state of many dying people, well-documented in the press and rightly causing public disquiet. It is being said that the only compassionate and realistic answer is for these people to have the right to die when they ask to end their intolerable existence.

Doctors are committed to the service of health and to the relief of suffering (World Health Organization, 1948). To prolong life by all means available to intensive care, regardless of its quality, is not to serve health but rather to fail to balance technical possibilities with informed clinical judgment. It has been said that to refrain from all possible active treatment is "passive euthanasia." This is a misleading definition, and one which the British Medical Association and the Church of England's Board of Social Responsibility Working Party have both refuted (British Medical Association, 1971; Church Information Office, 1975). As the Working Party says:

> In its narrow current sense, euthanasia implies killing and it is misleading to extend it to cover decisions not to preserve life by artificial means when it would be better for the patient to be allowed to die. Such decisions, coupled with a determination to give the patient as good a death as possible, may be quite legitimate. Nor should it be

used to cover the giving of drugs for the relief of pain and other distress in cases where there is a risk that they may marginally shorten the patient's life. This too we think is legitimate.

Such decisions have always been part of clinical judgment; no doctor is committed to preserving life whatever its quality, and to ease the distress of dying is undoubtedly part of medical treatment (Devlin, 1960).

The doctor has to serve health, and surely there comes a time for the very old and for people with such illnesses as we are discussing when it can be said truly that to die has become the "healthy" thing to do. The two extremes of dying in pain and being killed do not exhaust the possibilities for the stricken patient (Horder, 1936). There is another way, the way of giving appropriate and understanding medical care and compassionate and personal nursing care arising from true social concern.

The Working Party considered that:

> If all the care were up to the standards of the best, there would be few cases in which there was even a prima facie argument for euthanasia; better alternative means of alleviating distress would almost always be available if modern techniques and human understanding and care of the patient were universally practiced. It should be the aim to improve the care of the dying in hospitals and hospices and in their homes to as near this standard as the money and the staff available will allow.

It believes that, at present, ignorance and mistaken ideas are a greater obstacle than shortage of money and staff, and that to justify a change in the law to permit euthanasia it would be necessary to show that such a change would remove greater evils than it would cause. It listed among these evils: the pressure it would place on patients to allow themselves to be put away, recourse to euthanasia in many cases in which it was far from morally justified and performed for the wrong reasons, and grave weakening of confidence in doctors by a majority of patients.

Finally, the Working Party wrote, "that in the rare cases (if such there be) in which it would be justified morally it would be better for medical men to do all that is necessary to ensure peaceful dying and to rely on the flexibilities in the administration of the law which even now exist than to legalize euthanasia for general use."

What has come to be called "the Hospice movement" has set out to give such people all the care that will help them to die easily and at peace, to spread knowledge and concern of its potentials in special units or hospices, in general hospitals, and in the patient's own home.

"I WANT
WHAT IS IN YOUR MIND
AND IN YOUR HEART"

St Christopher's Hospice was originally founded in 1948 with a legacy of £500 given by a man who, having escaped from the Warsaw Ghetto, died of cancer in a busy surgical ward in London at the age of 40. During his last 2 months he made friends with the author (then a medical social worker), and the first ideas of a place that could have met his needs began to form as we talked. In his words quoted above he asked for the confident skill of the mind that would have relieved his pain and other physical distress; he needed even more the friendship of the heart, nearness to someone who saw him as another person, good to meet and to know, to laugh with and to commend with love to the God of his fathers. The anguish of a lonely, apparently unfulfilled life was eased, and he died in peace, leaving a heritage that went far beyond his £500—a vision of what could be done to help people like himself to die in peace and dignity.

When we talked about his legacy he said simply, "I'll be a window in your Home." Years later the name Hospice was adopted for that Home; its meaning, "hospitality for travellers." The name came originally from the resting places which grew up along the pilgrim routes of the Middle Ages, where religious communities welcomed the pilgrims until they were able to continue their journey. Hospices for the incurably sick, the destitute, foundlings, and the aged were established as the years went by, and the acutely sick were admitted to the new "Hospitals." Fresh life came to the old word when the Irish Sisters of Charity began to use it for homes for dying patients opened in the nineteenth and twentieth centuries. Throughout this time the main theme was that a hospice should quite simply be "given to hospitality," that it should welcome those whom no one else wanted to care for and give them the promise that this welcome would last as long as the need existed.

St. Christopher's grew from the gift of one man in 1948 and from the needs and achievements of many more over the years. It was planned to be something between a hospital and the patient's own home; combining the skills of the one with the warmth and welcome, the time available, and the beds without invisible parking meters beside them of the other.

After 7 years of training and planning, and working and visiting in those homes already set up in England, a small steering committee was able to form a charity in 1961. In 1967 St. Christopher's opened with nearly the whole of the £500,000 needed for the land, building, and equipment already given. The committee knew that the patients, families, and elderly residents for whom it was planned and built would come with problems which had often been overwhelming. Because of the very problems it set out to face, they did not expect the Hospice to come about easily, glibly, or just by waiting for things to happen. "How could we expect a smooth passage when we set out to help people to overcome hard things and make of them the very means of victory? That will be the nature of the work all through and we have no right to expect that such a project should be simple or easy, nor be surprised at struggle, set back or crisis" (from report of Annual General Meeting, 1966).

During its 8 years of existence St. Christopher's has continued to expand its services to those it cares for and to the staff, the students, and the many visitors. Its capital needs are met by gifts, the running costs of patient care, research, and teaching by various contractual arrangements with the National Health Service. The contracts leave an increasing deficit which so far has been met by gifts. Few patients pay for their care; they are admitted according to their need for what the Hospice can give, and any contribution they can make is discussed with the families after they have been admitted. Of the total running costs for 1974 they gave 2 percent, though many other gifts came from those who remembered care with gratitude. Giving care is St. Christopher's only way of fund raising.

The Hospice has 54 beds in its wards, divided into 4 or 6 bed bays, with 6 single rooms. It still has one more floor (used at present for visitors who are studying the work of the Hospice) which will form the fourth and final ward of 10 to 12 single cubicles and a large dayroom.

Patients are admitted at the request of the doctors treating them. Approximately 60 percent come in from their own homes, and most of these have been visited, often many times, by the Domiciliary Service of the Hospice. The original application may have been made by the hospital doctor or come directly from the patients own general practitioner at home. Most of the patients admitted suffer from terminal malignant disease, but a small number have neurological illnesses such as motor neurone disease or nonmalignant causes of pain. About 8.5 to 10 percent will be discharged home again; others who have improved return to their original hospital for further treatment, stay in the wards, or are transferred to the Drapers' Wing. A small group have achieved unexpected remissions of up to 5 years.

It has always seemed important that there should be a mixed group of patients and that "Hospice Care" should refer to the active relief of various types of distress and a personal approach to a patient and his or her family, at home as well as in the wards. A hospice is not only a place that "cares for the dying" but a community giving less technology and more personal care than the usual busy hospital ward. The welcome number of such units being opened and planned at the present time is adding diversity and fresh approaches to this fundamental concept.

The Drapers' Wing contains 16 bed-sitting rooms for a group of elderly residents who bring their own furniture and form a quiet but most important part of the life of the Hospice. Four of the original residents are still giving the contribution of a prayerful and secure old age to us all. Eighteen residents have died during the 7½ years, either in the wards or in their own rooms. Other people have moved there from the wards for periods up to 18 months after an unlooked for remission made normal living possible once more but who had no home to which they could return. Relatives and colleagues of the staff members are welcomed whenever possible, and at present the husbands of two patients are taking up residence, the first men to live there. The wife of one of them is still in the ward as a long-stay patient, and this is bringing increased traffic between the two parts of St. Christopher's. Separated from the wards and yet part of the life of the whole, the Wing plays an important part in bringing one end of life to the community, while the children in the Playgroup all the year and their elders in the School Club during the holidays bring the other into sight and sound. The children join in the midday meal with their mothers and meet the patients when weather allows them to visit the garden in their beds or wheelchairs. They take these encounters with cheerful interest and are so little disturbed that most continue to return frequently as they grow older.

The Hospice is generally well staffed. It has a staff ratio comparable to an acute medical ward, and it is usually up to full establishment. A considerable number of the trained nurses have returned to nursing in coming to the Hospice, often after some years at home with their families. More than half of the untrained auxiliary nurses started nursing when they came to St. Christopher's. Some are students working for a limited period before university or other study, others have family commitments which make training an impossibility for them. Many staff of all departments have worked for years at the Hospice, and the turnover is not high.

There are some who have decided to commit the rest of their working life to St. Christopher's, others whose home needs must take precedence but who often involve their whole family in the doings of the Hospice, a younger group who are using their time to help sort out their future priorities, and many part-timers, staff, and volunteers who help to knit the work into the wider local community and prevent it from becoming inward looking. Each group has its contribution to bring to the life of the whole, but perhaps special mention is due to the particular warmth of the non-European nurses and orderlies who add a quality of spontaneity to the atmosphere that is especially welcome to the very ill and their families.

Every individual part of the whole team has its contribution to make. Reception is conscious of its importance as the first welcome to patients and visitors, administration has a sizeable budget to deal with but has time to be the natural organizers of staff parties, and men of the maintenance team not only deal with Hospice engineering problems with cheerful speed but often offer to help in staff households nearby. Sometimes the mutual support that all need in turn seems to come only from their own particular group, but meeting across different "levels" also takes place and is revealed clearly in the response to a particular tragedy or celebration.

GIVEN TO HOSPITALITY

Men and women can fulfill their lives in passivity and weakness as well as in strength and activity. Those who welcome each patient to St. Christopher's do so with the conviction that he or she is an important person and that hospitality to a stranger is a prime necessity.[1] Those concerned take care to know the name of newcomers before they arrive, and a senior nurse joins the stewards at the ambulance to welcome them personally. The patient is lifted directly into a warm bed, and his family travels in the lift with him to the ward. It is impossible to overemphasize what such a welcome means to a mortally sick person who has so often felt alien and rejected. He has been the "failure" who cannot get better in the acute ward, feeling obscurely that it is his own fault, or he has suffered long pain at home which has led to despair of ever finding peace. A great deal has happened to bring relief to patients by the time the doctor comes to speak to the family—the nurses have already introduced them to their neighbors and begun to settle them in their own place. Patients will not be moved so long as they stay in that ward; their bed has their name on it instead of a number, and they are encouraged to put out small personal things on their locker. Everything is done to establish their identity, however ill they may be. Even those patients who are already confused or unconscious seem to show that they know they have been greeted as persons and not merely admitted as cases. "Our own name helps us to know that we belong." The first greeting by name and its repetition on each ward round and at every contact between a staff person and a patient emphasizes his relationship to the community. In one of the first annual reports after the Hospice opened it was written, "Every time we greet a new patient we see the colorfulness of the Hospice afresh and find that it is all very good." Each time it has been new also for the patient at the moment when we say, "Come just as you are—you are welcome."

Not all patients are easy members of the ward community they enter, and there are some who need to work out their way of living and dying in

---

[1] "I won't be forgotten *here*"—a patient on admission.

the privacy of a single room. But a hospice must welcome people simply on the grounds of their need and of their common humanity and has to find a way to enable each one to have his or her own appropriate way of dying.

Two people make a meeting. It cannot take place where one of them is obscured by a professional role. We are all acquainted with the superficial greeting of a patient which expects the gratified answer and is much taken aback by anyone bold enough to express his real feelings. Many medical students who meet hospice patients on teaching rounds ask how they can begin to transfer this experience back to their teaching hospitals. It is suggested that a simple beginning could be a resolution always to say "Good morning" to patients by name, especially to those who are dying. The student, like everyone else who feels that he is facing a situation where he has little to give, will feel tempted to pass by, feeling that they can be no better than a useless disturbance. If they can convey the attitude, "I am not only concerned with what is yours (your diagnosis, your response to treatment, and so on) but with you as a person (however despairing you are, however unattractive)," much can develop from this one moment of mutual recognition.

Neither students nor relatives can meet those patients who remain swamped by distress or become smothered by treatment. The result of the proper control of terminal physical distress, seen repeatedly in every place where this skill is practiced, is for the patient to go on living in relationship with those around him. So many of us have known bitter regrets that we have not learned love until too late; so many families find words to express their care only when the patient can no longer hear them. The extra time for such communication is frequently used for reconciliations or even new beginnings. As one daughter wrote, "I came to know my father better during these visits—as a man and not just my father . . . you at St. Christopher's helped us to look more honestly at ourselves and offered constructive help when we asked for it . . . to be aware of death without being afraid of it seems to make one that much more aware of life." None of this, nor the many encounters between families which it represents, would have happened if the patients had remained imprisoned in the distress with which they were admitted.

Much of the communication at St. Christopher's may at first sight look superficial. Visiting students find themselves busy serving meals and giving so much practical care that they do not feel they can sit down and have the long talks they somehow thought would make up their experience. But the part of life before death is like the rest, it is full of ordinary and exasperating things. Feeding a person who cannot even manage to get a spoon to his mouth can be a chore to the worker and a humiliation to the patient; it can also be a social occasion when the worker can just come as a neighbor. We all feel clumsy at times and must often say the wrong or hurtful thing, but as we keep coming for such simple errands we have the opportunity for a new beginning. The place to find meaning is so often in the ordinary, in the endlessly repetitive and insignificant. A true meeting between two people is a gift coming unbidden into the midst of such action.

Humiliation and exposure are the lot of many of the very ill. We can help them to feel valued in the way we give the things of everyday life. Few infusions are to be seen in a hospice—many people, families included, are to be seen giving food and drink, slowly and kindly. Patients do not feel thirsty, and do not look dehydrated, and the drink they need is given in a manner which draws them near to others. Drips and tubes may seem a quicker and more efficient way to keep up a fluid intake, but at this stage personal contact matters more than electrolytes and can give refreshment where, before, everything was drought and isolation.

When we visit a dying person we may meet the unexpected. Most people are honest as they face death, and they are likely to have dropped much of the mask we all tend to wear in our daily encounters with others. They will not let us be sentimental, and they are usually realistic and challenging, whether or not they *know* what is happening. If we can use our skills as vehicles to bring us close to the person we are trying to help, we may find we are uncomfortable, but we will surely gain from the exchange.

We have considered a patient's relationship with St. Christopher's as a person, for that is what first arrests the attention of both the patient and his or her family. But the staff would not be able to greet them with such confidence nor offer such immediate security if the personal meeting were not accompanied by careful coordination of all the Hospice can offer and by the efficiency of its treatment.

ADMISSION AND CONTINUITY OF CARE

About 40 percent of St. Christopher's patients are transferred directly from a hospital; the rest are admitted from their own homes. They are sent with uncontrolled pain and other symptoms, with emotional distress, and with social and interpersonal difficulties which those previously caring for them were unable to help. They are not a random selection of people dying in this part of London; they are a group who present themselves with unrelieved distress.

Every effort is made to enable them to stay at home as long as they wish, to come at the optimum moment for them, and to return home if possible. An admission meeting considers all applications daily, and patients come in according to their need. Those in distress at home have priority over those already in a hospital, and discharged patients are always readmitted immediately. St. Christopher's social worker may begin his or her contact with the family and with other workers involved before the patient comes in, and many families visit to see the place to which their relative is to be admitted. The Domiciliary Service staff go to assess the home situation whenever it is indicated, and report daily to this meeting.

Continuity of care has priority and may not be easy to establish with those previously treating the patient. Notes may be confusing. Liaison between the various departments of a hospital are not always good, and there may also have been much delay in writing to the family doctor on a patient's discharge. Letters and reports are held up and, when they come, little is said in them of what the patient or family has been told to expect. The Hospice doctors sometimes have to be most importunate in obtaining vital medical information. This is often more easily dealt with when the patient is seen first at home, but some admissions are urgent, as when the family doctor has only contacted the Hospice when the situation has broken down irreparably. St. Christopher's is usually able to offer help at once, for it can take over 550 admissions a year with a median length of stay of only 10 days.

THE HOME-CARE PROGRAM

The patient and his family may be referred by the hospital who has treated him or directly by the family doctor. In any case the latter will be contacted before a home visit is made, and he will continue to be involved with the patient's care, consulting and cooperating with the Hospice nurses and doctors. Four specially trained nurses and a part-time doctor with experience in general practice carry a case load of over 70 patients each month, covering an area of 6 miles or so from the Hospice, which is in a heavily populated area. Family doctors are now asking more often for assessment visits to be made early in the illness, enabling the home care staff to get to know the family before matters become desperate. Some patients are seen only once or twice at home before they need admission, but in that time come to terms with what many of them know is the final farewell to their home. Others may remain at home for many weeks or months, and a considerable number are able to remain there until they die.

The clinic staff reports in full to the wards as they hand over care of the patient when he or she is admitted. As far as possible, the problems that arise as one group of staff replaces another are faced and dealt with by direct consultation. Thereafter, clinic staff will continue to attend open ward meetings, and may continue to pay social calls on their patients in the ward.

Peggy and her husband lived in a first floor flat in a housing estate in Bermondsey. She was well known to all her neighbors and much loved for her warm and friendly nature. Two months before her death her doctor asked St. Christopher's for help in the control of her pain and St. Christopher's nurses became almost daily visitors to the flat. Peggy was a tiny slip of a thing with the spirit of a giant. She was determined to remain at home because her husband suffered from arthritis and found it hard to get about. The door of the flat was always open and neighbors came and went through the day. Nursing care was given by the District Nurses three or four times a day; a night nurse took over at dusk.

The role of St. Christopher's was to assess Peggy's constantly changing needs and to adjust her drugs accordingly. All the expertise gained in our wards was used to keep this young woman at home. It was a triumph of cooperation between the General Practitioner, the District Nurses and ourselves. Peggy died early one morning after a peaceful night's rest. She slipped quietly into eternity conscious to the last. The morning of her funeral was crisp and cold. Her body lay in her own home surrounded by masses of flowers, the narrow hall was lined with them and sprays and posies extended along the open balcony and down the stairs, spilling out in a cascade on to a forecourt below. Neighbors leaned over the balconies on every floor as the coffin was carried out; the traffic in Jamaica Road piled up in both directions as the cortege crossed the road to the church opposite; local shops closed their doors briefly during the funeral service and those who could not get into the church stood about on the pavement as the bell tolled. We are glad that we made it possible for Peggy to remain at home and to die surrounded by family and friends. (from the Domiciliary Service)

"YOU WELCOMED US AS WELL"

When patients enter the hospital, they leave their own community and much of their identity. We are all bound up in our homes and our possessions, our work and our hobbies, and we feel stripped and humiliated if our clothes and personal belongings are removed. The emphasis on possessions, clothes, and idiosyncrasies in a hospice is a way of maintaining identity. Many hospital wards do little to integrate their patients into a new community in which they have an active part. The way a patient is welcomed into the new life of a hospice can be a reaffirmation of his own home and community, even though he may never return to them.

People matter more than things, and a patient is, above all, part of a family and circle of friends. St. Christopher's tries to welcome the family as wholeheartedly as it greets the patient who is part of it. The staff in the wards as well as those in the Domiciliary Service frequently spend as long or longer with the family members as with the patients. Much of this is on a simple and friendly level, but many ward groups and discussions are guided by the social psychiatrist who has been part of the Hospice team from the beginning.

Patients are referred to the psychiatrist by the nurses as well as by the doctors, and his advice may be sought by anyone. Over the years he has found that he sees approximately 15 percent of all patients, and there are others whom he discusses with the ward staff but does not meet directly. He is involved in ward and general staff meetings and with a small senior staff group as well as in a regular seminar with visiting students and graduates. He also acts as consultant to the group working with the social worker to identify and visit those families in special need of support in their bereavement.

Two years ago he established a patients' group. It meets weekly for an hour's discussion, and friendships formed there may extend to other contacts during the week. The number attending varies from as few as 4 to as many as 15. The core is composed of long-stay patients who may come regularly for many months and who welcome and absorb into the group a number who only come once or twice before they are too ill to attend. Family members sometimes join, and a discharged patient returns faithfully. Various subjects are brought up; sometimes discussion is general, at other times it is focused on life and death in the Hospice. The loss of a member of long standing is faced and talked about because the members as a whole feel secure enough to grieve together and to look at the implications for themselves. On other days they concentrate on learning from or instructing those who visit them. It is a coveted honor for staff or visitors to be invited to join in one of the meetings, and although small in number, this group has an impact on the life of the Hospice as well as on that of its members.

Since St. Christopher's opening 8 years ago, Dr. Parkes, the psychiatrist, has carried out a number of psychosocial studies. He recently (1975) completed a comparative study of 34 families of cancer patients who died at the Hospice, matched with 34 families of patients who died elsewhere. Statistically significant differences favoring the group from the Hospice were:

1.   Greater mobility of the patient.

2.   Less pain rated as severe (but not bought at the cost of greater drug-induced confusion).

3.   Less anxiety among spouses during the period of terminal care with fewer somatic symptoms.

4.   Spouses spent much more time at the patient's bedside and much more time talking to staff, other patients, and visitors. They were more likely to have helped to care for the patient and more likely to know a doctor's name.

5.   Doctors and nurses at St. Christopher's were less likely to be seen as "busy" or "very busy" than staff elsewhere.

6.   Despite the fact that two to three patients died each week on each floor at the Hospice, only 6 percent were said to have been upset by the death of another patient. The same figure was given for those in other wards, none of which were for "terminal care."

7.   Twenty-seven from each setting completed a checklist which allowed them to agree or disagree with general statements regarding the hospital in which their spouse died. The statement which best characterized St. Christopher's was "The hospital is like a family," which was checked by 78 percent of the St. Christopher's families and 11 percent of the rest.

This family feeling explains why some relatives have returned to work as volunteers, often for several years service. For others, the connection continues informally; letters are exchanged, visitors come back to talk to the ward or reception staff they know, or they appear at Open Days, sometimes years later, to bring their friends to see the Hospice. Many respond to the card sent to all next of kin on the first anniversary of a patient's death. It is of one of the Resurrection pictures in the Hospice with the words "We are remembering you at St. Christopher's." The list of names put on the notice board outside the chapel each week makes this a fact and not merely a pious fiction.

A few relatives come regularly to the Sunday chapel service, others come for festivals or anniversaries. An increasing number come to a monthly social club which is also attended by members of staff and their families. This club has gradually built up until space is becoming a problem, and it expands into a large general party each Christmas and Midsummer. In many ways the life of the Hospice resembles that of a village, a place which shares the good and the sad and which does not lose its interest or attraction for those who once belonged. Nurses return to show off their new babies, students call back for a meal, and the friends who support the work by their prayer and gifts return each year at Open Days to see the new developments and to meet old acquaintances. The follow-up of the bereaved and the sad fits naturally into such a context, and surprisingly few of them have made dependent and clinging relationships with the Hospice.

Another of Dr. Parkes's studies (1975) set out to assess the reliability of the method developed to identify the wives and husbands who were likely to get into difficulties after bereavement. Of 17 spouses who had a "poor outcome," 13 had been correctly predicted. Those who were expected to need help urgently were all followed up, the next group were assigned at random to two groups. One was supported by visits from St. Christopher's staff or volunteers who were known to them, and the other was not. Both were visited 20 months after bereavement when the "unsupported" group were found to have almost twice as much depression as the "supported" group. They also had significantly more physical symptoms of anxiety.

A CENTER FOR
THE CONTROL OF CHRONIC PAIN

Mr. B. needed constant adjustments of his medication, especially during the last few days of his life. Specialized care was essential to ensure that his potentially great distress was anticipated and alleviated.

The Hospice has been concerned with the nature and management of chronic and terminal pain ever since the years spent by the medical director in St. Joseph's Hospice (Saunders, 1965). Ever since its first planning and through the development of the teaching program, the work has been based on growing experience and on a series of studies and clinical trials (Saunders 1963, 1975; Twycross, 1974). Every year the medical and nursing notes of all the Hospice patients are summarized by a doctor and analyzed by a nurse, neither of whom is involved with ward care. Only a small number (1.5 to 2 percent) are reported as continuing to complain of unrelieved pain during their time in the wards. A further study has been carried out by Parkes. His research worker has never worked in the Hospice, visits from the Tavistock Centre for Human Relations, and is not identified with St. Christopher's. She interviewed the families of 45 patients who had died in the Hospice and 100 who had died elsewhere in the area. Thirty-six percent of St. Christopher's patients were recalled by their families as having severe, unrelieved pain before their admission; the other families rated 20 percent. After admission the St. Christopher's families recalled pain in 8 percent while at the other hospitals the figure remained at 20 percent (see Figure 9-3). It is scarcely surprising to find that the figure given is higher than that rated by the staff. We must all have spoken

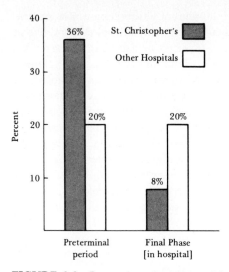

FIGURE 9-3 Proportion of patients with severe pain which was mostly unrelieved.

to families whose relative is lying quietly unconscious and heard them say, "We long to see him out of his suffering," and had to try to explain that so far as we can tell he is now no more aware of any movement or noise than when he was snoring in healthy slumber. The Hospice recognizes that there is still further work to be done in the control of pain and other physical distress, but there is reason to say that at present greater success is achieved than is usual elsewhere.

Hospice doctors and nurses recognize and consider the differences between acute pain which forms the basis of much teaching in therapeutics and that of chronic or terminal pain (LeShan, 1964). Orientation is that use of analgesics should be only a part of a multifaceted approach. Terminal pain needs to be considered as an illness in itself, to be diagnosed and treated with attention to detail, according to a rational plan of treatment and with an individual approach to the whole spectrum of a patient's distress, social and emotional as well as physical.

Eighty percent of the patients referred to the Hospice have pain sufficiently severe to need narcotics for its adequate relief. Many have had unrelieved pain for long periods, and it may take time before they learn to expect relief rather than distress. Both are self-perpetuating, and the doctor should so anticipate the onset of pain that the patient does so no longer. Drugs balanced to need and given regularly so that pain does not occur prevent the vicious spiral of pain, tension, increased pain, and a

higher dose of analgesic. The best treatment of terminal pain is its prevention. Of 108 patients admitted to a controlled clinical trial of two different
narcotics in the Hospice, 61 percent reported to the nurse observer that
they had no pain at any time when she visited them 10 days later. None of
the remaining 39 percent reported unrelieved, severe pain, although all
had been admitted to the trial because of pain. A series of studies being
completed has included a controlled clinical trial of morphine and diamorphine given orally in a cocaine elixir with a phenothiazine in which it
was found that there was no clinically observable difference between the
two opiates when given regularly. This study and further work on the
absorption of these drugs when given orally and retrospective studies of a
group of patients who received opiate drugs over long periods in the Hospice and in their own homes will soon be published. This work is at last
bringing objective science into a field too long confused by myth and
misconception (Twycross, 1974). Too many patients have suffered unrelieved pain because their doctors considered that the drugs which could
have given them comfort were virtually unusable.

Parkes's work quoted above has shown not only that the patients are
given better pain relief in the Hospice but also that this is not bought at
the expense of alertness or the possibility of living in as full a manner as
their physical condition allows. The proper balance of the analgesics and
the adjuvants to the patient's need will rescue him from the two alternatives that are usually offered, frightening pain or too heavy sedation.

TEACHING AT ST. CHRISTOPHER'S

Each development at St. Christopher's has grown out of need and demand. Teaching of several kinds grew from the requests for experience,
courses, lectures, and seminars. There has been a growing interest in this
field ever since the first groups of visiting nurses and social workers went
many years ago to St. Joseph's Hospice. The programs at both hospices are
constantly expanding, with an emphasis on multidisciplinary groups and
staff learning together.

St. Christopher's, like other such centers, has more requests of all
kinds than it can accept. It has to keep the priority of patient and family
care and refuses to disturb their peace by too many invasions by visiting
groups. Special days are set, a ward or a bay may be omitted for a season,
and a general rule throughout the house, (first promulgated at St.
Joseph's), runs as follows, "If you don't feel like talking with a stranger
shut your eyes and pretend you're asleep." No ward rounds, not even those

composed of medical students, examine patients or are taught round the bed. The emphasis has always been to enable individual visitors to talk with the patients, many of whom are glad to meet people and to think of themselves as hosts and teachers.

A complex program involves most of the Hospice; ancillary staff, doctors, and nurses all go out to give lectures and are frequently involved in talking with visitors. The aim is to pass on an attitude of attention and respect to patients and such general principles as can be interpreted in different settings. Much emphasis is placed on the skill and analysis of terminal pain and its relief, for this is something which should be eminently transferable to any situation.

Nothing can take the place of a meeting with a patient and his or her family, however brief. At times the conflict between the need to enable such meetings to take place and the need of the patient can be difficult to resolve. From time to time the ward staff may say that their patients have had enough visitors; far more often they recognize how much it means to the sick person to know that they are the most important educators in the Hospice.

Some 2000 day or half-day and 90 to 100 resident visitors call for great powers of organization and assimilation in a relatively small place. Of course some go away unsatisfied, either with their experience or with St. Christopher's. The remarkable thing is that this happens to so few. Some undoubtedly bring their own problems and do not allow sufficiently for the cultural shock of another country and its ways, while others helpfully share their insight concerning a weak spot.

Those in courses in St. Christopher's are asked to present a case study in a seminar before they leave. Nearly all of them emphasize as they do this the honor that meeting with the patients has been to them. It is indeed the highlight of their stay. The constant theme in their final evaluations shows that it is as part of a ward team that they find their best experience. It is also in the wards, where death and bereavement are so closely and constantly encountered, that they also find threat and hurt. Regular seminars with the psychiatrist help these feelings to be expressed and worked through. Staff at all levels find they may also be involved, and teaching is a demanding part of their commitment to the Hospice. It is far more often a rewarding than a negative experience in spite of its potential for focusing on any discontent or feeling of lack of communication.

This program, like the Clinical Studies and the Domiciliary Service, are all funded by the Department of Health and Social Security with small supplementary grants from trusts. A limited number of places are available for overseas residents, but these now have to be restricted to those working in the field already, or for those who are planning new centers.

ST. CHRISTOPHER'S HOSPICE
AS A CHRISTIAN FOUNDATION

> It is planned that the staff should form a dedicated community, unit-
> ed by a strong sense of vocation with a great diversity of outlook in a
> spirit of freedom . . . each giving in a spirit of quietness . . . that
> each person who serves must give his or her special contribution in
> their own way and that the service must be group work, open to
> further light and expansion as the Holy Spirit may lead. This free-
> dom to be held in a foundation based on the full Christian faith in
> God, through Christ. (From the statement of St. Christopher's reli-
> gious basis)

St. Christopher's Hospice has a long prehistory. Much of it belongs to
individual experiences, but a foundation group composed of future staff,
council members, and friends met regularly for 5 years before it opened to
discuss plans and to pray together. Some of the original group and others
who have joined since form one of the many meetings, formal and informal, which make up such an important part of the life of the Hospice. At
one of the first meetings a statement was drawn up by one of the members
and put forward for discussion as the "religious basis." At that time the
group did not feel ready for such definition, and it was put aside until the
Hospice had been working for 3 years. The group was then greatly reas-
sured to find that the Hospice had begun to grow into the pattern that
most of the staff had never seen expressed in writing. Each time it is
discussed it is felt that this statement has come new to the occasion, full of
depth and immediacy. Nevertheless, each time the group has decided that
it should be kept for referral and not be published or in any way imposed
on those who come to work in St. Christopher's. It belongs to those who
are already working out their commitment.

In its work as in this statement, the Hospice is committed to the
Christian faith "in a spirit of freedom," to giving service, "in a spirit of
quietness," and above all, to the belief that "love is the way through." For
many of those who work there this love is first of all expressed in the love
of the God who has himself gone through death to resurrection and "in
whom all are made alive" (Corinthians Chapter 15, verse 22).

No one can impose a faith or a philosophy upon others. Long ago the
first patient said to the writer, "I like you too much to say 'I believe' just
because I like you," as he returned to the faith of his Jewish forebears. But
those who have some conviction and confidence can help others to find a
map in their bewilderment and to move trustfully towards what they see as
true. Most of St. Christopher's staff show, by the way they care, a confi-

dent hope concerning the unknown that the patients face, and this is able again and again to give substance to their belief that death is not the end.

The many different pictures of heaven in the Bible include a wedding, a banquet, a city, a kingdom, and a concert. Individuals are promised the security of being a pillar in the House of God and that they will receive the seal of freedom and a unique name known only to God. Individuality in community, peace and nourishment and the service of love can be offered here and now. In the Hospice they are shadows of the realities to come.

One day a man was being shown some pictures of himself at a Christmas party in the Hospice. He wanted to pay for them; the writer wanted to give them to him. In fact we both wanted to give, neither wished to receive. I held out my hand and said, "I think life is about learning to receive." He held out both his, palms uppermost, next to mine and said, "*That's* what life is about, four hands held out together." Such mutual giving, with all its reconciliation and new life, seems to be the way in which the Hospice is experiencing the life of the Resurrection, made present once again. The way to reach out to it is simple but costly.

A condition of complete simplicity
Costing not less than everything. (Eliot, 1944, p. 59)

David Tasma, the first patient, found peace in his own way. A Jew with little relation to his faith for years, he had memories of long hours of discussion with his grandfather, who had been a rabbi. When he came back to this faith, his clenched, anxious, fighting fists relaxed into open, accepting hands. The main challenge of this Christian foundation seems to be for openness and simplicity and the symbol of the open hands.

Much of the atmosphere of St. Christopher's comes from the architecture and from the colorful pictures that fill the Hospice. These are all the work of one artist, Marian Bohusz, a Pole who spent the war in a prisoner of war camp and who has lived in the West since then. He paints light out of darkness again and again in glowing images of conviction. His triptych in the chapel illustrates the dependence and vulnerability of incarnation, the making of sin, loss, and death into the means of their own defeat in crucifixion, and the sudden glory and restoration of all loss in resurrection. All are contemporary experiences in St. Christopher's. For many of the staff these are living images which open up the happenings of everyday life into a realm of hope that is perhaps all the stronger when no words are used.

Those who work in the Hospice are of various denominations and of a "great diversity of outlook." All are made to question their beliefs in the face of the griefs and problems of those for whom they work. At any time some may be finding their way through doubt to faith, while others feel they can only go on waiting for the answer; all find the strength of being with others who also are searching. The fact that many of them share a Christian faith does not exclude members of staff and volunteers who have other faiths or no faith from being important members of the family. They feel accepted, and some have come to belong to their own traditions more fully.

It has been said that a society consists of those who are united in the service of a common purpose, focusing first and foremost on the work to be done together. Whereas a community exists where the members are united in sharing a common life, where the prime motive is in being together, though this too may issue in a common service (MacMurray, 1950). These two are not mutually exclusive, and each is faced with the challenge of organization and authority. As the real meeting with a patient is a gift, so too is the true meeting of those who work together. This cannot be claimed or grasped as of right, and any developing group will have problems and vicissitudes in this as in other areas of its life. St. Christopher's has not been exempt, but takes heart from the words of T. S. Eliot:

> Who are only undefeated
> Because we have gone on trying. (Eliot, 1944, p. 45)

"EVERYTHING THAT WENT BEFORE AND ANYTHING THAT MAY COME AFTER WILL BE WORTH IT FOR THAT DAY"

Mr. B. died 5 days after the photograph in Figure 9-4 was taken at his birthday party. His wife had prepared a small celebration and came in to find that, according to Hospice custom, a birthday cake and party had been organized by the ward. The party continued for much of the day. The writer was away but was told about it afterwards by Mrs. B. She said, "Everything that went before and everything that may come after will be worth it for that day." Just as Figure 9-1 shows how much suffering had "gone before" and the discomfort Mr. B. still had to contend with, so Figure 9-4 shows the achievement of joy that summed up their lifetime together.

This photograph also shows much of what St. Christopher's means for the staff and is an illustration of what enables them to continue with such work at the level of caring demanded and given. "Efficiency is very comforting," said one relative. It is comforting to the family and also comfort-

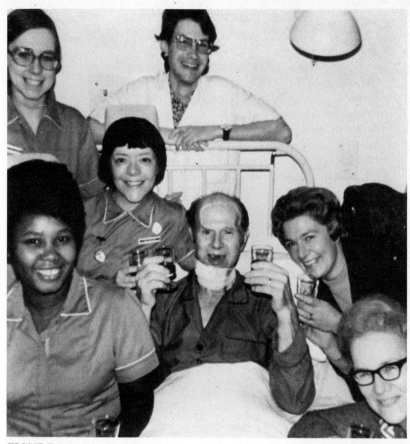

FIGURE 9-4 Mr. B., 5 days before his death, at his birthday party with his wife, daughter, nurses, and students.

ing to the staff to see pain relieved and relationships reaffirmed. Much weariness and mental suffering may still remain, but it is deeply rewarding to meet people who are making such achievements of life's pattern and to join in such occasions. We cannot take away the whole hard thing that is happening, but celebration is still an important part of life, and each Hospice occasion is a salute to this kind of courage. There is no need for the staff to idealize their patients, the daily reality of troubles accepted and overcome is enough. Neither patients, families, nor staff are protected from sadness, but in sharing it as they do they find that living and dying well are linked together and are constantly opening up new and creative possibilities.

IN THE MIDST OF LIFE[2]

Death and I are only nodding acquaintances
We have not been formally introduced
But many times I have noticed
The final encounter
Here in this Hospice,
I can truly say
That death has been met with dignity
Who can divine the thoughts
Of a man in close confrontation?
I can only remember
One particular passing
When a man,
With sustained smile
Pointed out what was for him
Evidently a great light
Who knows what final revelations
Are received in the last hours?
Lord, grant me a star in the East
As well as a smouldering sunset.

REFERENCES

British Medical Association. *The problem of euthanasia.* London: British Medical Association, 1971.

Cartwright, A., Hockey, L., and Anderson, J. L. *Life before death.* London & Boston: Routledge & Kegan Paul, 1973.

Church Information Office. *On dying well.* An Anglican contribution to the debate on euthanasia. London: Church Information Office, 1975.

Devlin, Lord Justice. Lecture to the Medical Society of London, 1960.

Eliot, T. S. *Four quartets.* London: Faber & Faber, 1944.

Horder, J. Parliamentary debates, House of Lords, 1936, **103,** 466–506.

LeShan, L. L. The world of the patient in severe pain of long duration. *Journal of Chronic Diseases,* 1964, **17,** 119–126.

MacMurray, J. *Conditions of freedom.* London: Faber & Faber, 1950.

Parkes, C. M. P. *Evaluation of family care in terminal illness.* Alexander Ming Fisher lecture, Columbia University, New York, 1975. To be pub-

---

[2] By Sidney G. Reeman, (a patient in the Hospice who died on March 3, 1975, and who wrote over 50 poems during his 4-months stay).

lished in *Man and medicine,* New York: Columbia University Press, 1977.

Saunders C. M. The treatment of intractable pain in terminal cancer, *Proceedings of the Royal Society of Medicine,* 1963, **56,** 195–197.

Saunders, C. M. The last stages of life. *American Journal of Nursing,* 1965, **65,** 70–75.

Saunders, C. M. Alexander Ming Fisher lecture, Columbia University, New York, 1975, in press.

Twycross, R. G. Clinical experience with diamorphine in advanced malignant disease. *International Journal of Clinical Pharmacology, Therapy and Toxicology,* 1974, **9,** 184–198.

World Health Organization. *The declaration of Geneva,* Geneva, Switzerland, 1948.

10

MAKE
TODAY
COUNT

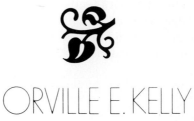

ORVILLE E. KELLY

The date was June 15, 1973. It was a cloudy day in Burlington, Iowa. I remember these details because I was about to enter a hospital to have one of several tumors removed surgically to determine if there was a malignancy. In other words, I would know in a few hours whether or not I had cancer.

I slept little the night before the operation. I couldn't talk with my wife, Wanda, or joke with my children as I would normally do before retiring. I was terribly depressed and afraid. Several physicians had looked at the growths beneath my arm and in my groin, but only the last one suspected cancer. I just couldn't believe it was happening to me. I knew things like cancer—and death—occurred, but I guess I always thought such things happened to someone else.

I had never faced a serious illness during my lifetime, until now. I had only been in the hospital twice—once for an operation and once when I contracted pneumonia. Both were relatively short confinements.

In the past, I thought little about the prospect and inevitability of death. Several times during our marriage, Wanda tried to talk to me about funeral arrangements, what I wanted her to do in case I died before she did, and related subjects, but I brushed aside any attempts she made to converse with me about these things. I didn't like to think about dying. Of course I knew I would die some day, but I didn't want to worry about it until I grew old. After all, I had a lot of living to do and death was not on the itinerary.

As a newspaper editor, I would publish articles about cancer when I received them, but I knew little about it. Once, an elderly and distant relative lay dying of cancer, and I went with my grandparents to visit her. I was 11 years old. I vividly recall a stench in her room and bloody bed sheets. The scene terrified me, and I fled from the room. Cancer has always been synonymous with death in my mind.

I consider myself an average individual who had a normal, but somewhat hectic, childhood. I was born in 1930 and was raised by my grandparents. I spent my boyhood years on farms in Iowa. In 1948, I joined the U. S. Army. I became a sergeant major, and in 1959, I met Wanda Klossing in Burlington, Iowa. We were married 4 days later. I left the Army in 1960 to become a husband and father and to build a family of my own. My plans were that my wife and I would raise our children and then travel. Meanwhile, I became a newspaperman in Illinois, going from reporter to editor in a few years. Looking back on those days, I would consider them happy ones. I loved my wife and children. We lived in a nice house, with two late model automobiles parked in the driveway. Typical middle-class Americana. Barbecues, cocktail parties, and vacations once a year.

But in 1972, I noticed I was growing tired before the day at the newspaper was finished. I didn't feel well many days. Bad health was something new for me. One of my hobbies had been weightlifting, and I was proud of the fact that I had lost few arm wrestling matches in the past. I couldn't cope with what was happening. I went to a physician for a physical examination. He could find nothing wrong. I was convinced nothing was seriously wrong, and whatever it was would go away. But it didn't. Some days I couldn't get out of bed. Soon, I had to give up my newspaper career. Wanda and I and our children, Mark, Tammy, Lori, and Britton, returned to our hometown, Burlington, Iowa.

It was September, 1972.

We managed to exist as a family, with me doing odd jobs and Wanda working in an electronics factory. It was quite a contrast to the beautiful home we had left. Most of our furniture had been sold. Often, I didn't feel like getting up in the morning. By this time, I was bewildered. I had been to three other physicians, and none had found anything seriously wrong. I even thought perhaps I was imagining my problems. I still thought everything would turn out all right and I would return to work as a newspaperman.

In May 1973, I noticed a lump under my left arm. Upon inspection I discovered there were actually two lumps. And I soon discovered another lump, about the size of a golf ball, in my groin.

That is when I went to still another physician.

"You don't know how I hope I'm wrong," the doctor told me after the examination, "but I think you might have something called lymphoma."

"Is that bad?" I asked him.

"It depends. Depends on how long you've had it . . . how far it has spread."

"Can it be cured?"

"We won't know until I remove one of the tumors and find out if I'm right. Then, you'll have to undergo a series of tests."

I didn't ask him that day if lymphoma was a type of cancer, but I knew it was. I just couldn't accept the fact I might have cancer. It was impossible. Elderly people died of cancer, but I wasn't old. I couldn't even stand to think of the word. Lymphoma sounded cleaner and easier to live with. During the course of our conversation, the doctor mentioned "carcinoma." That sounded even better. Then I looked the word up in my dictionary at home: "a malignant tumor; cancer." I slammed the dictionary shut. Well, I still didn't have to tell my wife and children or my friends and relatives.

So there I was, on that cloudy Friday in June, lying on an operating table in the hospital, while the doctor sliced into the flesh beneath my arm. As the nurses flitted in and out of the room and the doctor worked to get at the tumor, I thought of my wife waiting for me in the lobby of the hospital. My oldest son and my mother-in-law were with her. I thought about our plans for the future. Our love for each other. I felt tears in my eyes. I quit thinking about my family. I had always been careful never to show my emotions too much. A man, I thought, should never cry.

I saw the tumor in the forceps when it was removed. I was trying to be optimistic, but I just knew it was malignant. The doctor told one of the nurses to take it to the pathologist for diagnosis. That was the longest 20 minutes of my life.

The report confirmed my fears—"Malignant!"

Then the doctor was asking me if I would tell my wife or should he do it for me. I knew I couldn't look into Wanda's eyes without losing control of myself emotionally. I just couldn't do it.

"Would you please tell her?" I asked.

I could see her standing in the corridor, outside the operating room. The doctor was talking to her. Now she knew. And I knew.

The nurses helped me dress. I had never felt so depressed in my life. I had cancer. And I was going to die. No one had to tell me I would die. I just knew it.

I spent a week in the hospital at Burlington, undergoing tests. Then my doctor sent me to the University of Iowa Hospital in Iowa City, Iowa. I spent several weeks there. I used to read my medical records as I went from floor to floor for the tests and examinations. I knew things were not good, but I wanted someone with authority to tell me the truth. I couldn't yet believe all this was happening to me, but I had to know the truth. I kept asking the doctors what was going to happen to me. Would I die of cancer? How long could I expect to live? Would there be a lot of pain? Would I be confined to a bed?

One day a doctor entered my hospital room and closed the door. When he closed the door, I knew he had something to tell me that would not be pleasant.

"I think it is time we had a talk," the doctor said. "You do have advanced cancer. We don't think we can cure you, but we can treat you. I can't tell you how long you might live. No one can do that. But I can tell you about some other lymphoma patients who have lived for several years."

I had never been in shock, but I guess I know what it's like. I felt my whole world had fallen apart that day. But no one will ever know how grateful I am that the doctor told me the truth.

When the doctor left, I knew I had to call Wanda. She and the children had stayed in Iowa City, in a motel, for a few days. But I wanted them to be at home. I had the strangest feeling that something was going to happen to all my family. I wanted them home, where it was safe. I didn't want my wife driving on the highway. It was too dangerous.

When she answered the telephone, all I could say was, "Wanda . . . Wanda . . ." The words just wouldn't come. How do you tell a wife you are going to die of cancer? The doctor wouldn't commit himself, but when I pressed him for a time limit, he gave me the statistics, in his opinion—6 months to 3 years. There was no future for me.

"What's wrong, Honey?" my wife asked.

"Nothing. I just wanted to tell you I loved you."

I just couldn't tell her the truth. I didn't want her to suffer any more than she already had. I decided to never mention the word *cancer* again. We would never talk about it.

Back in my room, I tried to think about something other than my problems. But I couldn't concentrate on the magazines at my bedside, or on the television programs. I had always wondered what thoughts were in the mind of a condemned prisoner on death row. Now I knew. I had received a death sentence of my own. But there was a defense mechanism in my mind. Whenever I started thinking about death or cancer or any of my problems, I would start thinking about the past, when everything was "all right," crowding all other thoughts from my mind.

Sometimes I could leave the hospital for a weekend pass at home. I should have been happy to be home, but I wasn't. I couldn't tell my wife how I felt. She was trying to protect me. The children knew something was wrong, but since no one was being honest with them, they could only remain quiet and never ask questions. Our home life had changed. There was no laughter in the house. I quit disciplining the children. I didn't want them to remember me as a harsh father.

One weekend my wife asked if she could discuss something with me.

"What is it?" I asked.

"Can I talk to you about the children? I've got to know how you feel about some things."

I knew what was coming next.

"I don't want to talk about it now."

My wife had talked to the doctors at the hospital. She knew the prognosis. But I was still trying to convince her everything was going to be all right.

I began to realize I desperately needed to talk to someone. But there was no one. The nurses at the hospital were friendly but cautious about answering my questions. The doctors were efficient but very busy. I couldn't talk to my wife because I didn't want to upset her. I tried to talk to some of my friends, but I saw it was bothering them. Some told me not to worry because everything was going to be all right. The doctors certainly knew more about my prognosis than they indicated, so I knew they were just trying to evade the issue. Some of my other friends were affected emotionally by what had happened to me, and they didn't make very good listeners. They were concerned but couldn't bear to discuss anything with me.

I began to feel as if I was the only cancer patient to suffer these emotional problems. I started to feel sorry for myself. I had nightmares, with me walking toward a casket in an empty room. Upon approaching the casket, I could see myself in it. I would awaken suddenly, sweating and terrified.

I knew what was wrong. I was afraid to die. I couldn't face the fact I would probably die of cancer some day. I couldn't stand to think about the future, without me a part of it. I couldn't visualize my family going on without me. I was afraid of the finality of it all. What would happen to me? Was there really a God and a heaven? I had cursed God during the early weeks of cancer, blaming him for all my troubles. Would I go to hell now, because I had sinned? I didn't know.

I found that most people were willing to accept the fact that I was a terminal cancer patient and then ignore me. They weren't trying to be cruel, I'm sure. They offered no comfort or understanding to me, though. Even my family was careful not to talk about the "wrong things" when I was present. My friends and relatives, I found, were ill at ease around me. One evening a friend called me on the telephone.

"I'm just dying to see you again," she said. "Oh, I'm sorry!" she exclaimed. "I didn't mean to say that."

I hadn't noticed. "What is it you're apologizing for?" I asked.

"Oh, never mind."

It took me 5 minutes to satisfy my curiosity by finding out what she had said.

My family's attitudes toward cancer in our family grew worse. They couldn't talk to me about my problems, or their own dilemmas. It never occurred to me they were suffering just as much as I was. After all, it is not easy to watch someone you love die of a disease which cannot be cured while you are helpless to do anything about it.

In August, I was released from the hospital to await my first chemotherapy treatment. The treatments prescribed for me sounded nearly as bad as the cancer. I was told to return to the hospital in 3½ weeks. The thought of what could happen from the onslaught of drugs tormented me. It all seemed senseless. Why fight to keep alive for a few more months? I was going to die anyhow. Why not get it over with? I thought about suicide, but then I knew I wanted another Christmas with my family. Suicide was not the answer.

On the day I had to go to Iowa City for the chemotherapy treatment,

I nearly convinced myself I should stay home. I didn't want any more suffering. But I went, and the fear of the treatment was much worse than the actual treatment. I have discovered since that fear is often worse than that which you are afraid of and it is also harder to live with.

On the way home from the hospital that day, Wanda and I were in the front seat of our car. I was driving. My youngest son, Britton, was asleep in the back seat. I forgot my troubles for a moment. It was great to be alive. And, by gosh, I *was* alive! Cancer hadn't killed me yet.

It was a beautiful day. The fields lay like a gold and yellow blanket in the sun. I was driving through the countryside where I was born, 43 years ago.

I looked toward Wanda. We hadn't spoken since we left the hospital. I cannot describe the look on her face—dejection, depression, hopelessness.

I knew something had to be done. I could stand it no longer.

"Wanda, let's talk about it," I began. "I don't want cancer, but I have it. I can only try to fight as long as I can to stay alive. I will probably die of it someday, but I'm not dead yet. We really don't know how long I will live, but let's not waste the time we have left. Let's tell the children when we get home, then let's have a barbecue."

We told the children, and we had the barbecue. It wasn't easy then, and it's not easy now. The children were very upset by the news, but at least it was out in the open. There wasn't anything to hide any longer. I could try to cope with it now.

Although life will never be normal for our family again, we are living once more. Before, it was like a funeral every day. We acted as if I were already dead.

But I had one thing to be thankful for—I had some time. Statistically speaking, I had some time.

I quit measuring time on the calendar. What is a day, a month, or a year, really? Only words in a dictionary. For those who die tonight in this world, one day more would be a lifetime.

I wrote an article for the local newspaper about my experiences as a cancer patient who knew he was terminal. People began to call me, and I found that my problems were their problems. Although each family has its own unique problems when there is cancer or a terminal illness involved, some are common to all.

It took the specter of death to really make me aware of life. I began to write again. One of the first results was a poem for my wife, written one night when I couldn't sleep because of drugs:

Spring, and the land lies fresh-green
Beneath a yellow sun.
We walked the land together, you and I

And never knew what future days would bring.
Will you often think of me,
When flowers burst forth each year?
When the earth begins to grow again?
Some say death is so final,
But my love for you can never die.
Just as the sun once warmed our hearts,
Let this love touch you some night,
When I am gone,
And loneliness comes
Before the dawn begins to scatter
Your dreams away.

Summer, and I never knew a bird
Could sing so sweet and clear,
Until they told me I must leave you
For a while.
I never knew the sky could be so deep a blue,
Until I knew I could not grow old with you.
But better to be loved by you,
Than to have lived a million summers,
And never known your love.
Together, let us, you and I
Remember the days and nights,
For eternity.

Fall, and the earth begins to die.
And leaves turn golden-brown upon the trees.
Remember me, too, in autumn, for I will walk with you,
As of old, along a city sidewalk at evening-time,
Though I cannot hold you by the hand.

Winter, and perhaps someday there may be
Another fireplace, another room,
With crackling fire and fragrant smoke,
And turning, suddenly, we will be together,
And I will hear your laughter and touch your face,
And hold you close to me again.
But, until then, if loneliness should seek you out,
Some winter night, when snow is falling down,
Remember, though death has come to me,
Love will never go away!

Some of the wire services picked up the story of a man who was trying
to learn to live with cancer instead of just going home from the hospital to

die. The letters began pouring in. People felt they had someone to talk to, even if it had to be by letter. I began to receive telephone calls from the United States, Mexico, and Canada.

"My problem really isn't my cancer, it's my friends and relatives who refuse to admit I have it," a lady from California wrote.

"My sixteen-year-old daughter died of Hodgkin's disease last December," wrote a mother. "She died alone because her friends were too depressed to come see her."

"Would you please teach me how to die?" wrote a teenage girl from Michigan. "No one wants me to know about it, but I think I am dying of cancer. I haven't even been to a funeral and I've never seen a dead person. What is death?"

I try to answer all of the letters I receive, although due to the volume received, I always seem to be behind in answering them. Many of the people who write to me are dying and want to talk to someone or tell someone how they feel. They don't want sympathy—only understanding.

Sometimes I am too late. The other day I came across a letter I had received some time ago:

Recently, I turned 24 years old with the certain knowledge that I would be a widow within the next month, or possibly two. My husband is 27 years old and we have a five-year-old son and a two-year-old daughter.

The young lady went on to tell me that her husband had malignant melanoma. The cancer had spread quickly.

My husband began to wake up each morning hurting in a different place. It was a race which would be destroyed first, his liver or his brain. We finally talked about death together. When he discovered I had known this for some time, he was so sorry I had not been able to share the burden with him. Had we shared this from the beginning, we could have made many more days count.

All we can do is ease his pain. He cannot swallow. I am ready for my husband to die. I even wish it. Actually, the man I loved died about a month ago. Tears roll from his one eye and you wonder if they are tears of pain or frustration.

Thank you for reading our story. This is the first time I have ever written it down. So many times we look back and wish we had done this or that. I sometimes wish if only we would have had a little more time, a few months, or weeks, or even days. But, we have said our 'I love you's' and now we have said our good-byes.

I called her immediately after reading this letter. Her husband had died 5 days after the letter was written.

No, there is nothing good about cancer. But life must go on. My wife some day will have to send the children off to school, cook meals, and do all the things a mother has to do.

Most people I hear from just want someone to talk to and write letters to—someone who understands or who will listen. One lady who resided in a nursing home and who had bone cancer told me she was getting ready to celebrate her wedding anniversary (her husband would not be with her, he was in another nursing home). She wasn't bitter about the cancer or the isolation, but she wanted to tell someone about her anniversary.

I wrote back, sending a card. She sent me another letter, saying, "It's so nice to have a friend." Not long afterwards, she died. But for a moment in time, our lives touched, and I could reach out to her.

I think it is so important to be a human being, to have compassion.

It may seem strange, but I don't really consider myself a *dying person* at all. I think I am learning to live again. I think how tragic it would have been if I had committed suicide or had just given up. Yes, I may be dying of cancer, but we are all dying of something. Of course, there is a difference. I am more aware of my impending, probable death from cancer. But we all die. We don't all live to be 70 years old nor do we all live to be a 1000 years old. Death is a natural occurrence in the lives of all persons.

For me, the days and even the nights are more acceptable now, but I still have moments—and even days—of depression.

Sometimes I awaken and think for an instant it has all been a bad dream. . . .

I open my eyes. It is early morning. My wife is asleep beside me. First I thought about death, and now I think about cancer. No, it was not a dream. I do have cancer. But for just an instant, I thought things were "all right" again. No sentence of death, no chemotherapy treatments, no nightmares, no sleepless nights, no worrying about low blood counts, no pain. But I realize things will never be the same again for myself or my family. This would have happened, though, without the presence of cancer. Yesterday never happens again. The "good old days" are a part of the past, terminally ill or not.

I realize, as I lie thinking, that nearly 2 years have gone by since the cancer was diagnosed. What has been the worst of all? Fear. The fear of dying, fear of operations, fear of pain. Fear has been worse than what has actually happened. I haven't died yet, the tests are over for now, and the pain has been bearable.

What has changed it all? Perhaps the difference is that I can now live with this fear of death. It has always been the silent stranger at my side. Now I am afraid, but not terrified.

And the thought of the chemotherapy drugs terrified me, too. Then, I take other drugs—for a high uric acid content in the blood, hypertension, and a few other medical problems. At night, I take sleeping pills, and when there is pain, I take more pills. I take pills to counteract the side effects of pills. Sometimes, I take as many as 57 pills a day.

Each week, I go to the hospital in Burlington for a blood count. Platelet, white cells, hemoglobin, and hematocrit . . . they all tell the story of the cancer's progress through the body when read by a doctor.

Not long ago, my potassium count was extremely low. Two-tenths of a gram from the danger point. The drop was caused by one of the drugs I was taking. My doctors stopped the drug and administered medication to raise the count. It rose to normal.

Then, I contracted pneumonia. Three weeks of bed rest. The fever wouldn't drop. I had difficulty breathing. I realize many cancer patients die of complications, not the cancer itself. My white count started dropping. Not much left to fight the infection. Then one night the fever subsided. I could breathe again. Another crisis met and still I lived. Hope, the will to live; I just wasn't ready to die.

"I'm too busy to die," I told Wanda.

There is a battle going on inside my body. The chemotherapy drugs fight to stop the growth of the cancer cells and kill them. The cancer cells fight to conquer my body. As the drugs fight the cancer, they also destroy healthy tissues. Damage is slowly being done to some of the vital parts of my body. There will be a victor some day, but it cannot be me. But I still have hope—for more time, for a remission. I will not retreat yet.

"You look healthier than I do," a doctor told me not long ago.

Is this a compliment? It is to me. I refuse to be cast in the role of a dying cancer patient. Yes, I am realistic. I know we save one out of three cancer patients, which means we lose two out of three. But I am not dead yet and I refuse to give up. . . .

My family still sleeps. I pull aside the curtains of my bedroom window and look outside. The sun is ready to leap from its hiding place below the horizon. I can see the Mississippi River, silent in the morning light. As I look across the rooftops of the houses, I see my city slowly come to life. A light is turned on inside a house. A laborer is walking to work. A factory whistle shatters the solitude of the morning. A freight train winds its way through the city.

I get out of bed and turn on the shower. My son, Mark, greets me with a "Good morning, Dad." I find it hard to believe he is nearly as tall as I. Once I could hold him in my arms, and at nighttime he would fall asleep on my stomach as I rubbed his back. Time has moved faster than my thoughts.

My two daughters, Tammy and Lori, are still asleep. My youngest son, Britton, is curled in his bed, his arms wrapped around a worn, stuffed bear. Just the other night, he climbed into my bed and asked me, "Daddy, do you have cancer?"

I assumed one of the three older children told him. He is only 5.

"Yes," I replied.

"Are you going to die?"

"Maybe . . . some day. Everyone dies. Do you remember when the cat got run over by a car? Now it is dead. But I'm not dead yet."

God, let the world be kind to my wife and children. There has been enough suffering in the Kelly family. . . .

Wanda enters the bathroom. Her eyes are still filled with sleep.

Sometimes I wonder if she still cries at night. Is she really happy once again, under the circumstances?

I hope so.

Once I wrote these words to explain how I really felt about my wife:

I have spent 15 of the happiest years of my life with this incredible woman. We have shared thousands of beautiful moments growing and learning together and I somehow knew our children would be like her.

She is a woman whose name will never be included in a book of outstanding achievements, but she has more compassion, character, and plain common sense than anyone I've known in my lifetime.

If I had been a Pharaoh in ancient Egypt or a king of the past, I would have erected a great monument in her memory. But I am just an ordinary man and that monument is in my heart.

Sometimes at night, when sleep comes hard, I awaken her to talk to her for just a little while. She is always there willing to help, or just to listen to me.

My hopes were that we would grow old and watch the seasons pass together, but as we all know, life is a fragile and unpredictable thing.

I take a shower and then start taking my medicines. The bottles are lined up like a platoon of soldiers on my dresser. I swallow 20 prednisone pills, 3 Cytoxan tablets, 1 allipurinol, 1 Valium, 2 aldactazide, 1 reserpine, 1 tetracycline, a dose of kaon for the low potassium count, and some medicine to help my intestines withstand the onslaught of the drugs.

Now I am ready to tackle this day. I wrote a poem to explain how I feel about life:

Let me touch the green of Spring once more,
And caress the eager dawn.
Let me hear the midnight thunder

And see the skies explode again.
Let me be there when the snow begins to fall
From darkened skies some silent night,
And let me dream once more
Of sunlit days and silver nights,
Before I die.

11

TERMINAL CANDOR AND THE CODA SYNDROME: A TANDEM VIEW OF FATAL ILLNESS

LOIS AND ARTHUR JAFFE

N ARTHUR

Night, especially around 2 A.M., seems to be the time Lois selects to talk about death, particularly her own impending death from acute leukemia. Perhaps it is the darkness of the night which accentuates the loneliness of dying. Or then maybe it is the silence, creating an ambience of intense intimacy—or possibly suggestive of death itself—which stirs her restlessness.

The night I'm remembering, she suddenly brought up the matter of her funeral. She talked of the pine coffin she wants, to be made by a carpenter friend of ours, not store bought. Lois wants no traditional eulogies, but readings from her favorite poetry, and a long silence in which friends can ponder the meaning of their own lives or reflect upon their connectedness with her, should that enter their thoughts. Mostly, she wants whatever would have meaning for the living, especially for me and our children.

As Lois went on, I protested that it was getting a bit too heavy, and that at the moment, I felt victimized. Obviously shocked by the word *victimized*, and above all, curious, she asked "Victimized? How?"

My answer stunned, delighted, and sent her into an almost uncontrollable fit of laughter.

"I feel I'm a victim of terminal candor."

Such has been our relationship throughout this 2½ year period of Lois's fatal illness: a relationship laden with sadness, tenderness, and caring. Furthermore, a forthrightness about our mutual feelings and thoughts permits anxiety, anger, and fear to be defused by the use of "gallows humor."

The use of candor, combined with humor, has become my main way of coping with permanent uncertainty.

LOIS

As Art and I talked that night for hours on end, we began to realize how "terminal candor" had indeed infused our lives with a special intensity, richness, and intimacy that neither of us had experienced prior to my illness. It also pinpointed an issue that is rarely discussed between the terminally ill and their families and even more rarely appears in print— the problem of often being "out of sync" with each other in regard to every family member's experiencing of various "stages of dying" (Kübler-Ross, 1969).

Certainly this issue of "synchrony" has been our main problem during my prolonged 2½-year remission, when I was originally given approximately 1 to 1½ years to live. Art, our four children, and I have had to contend with our feelings of denial, anger, bargaining, depression, and acceptance, each at our own emotional pace. We have not been able to progress neatly through these five stages, arrive at acceptance, and stay there. Instead, each of us tends to flow back and forth among all the stages at different times, our individual rhythms often depending on events in other facets of our lives.

The longer I have been in remission and able to attend to so much of my unfinished business, the more I have been able to confront and accept my impending death. On the contrary, the longer I have been in a healthy, vital state of remission, the harder it is for Art to accept the fact that I have a fatal illness, and the angrier he gets about my illness.

I find that this permanent uncertainty about time limits has created a state of emotional and cultural limbo for me, and for other fatally ill people like myself whose prognoses have been based on statistical norms. Yet no individual is a statistic. Furthermore, statistics have become quickly outdated due to current medical research and experimentation which have prolonged lives beyond anticipated time limits. Many patients and families experience great emotional discomfort and dislocation when they have been psychologically prepared to accept an earlier death which then does not occur.

This "limbo position" poses a paradox. On the one hand, the lives of the fatally ill are often richer and more meaningful because we *are* confronting time limits. On the other hand, it imposes a tremendous strain. I cannot plan for the future. I must constantly restructure priorities in the immediacy of knowing my life is time-limited. I must keep in touch with my own body processes and the reality of the diagnosis when I may feel, look, and act healthier than ever. I must go back into the hospital every 6 weeks for 5 days of chemotherapy at a time when I usually feel my best, only to be made sick again and vomit for 48 hours and run fevers. Our home life, my work, our social life, and my family's routine are fractured by this interruption. Often the very state of being in a full remission— looking and feeling and behaving "normal"—prompts everyone involved to slip back into denial and proclaim that the diagnosis must be wrong, or that a miracle has occurred and the patient has been cured.

I find one of the most difficult things for me is to keep my own body and psyche "in sync" so as not to be tempted to avoid treatment or to invest unrealistically in the future. This often means being out of sync with others around me who are convinced that I no longer need treatment since I am in a prolonged first remission.

Being out of sync is further exacerbated as both the patient and family struggle to invest as fully as possible in life and each other, in spite of their knowing intuitively that dying must entail a certain amount of mutual disengagement. The terminally ill person and those who will be left behind must, of necessity, prepare to head in two different directions.

Because of this need for a certain amount of disengagement and Art's anticipated reinvestment in other people and activities, we find we seek more time to ourselves—more emotional space—as do our children who range in age from 17 to 25. Instead of a huddled state of togetherness to assuage our anxiety, we often need private time or an opportunity to be with peers in order to dilute the intensity of ongoing terminality.

The main coping devices for me these past 31 months have been to talk openly about my illness and impending death, to read about it, to talk to other terminally ill patients and their families, and even to teach about it. Is this a counterphobic way of dealing with my fears? Probably, but it is also a detoxification process, for the more I encounter death, the less I have come to fear it.

From the beginning, Art and I chose to be open with each other, our children, our friends, and our community about my impending death. We have released enormous energy that would have been dissipated had we played the fruitless charade of "protecting each other" by keeping my terminality a secret. Instead, our energies have been used to fight my illness and to live life as fully as we can.

But this "terminal candor" has now become interminable. The problem is now: Can we withstand this intensity, this constant open communication without burning out, and without burning out others in our wake?

As this process of ebb and flow continues, it becomes more and more apparent that I alone am not the patient. Rather, my whole family is.

ARTHUR

Dying, as I have discovered, is very much the same as living. The longer one dies, as in Lois's case, the more complex becomes the process; the story gets not only longer but more involved. The story should be coming to an ending, but it continues almost beyond its "natural" conclusion. We seem to be in a phase of coda which has more melodic line, tension, and counterpoint than its preceding symphony.

Usually a coda is the short, final, concluding passage which brings a composition to a proper close. I was prepared 2½ years ago for this coda phase when I was told that Lois's leukemia was terminal. But a 2½-year coda starts to seem interminable. One might call the symptoms a "coda syndrome."

Intensity by definition implies straining to the utmost, and intensity, as Lois accurately recounts, has been the major element of our relationship during this period of remission. Yet people were not made to withstand intense sun, intense cold, or intense feeling. Yes, gallows humor is one way to get relief. But it is just a sort of ice cube that gives instant relief, and then quickly melts away.

Perhaps this getting out of sync is a more natural and effective way of surviving the coda syndrome—a sort of counterpoint—allowing us to live our individual lives. Simultaneously, recognition that we are out of sync provides a contrapuntal theme which continues and enriches our relationship.

The coda began on a low, quiet note: "Your wife has acute myelomonocytic leukemia," followed by a rather startling, even lower note: "that should last 18 months perhaps." A long, silent pause . . . a gasping for breath to survive the moment.

Now the full development of the coda line commences. The first note of this phase is perfect synchronization: that moment when Lois and I see each other for the first time, cry together, and for that short period in time we are in perfect harmony. We know we will never again have this moment to express our unity of feeling, love, and concern.

Now the coda loses its great swell of line and becomes more earthbound, grounded in our children, parents, friends.

Telling our children was not difficult. I took a page from the doctor's book and talked medically rather than emotionally about what Lois's illness might mean to our individual lives. Now that I think back on this technique, I'm not sure it wasn't right, and I'm not sure it was, either. I didn't know then, and I'm not sure I know now, how this illness will affect each of us. I did not suggest any additional concerns to them at the time because I thought they had enough, and that they would probably consider their individual aspects at their own time and pace.

I described to the children how the disease would express itself, how Lois would feel and be treated, and the prognosis itself. I tried to demystify the illness so they would not have to fill in gaps with fantasies and projections. I suggested that they keep in touch in a routine manner (weekly phone calls, frequent visits home since they were away at school), and that they relieve Lois of household duties when possible. Above all, I urged them to pursue their own studies and careers so as to relieve Lois of any anxiety she might feel about delaying or upsetting their routines. The need, as I saw it, was to keep things at home as normal as possible during this abnormal period. And, in fact, the children's response to this traumatic new event was to show more stability in their life-styles and studies than ever before.

Now a note of anger sounds. I begin to hate the house we built where our lives have been lived, the house filled with all those birthday, anniversary, or "just because" gifts and remembrances. I hate being alone, especially there, and while I gradually got over the feeling of hating the house, I have never gotten over the feeling of loneliness each time Lois enters the hospital. I suppose it is because it gives me a bitter foretaste of her terminality and my own aloneness.

The first time we discovered we were out of sync was resolved with a light touch of gallows humor. During Lois's first hospitalization of 7½ weeks while the doctors were still struggling to bring her into remission, I often stayed overnight in Pittsburgh as our home was 45 miles away. By so doing, I could spend late evenings at the hospital and be there again early in the morning.

During this period, I had stayed the Friday night in Pittsburgh and returned to the hospital early Saturday morning to be with her. At about 11 o'clock, I informed her that I was going back to Butler. She did not want me to leave and demanded to know why I could not stay.

I reminded her that I had checks to sign and certain instructions to deliver. Besides, it was Saturday, and as the wife of a retailer, she knew it was the busiest day of the week. Her plaintive question was, "And what if I were dying today?"

I answered, "Never on Saturday. You know better than that!" She laughed through her pain for a full 5 minutes.

But we were out of sync. She had her schedule, and I mine.

LOIS

Art has described our period of perfect synchronization when our grief, our love, our fears, our concerns were as one. In retrospect, this is when I most needed that empathy and harmony. Art must have known intuitively for, after we had talked and cried together, he turned to me and asked the most important question he possibly could have put to me: "What do you want to do with the time you have left?"

It was important because it immediately put me in touch with the fact that I had been extremely happy and fulfilled in my life. I really wanted to continue with exactly what I had been doing: teaching, therapy, being a wife, a mother. I had no desire to hop on a boat to Tahiti. I simply wanted to get into remission and return to what I had enjoyed for so many years. His question not only gave me hope for remission but also gave me permission to focus on what I wanted for myself.

This brief synchrony was broken by the grueling treatment and my garnering all my energies to battle for life. Often when Art and the children came, I was too drained and sick to do much talking. I felt guilty about Art having to drive back and forth, handle the children, our home, and his business as well. So, at times, I would urge him to remain at home. At other times, when I was feeling more energized, I would become resentful that he couldn't spend more time with me. I was angry, too, that no one was around to give *him* the support I felt he needed.

The bulk of my anger became displaced on my hospital environment, particularly those aspects that threatened my own sense of control. These aspects included having to endure endless waiting in the x-ray department when I was racked with chills and fever; experiencing the traumatic loss of my hair that became symbolic for all my potential losses; seeing my body waste away and having no appetite to combat it; vomiting perpetually and continually; feeling trapped in a bleak, grey room that overlooked the barren rooftops of the city. I felt like Sisyphus pushing the damn rock up the mountain each time I had a round of chemotherapy, only to have the rock come crushing down again, draining me of every drop of energy. Yet I knew that I had to keep on pushing if I were to live. As the chemicals gradually began to combat the invading leukemia cells and it seemed as if I might soon get into remission and return to my family, I began to panic at the thought of having to take care of myself at home. However uncomfortable, I felt safe at the hospital. Because of the perpetual openness, honesty, and compassionate care of my medical team, I had come to trust my hospital environment completely. Art wanted me home in the worst kind of way; I wasn't sure I would feel safe there.

I suppose on a deeper level my fears were: Can I function as a wife again? Will I have energy to function as a mother? In all the 7½ weeks of my hospitalization, there had been no opportunity for physical intimacy between Art and myself. The cold hardware of the hospital room, a room that I had come to associate with pain and nausea, provided no incentive for sexual rehearsal. On the hematology unit, there was no quiet, "non-medical" room for intimacy of any sort. In my depleted state, I wondered, could I function sexually again? My only sexual fantasies in the hospital involved my doctors, who had most frequently touched and tended to my body for weeks on end. My feelings of dependency and emotional attachment seemed quite naturally to transfer to those whose care was sustaining my life and soothing my ills.

Coming back home meant reinvesting in life again, and for others it meant reinvesting in their attachment to me. Could we take this mutual risk when it would mean suffering separation and loss all over again?

In reality, returning home was a shock of another kind. My senses were stunned by the feel of textures and the startle of colors. My eyes filled with joyous tears when I saw green grass and real growing flowers out my glass bedroom door.

I noticed that our youngest daughter, then 15, had moved into my role as "keeper of the house" and was doing a better and neater job than

I ever had. Yet neither Art nor my children ever felt the need to overprotect me; but rather they "made space" for me to move back and take over my household activities as I was able. As they helped me maintain my sense of self-worth, I in turn encouraged each of them to move ahead in his or her own life pursuits. I just wanted to be myself again, and I didn't want them changing themselves. In this respect, we seemed to be a family very much "in phase."

Art and I took a second honeymoon and headed south into the sun where we spent 2 weeks walking the beaches, bathing in the ocean, and coming to life and love again. Art was hesitant to approach me sexually at first. He somehow felt it might be indulgent of him and overtaxing to me to seek sexual gratification when I still appeared so frail and debilitated. I, on the other hand, felt a need as never before to assuage my own anxieties, for I had become heir to the generally accepted myth that a terminally ill individual will be neither interested nor able to function effectively in sex. With the aid of much loving communication, patience, and leisurely responding, we were able to regain the fullness of relatedness as well as the freedom of release that lovemaking in its richest sense affords.

When I first came out of the hospital, I felt an inordinate need to talk to each one of my children about our mutual feelings. But I found that the intensity was too great and that I had to wait for each one to take individual initiative in dealing with my impending death.

Our older daughter, who was 23 at the time I first became ill, was attending a university in Pittsburgh. She visited me almost daily during those first 7½ weeks in the hospital. From the very beginning, she was able to express a lot of anger about the disruption in her life which my illness had caused. When she subsequently transferred to another school in Philadelphia where her fiancé was obtaining his master's degree, she asked me to join her for several sessions with a therapist she was seeing. She was dealing with anger, grief, and fears of separation and loss that were preventing her from moving into marriage.

Expressing anger had become a dangerous risk, as she feared her anger might hasten my death. I, on the other hand, felt a need to express and receive only love during this precarious period of my life. But I could not have it both ways. I could not advocate open communication in relation to some feelings and not others. An accumulation of angers that had not been expressed over her lifetime were acting as a barrier and protection against the deep feelings of love that were equally painful to confront at this time of impending loss. This was the epitome of being out of sync: her needing one thing, my wanting another.

With the aid of a neutral and sensitive therapist to dilute the intensity, we were both enabled to express our resentments as well as our appreciations, both of which need to be said before a loved one dies so one is not plagued by these deep, unexpressed feelings after death, when it is too late. Happily, she was able to resolve many of her feelings and finally married this past spring, to the joy and delight of all concerned.

Our boys have found it much more difficult to tackle the emotional aspects of my illness, yet each has found ways to share his concerns. Our 23-year-old son's way of confronting my terminality was to announce to Art and me last year that he had decided to change universities from Louisville to Pittsburgh so that he could be of more help to us both, and also to cut expenses during this critical period. His more direct way of expressing synchronization with me was an offer to teach me how to smoke marijuana. He had read about recent research which indicated that smoking grass had abated nausea for many chemotherapy patients who could get relief from no other source. He felt I shouldn't neglect any aspect of scientific experimentation that could be of help—as well as enjoy myself at the same time!

Our younger son, age 21, is attending Penn State and majoring in human development. Last year he asked if he might come home to do a taped interview with me as part of a communication course assignment. He had always assumed the role of the family comedian and up to this point I had found it very difficult to talk to him about our feelings, as he would always turn me off with a flip comment. I suspected he was choosing a way where *he* could be in control, on his own terms, to discuss my impending death. I guessed right, and our encounter turned out to be one of the most moving and meaningful exchanges I have ever had with anyone near and dear to me. He wanted to know how it felt to be in my position and, in turn, shared his own feelings. More importantly, he wanted to know how I felt about the way he had turned out and expressed his feelings about how I stacked up as a mother.

Spurred on by a new sense of confidence and freeing of self, he next interviewed Art about his plans after I die. Did he plan to sell the house? Would he remarry? He did a magnificent job of dealing with anticipatory grief—my husband's as well as his own. He wrote a narrative for class, describing the process of what had occurred and his own reactions. In it he noted how good it felt to help me, when I was usually the "professional helper," and how meaningful it was for him to be able to ask his father about his future plans, when usually it is Art who asks *him*, "Well, what are your plans for the future?"

Both boys have found ways to become "the parent" when they feel we may need their support.

Our younger daughter, who is now 17, has been the only child at home during these past 2½ years. At the beginning of my illness, she found it hard to visit me in the hospital and would always bring a friend along to dilute the intensity. Little by little, she has been able to talk about my illness and death openly. She has invited me to discuss death and dying at her high school psychology classes and at a regional Jewish youth conference. In this way, she builds up her own peer support, while providing herself with a "defused" situation to confront her concerns. She has even picked up Art's gallows humor way of coping with ongoing intensity. When Art recently told her I was to appear on another television show, her retort was, "Don't tell me that mother is dying again!"

These episodes illustrate points at which the children have confronted my illness. However, my terminality is something we rarely discuss now, but rather, have come to treat as a "given." Like any subject that is overdone, death can become a bore.

ARTHUR

Of course the concept "out of sync" implies a condition of being *in sync*. The main force for synchronization at the time Lois first became ill was our realization that we had reached that state announced at the beginning of our marriage: "until death do us part." Since our marriage had been well knit from the beginning, the threads held together under the stress of terminality. The threat of death itself became and remains the greatest force for being in sync, but it has a pressure cooker quality that needs the lid lifted frequently. There is a kind of unnatural aura about constant synchronization, as romantic and sentimental as it is often made to appear.

If death is indeed not far, one can manage "in syncness" over a brief period, living only day to day—no next week, no next month, no next year to anticipate. This process becomes a sync force in itself, because the minutes and the hours are to be accounted for, to be spent together, or, at the very least, to know each other's whereabouts at all times. To keep in close touch is to be in sync because of a sense of imminent closure.

But life which continues on, not only for those around Lois but for Lois herself, becomes insistent, demands attention to birthdays, anniversaries, visits, and other functions. Thus one begins tentatively to make little plans, little bargains—dinner out next Saturday night, a visit to a friend next Tuesday. But no more plans until after the next hospitalization in 2 weeks. . . .

However, as the days stretch out, the time that once seemed so constricted expands to months and even years. One begins to fill the calendar on a monthly or even a 2 or 3 month basis with new bargains—a wedding 2 months away, a trip to Florida next month.

Nevertheless, Lois still plans for a promised death, and all her personal and professional commitments are related to this prospect. I also must continue my present activities in business, with family and friends, as well as think about the future, albeit without Lois.

Lois has chosen to use her terminal experience to help others in similar situations, while at the same time helping herself. These activities are revitalizing to Lois, adding meaning to her life as well as to her impending death. While we are proud of her magnificent efforts, her work nevertheless consumes great amounts of her now limited time—time away from me, the children, the family.

Here lies the crux of the dilemma: Wanting Lois to continue to fulfill herself, and simultaneously wanting more of her limited time for ourselves. Yet we feel a kind of guilt at making such a request.

Being selfish as we all are, and being those most close and constant to her, we often feel neglected and hurt that at this critical point in her life, Lois does not choose to share all her remaining time with us.

The tensions created by the swings from being in sync to being out of sync compose the one constant theme of the coda syndrome and the one that is the most debilitating and exhausting, leaving me always tired, never completely rested.

The longer this coda syndrome, the more one finds relief in allowing all who are involved to pursue their own way, without such striving to remain in sync.

Since Lois is going in a different direction, one in which we can accompany her just so far, differentiation for each of us during this coda phase is not only natural but an absolute necessity.

There is a definite rhythm in the coda. Every 5 weeks Lois enters the hospital for 5 days of chemotherapy. These regularly scheduled treatments serve as harsh reminders that no matter how "normal" Lois seems, she remains terminal.

For several days before her hospitalization, the coda notes are anxious and depressing. There is anxiety about the test results, waiting to find out whether the leukemia has returned. There is depression in anticipating the harshness of treatment which Lois will have to suffer. Furthermore, there is the interruption of our entire domestic life, not only for the 5 days but for several days prior and after the chemotherapy. Everything from social engagements, food shopping, laundry, feeding the dogs, to our sex life is either in limbo or disrupted. Then, there are the high notes of elation when Lois returns home—a pervasive ambience of warm affection and thankful closeness.

These hospitalizations serve to return us to the close, "sync" feelings of Lois's initial diagnosis, and to prepare us for the final time when we will want and need as "full a sync" as possible to meet the end.

Acute leukemia is a dreaded disease, a tragedy for the victim as well as those who are emotionally close to the victim.

For us, acute leukemia has also meant discovery, love, excitement, family unification, and many other things yet to be understood.

All of us—Lois, myself, the children, my family and her family—when faced with death itself, had to look into ourselves deeply and ask What is life? What is important? What are our priorities? To my mind, all of us became more compassionate, more concerned about each other, less concerned about material things, more now-oriented, and less future-oriented. We learned to value the moment and to demonstrate our love for one another.

These intensifications of feelings and discoveries also proved exhilarating, giving us hints of exquisite possibilities within ourselves we did not know existed. The children, and perhaps even myself, have discovered self-reliance more quickly and the self-respect which it engenders.

As a by-product of Lois's illness, family reunification took place. Relatives who had not talked to each other for a long period of time were brought together again.

Since leukemia is a sudden disease, we became increasingly aware of the present and that today is the time to plan for the future, for the sudden events we all know are possible, if not inevitable.

Above all, death no longer looms as some fearful monster from whom we must run. Instead, death has become a part of our living—more like a known acquaintance that one day may present itself as friend.

Terminal does not mean the end; rather, it means reaching our destination, after the journey.

LOIS

Prompted by Art's definition of terminal, I have sometimes wondered, "Did I catch the right train? Am I on the right track? Should I have spent far more of my time at home with my husband and family? Should I continue conducting seminars and workshops on death education and working with the terminally ill and their families? Has this been a surfeit for myself, however well it may have served to channel my ongoing death anxieties as well as those of others?" By having peer groups with whom I could talk, I could reduce my tension, gain rehearsal, share coping devices. I know that by starting "on the periphery," where emotions are less directly charged, I feel I have coped better with the more intense feelings in my own family system.

I often feel guilty about time away from home. Yet until the confrontation with death began to compress time for us all, this pattern had been most functional for 26 years. I now must constantly contend with preparing to separate from all those I have come to love—my family, my friends, my colleagues. My family is preparing to lose only me. Is this my way of diluting that final pain of separation, of preventing engulfment by too many painful stimuli? Or is this my way of keeping a foothold in life all around me? I have had to overcome a fear of living an incomplete life by striving for goals important to my self-esteem and by expressing myself as fully as possible. By trying to bring some meaning to my particular finality, I am attempting to handle the absurdity, the "why me?" of a premature death. The way I have chosen to relate to my death has become more important than death itself.

I, too, have had my own coda, filled with alternate swelling and subsiding phases. Immediately after my return home from those first 7½ weeks in the hospital, revitalized from our "second honeymoon," I felt an enormous need to become active again. I had to prove to myself and others that I was as competent as ever, could work as hard as ever, so as to warn people not to write me off, not to bury me before my time. I could not allow my self-image to change. All my life I have had to *do* in order to prove my worth. The threat of social and physical death intensified this drive, in spite of my depleted energies.

For about a year, I denied the implications of my illness. In spite of my frequent hospitalizations, I returned to teaching and doing therapy full time. I went back to pushing that rock up the hill again, only this time it was emotional drivenness, rather than medical necessity. I became obsessed with *deadlines* (a word that is not accidental in its connotations), of having to complete anything I started for fear that my time would run out.

One night I had a dream which had profound impact and portent for me. I rarely remember a dream, but this time I awakened in the middle of the night and wrote it down. In the dream, I was giving a party. I had already served, and the guests were about to leave, when I remembered I had more food warming. I went into the kitchen, peered into the oven, and saw white plates filled with spinach soufflé, fluffy scrambled eggs, and chicken breasts. I began to offer the plates to my guests, explaining I had more to serve. But the guests declined my offer, saying they had had quite enough, and proceeded to leave. I woke up with tears in my eyes. Being in that state of twilight sleep, I immediately went back to bed to finish my dream so I might understand my sadness.

In my dream, I realized I was sad not only because people were *leaving* me, but also because I had been so busy serving that I had not had time to enjoy my own party.

The next morning I decided to give up working full time, and to enjoy more of life around me. Thereafter, I explored a part of my life never fully experienced before, the need to *be*. Slowly, I began to feel that

I was worthy of just being, that I need not *do* all the time. For about a year, I slowed down; I stopped to smell the flowers. I shifted my "gotta's" to "wanta's," doing more of the things I really desired without a sense of deadlines. I spent more time with family and friends. I followed my body's lead—resting when tired, practicing yoga. As I relinquished more of the external controls, I gained the strength of inner control.

This coda had stretched for 2 years. In this time of "being," I wrote publicly about many of my thoughts and feelings, and thus touched the lives of many others. The momentum created by the workshops, seminars, and self-help groups for cancer patients and their families catapulted me into another phase of increased activity, albeit at my own pace this time.

Another paradox has emerged during this "swelling phase." The more I have turned onto life, the longer my remission endures; and the healthier I look, the more I begin to lose my credibility as a terminal patient. Now I feel an urge to move on to other things. But what? And for how long?

People ask me if I plan for the future. As Art has suggested, we are always in sync in our bargaining. For the first time, we are tentatively planning a trip 4 months away. Yes, I plan for the future—but only with my head. My heart and soul are in the present, in what I'm doing today.

I no longer undertake only projects which I feel I have a chance of finishing. It is enough to enjoy and value what I'm doing at the moment. I am reminded of a Talmudic saying from Ethics of the Fathers: "It is not up to you to finish the job, but neither are you allowed to desist from doing it."

I believe that Art's and my commitment to the basic tenets of Judaism has helped provide a key melodic line throughout this coda. Significantly, Judaism concentrates on life and survival. Although belief in a life-after-death exists, it is far from being dogma. The focus is on deed, rather than creed; on doing, rather than believing. The premise is that we create by our deeds our own heaven or hell here on earth. There is also the belief that our physical being dies, but our spirit lives on within the hearts and minds of those we have touched, those who are left behind. This belief system has given us harmony even during times when we are out of sync. For the first time, Art has begun to muse about how nice an afterlife would be, for he would like to see me again. I, on the other hand, am thoroughly grateful that I have had 26 of the best and richest years of my life with him. For me, this is really enough.

And so the melody continues to linger on. . . .

CODA

What have we discovered from this terminal candor and interminable coda?

Leukemia, like other cancers, often portends a slow leave-taking. This coda phase has put us both in touch with an important distinction between terminal illness and fatal disease.

Now we think of terminality as the last throes of dying, a matter of days, hours, and minutes. We also think of the critical time before remission is attained, or when remission ends with the reassertion of the imminent threat of death. Synchronization at these moments is most vital for the patient and family. Denial must often be confronted. Mutual feelings of anger, sadness, and love need to find expression. Family members must learn to let go, allowing the patient to die in peace without a sense of isolation or abandonment.

To live with an ongoing fatal disease constitutes the coda syndrome, a period qualitatively different from actual terminality. In the coda of prolonged remission, one must learn to reinvest in life, for however long it may last. While an acceptance of death enables one to take charge of one's life, a constant focus on death begins to deny that very life force. This is as true for the family as it is for the patient.

During the coda phase, differentiation and pursuit of one's individual emotional pace become most functional. To remain continually in sync is to become fused with the other person, to lose one's own sense of self. This is especially true when anxiety is pushing everyone in the family to think alike and feel alike. Thus, we have found it not only natural but also necessary often to be out of sync during this phase. Giving permission for such separateness has assuaged much guilt. By discovering new role and identity potentials, our family members have been liberated to move in different directions while still keeping in contact. In this freeing process, each has been able to demonstrate concern for the family as a cohesive unit in a way which did not exist before.

A 13-year-old junior high school student recently asked me: "What problems would you face if doctors found a cure for leukemia?" My reply after a long, breathless pause: "I would have to find a new identity."

Being leukemic is as much a part of my identity as being a woman or being Jewish. It is a part of myself I cannot slough off, no matter how hard I might try. I could conceivably lose my husband and children, and thus cease to be a wife and mother. But as long as there is no cure for leukemia, being a leukemic woman remains an integral part of my identity.

Should a cure be discovered before my death (and I do not expect this), I would most certainly confront an identity crisis. There are many secondary gains in having a fatal illness. I am excused from many mundane activities, and can easily extricate myself from involvements which I find draining. Even more important are the primary gains. Would this intensity of giving and receiving love continue? Would the sky seem as blue, the flowers as sweet, the senses as keen? Would the excitement of being in touch with all the nuances of this final stage of growth persist?

Paradoxically, there could be a certain sense of loss in giving up a fatal diagnosis, comparable in some ways to confronting death.

Since there is no cure for acute myelogenous leukemia at present, the internalized identity of "leukemic woman" prevents me from denying my illness. To slip back into denial would be to lose a part of myself, thus catapulting me into an identity crisis.

A sixth stage of dying, responsibility, may well follow Kübler-Ross's fifth stage of acceptance. Acceptance conveys passive assent, whereas responsibility implies an active state of doing something about one's situation. I have often talked about the time I "took ill." "Taking ill" assumes that we participate at some level in our illness. As with so many words we use out of awareness, I believe we unconsciously coin phrases that reflect the intermeshing of mind and body.

Hans Selye's (1975) experimental studies demonstrate that many diseases have no specific single cause, but are the result of a constellation of factors, among which nonspecific stress may play a decisive role. It has been postulated that leukemia may be a disease in which immune mechanisms break down, making one vulnerable to the invasion of cancer cells or viral infection. Certainly psychosocial stress might be one of the multicausal factors. I shall never forget that my first reaction to being told I was seriously ill was: "Thank God, I can rest now."

Art has referred to me as a victim of leukemia. I do not feel myself a victim. If in some way I have participated in taking ill, then I can assume some responsibility for prolonging my life.

To feel that one can *do* something to affect one's longevity is life-promoting. This active responsibility may take several forms, whether it is working at something one loves, participating in medical experimentation, or learning relaxation and meditation techniques to help master the tension of living a coda phase. Leaving no stone unturned in the push for longer survival, while quality of life remains, diminishes one's sense of helplessness and hopelessness.

Hope, for me, is not finding a miracle cure. Rather, it is being able to live as full and rich a life as possible in whatever time is left. I am determined to do all I can to achieve this end.

Art has written about his desire for me to be at home more, since we are living with such uncertain time limits. However, I believe that turning completely to my family for fulfillment of my needs and drives would create a climate of emotional intensity that might burn them out prematurely. When I die, I want my family to be close at hand, whether my last days are in the hospital or, hopefully, at home. My greatest fear is of a lingering death, a prolonged terminal phase. From my own observations I know that families burn out under this pressure in a way similar to medical staff who must contend with continual, lingering dying.

Neither biological nor social systems are built to endure excessive stress on the same part over a prolonged period. Both the body and the family need diversion from the impact of a constant stressor. Differentiation, active responsibility, candor, and humor have been crucial in enabling us to cope with the stress of this coda syndrome.

Art and I have found a quality of loving and living that alleviates our sadness over the prospect of an abbreviated life together. I have often wondered whether it is not this very love and care from my husband, our children, families, friends, and the medical team that have prolonged my life, every bit as much as the chemotherapy.

More than anyone else, Art has been my main source of support, as well as my most severe critic, throughout this period. He has helped change the tempo of this coda syndrome from a dirge into a dance of life by encouraging me to pursue my own life rhythm, thereby freeing himself to do the same.

> Once the realization is accepted that even between the closest human beings infinite distances continue to exist, a wonderful living side by side can grow up, if they succeed in loving the distance between them which makes it possible for each to see the other whole against the sky (from *Letters* by Rainer Marie Rilke).

REFERENCES

Kübler-Ross. E. *On death and dying.* New York: Macmillan, 1969.

Rilke, R. M. *Letters.* New York: Norton, 1945.

Seyle, H. *Stress without distress.* Bergenfield, N. J.: New American Library (Signet Paperbacks), 1975.

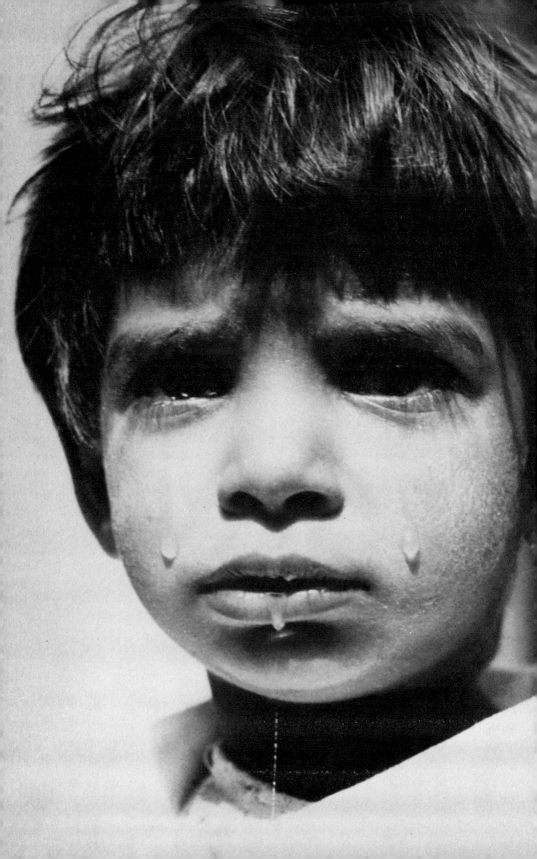

PART FOUR

THE SURVIVORS

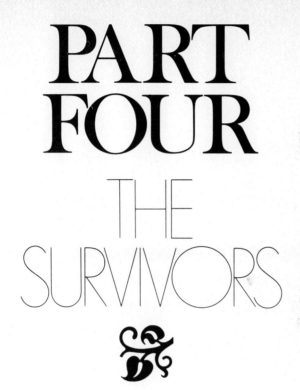

12

DYING AND PREPARING FOR DEATH: A VIEW OF FAMILIES

RICHARD A. KALISH

My aunt died 3 hours ago. At 81, she had been losing ground to heart and lung conditions for several months, a slow downhill path (somehow the term *trajectory* is too impersonal for me to use) in which periods of confusion and unawareness had become more numerous than those of alertness. Certainly uncomfortable, but not in great pain, she had remained in the apartment she shared with my uncle until her medical needs required that she move to a convalescent home. There my uncle attended her as much as his 86-year-old strength would permit.

She died in Tucson, Arizona, where she had lived for 30 years; I was called in Berkeley 1 hour later, and I confirmed my previous plans to visit Tucson a week later. (Better, I felt, to provide my uncle with some support at about the time that their many friends and neighbors might begin to fade away, and I took my 10-year-old son with me.) My mother has made plans to fly from Berkeley to Tucson for the funeral; one cousin will fly in from Cleveland; another cousin will fly down from Chicago; the only other surviving relative is a brother in Florida who—at 82, with his own health problems—will find it extremely difficult to make the trip, but will come nonetheless.

The funeral is being planned to coordinate with flight arrangements, work schedules in Ohio and California and Illinois, and other family demands. Friends are opening their homes to the visiting relatives, meeting them at the airport, caring for my uncle, arranging for the funeral. The rabbi had arrived at the apartment while I was still on the telephone and made a point of speaking to me.

When I talked with my uncle a week ago and 2 weeks before that, he referred again and again to how isolated he felt from his family, how alone (not lonely—that's another concept), and how important the constant flow of calls and letters were that he had been receiving. When I spoke with him 3 hours ago, he was unable to say anything without tears clouding his voice.

The images are not those we have sanctified, of a person dying peacefully, surrounded by loving relatives, nor are the images those we have condemned, of a person dying in isolation, cut off from human contact by an impersonal health-care system and its technologies. The images are probably much more representative of dying in the United States: an elderly woman, kept home as long as possible and cared for by a member of the nuclear family, finally going to a convalescent care center when medical needs and husband's fatigue combine to make additional home care impossible. Kept alive by an oxygen machine, her husband visiting constantly, and other family members in close touch by telephone, her time finally runs out. Family members are summoned by telephone, arrive by airplane. The extended family is briefly reestablished.

All of us are truly sad—we did love her. But when a woman is 81, her death is not unanticipated. Our lives, our children's lives are minimally affected. Because of geography, she does not leave a vital gap in our lives, except the gap that the loss of a beloved person inevitably leaves. She left no vacant roles that someone else will need to fill—except for my uncle.

But who will care for *him* when his health and energies ebb, when *he* needs someone to walk him to the bathroom at night, when *he* wants to feel the caress of tender love, when *he* wants to know that someone in the apartment really cares what happens to him, when *he* needs to feel less vulnerable? There is now no one to care for him; there is now no one for him to care for. "I always thought she would die before me," he said to me recently, and there was little doubt that that was both wish and assumption.

What if he wants to move to Berkeley to live near me? Or back to Cleveland, which is where he had lived his first several decades, to be near my cousin? Or to Florida, to be close to his brother? Will they welcome him? Will I? Am I my uncle's keeper?

THE FAMILY AND DEATH

"There does not seem to be any society—as distinguished from special, subsocietal religious or military orders—in which death is not normally the concern of the next of kin in the *first* instance. Even in a society such as ours, in which the important associations of an individual generally ramify very far beyond kin, close relatives almost always take the leading role in, and hold primary responsibility for, the arrangements that must be made after a death" (Parsons and Lidz, 1967, p. 141).

"Uniformly, one meets the flat assertion that the funeral is the single most significant family ceremony among Mexican Americans" (Moore, p. 277). Whether viewing the entire culture or subgroups within it, death in the family is a first-order concern.

The loss of a family member may be the single most upsetting and feared event in the life of an individual—at least that is what people say when they are asked. College students listed this as their greatest fear among 50 possible causes of fear, with their own death near the middle of the rankings (Geer, 1965). The well-being of survivors is considered more important than five other death-related concerns (e.g., fear of pain, anxiety over cessation of experience) by a wide variety of age, socioeconomic, and ethnic groups (Diggory and Rothman, 1961; Kalish and Reynolds, 1976). Further evidence comes from some very important work done on psychological stress, in which the death of a spouse was found to be the most significant life-change in terms of the amount of stress produced

(Rahe, McKean, and Arthur, 1967). The previous research has measured, of course, only what people *say* causes them the most fear—no one has yet been able to compare the amount of fear actually generated in the situation of facing one's own death as opposed to facing the death of a loved one.

The dying process of family members produces an immense range of emotional reactions, from guilt and anger to money worries to fear and anxiety. Also, the death of someone close to us is a reminder of our own vulnerability, which is fear-evoking in itself. For example, when the parents of a middle-aged man or woman have both died, that leaves the middle-aged person as the next logical one in the family to die. It is as though a buffer, a protection against death, has been removed. It is like saying, "As long as one of my parents was alive, I couldn't die because it doesn't make sense for someone to predecease his or her parents, but now . . ."

The media and the academic journals are both filled with articles about the failure of the family as a viable institution: nuclear families place too much pressure on their members, marriages are unstable, too many miles separate adult children from their parents, and so forth. This may be. Family structure is very likely changing in terms of sex role, social interaction among family members, power relationships, forms of discipline, geographical stability, and perhaps even permanence. Nonetheless, the family still provides—and will for the foreseeable future—the basis for the most intimate, most rewarding, and most trying relationships that people have.

In this article, I will explore what takes place within the family as members plan (or do not plan) for an eventual death and what happens as the process of dying takes place. I will focus on two pairs of dimensions: financial-legal and psychological-social. I will not discuss the time of death, the death and postdeath rituals and ceremonies, or the immensely important matter of bereavement—these are grist for another mill. First, however, I shall touch briefly on the meaning of death and the dying process for persons of differing ages.

The Dying of the Old

On the whole—and without wishing to debate some of the obvious exceptions—the death of an older person is seen as less tragic than the death of a person of any other age group, with the possible exception of newborns. This is the case whether the person responding is a man or a woman, is young, middle-aged, or elderly, is black, Mexican-American, Japanese-American, or Anglo-American (Kalish and Reynolds, 1976).

The issue that arises, then, is why? There are a number of probable answers. First, older people are likely to have diminished social responsibilities and fewer societal roles limiting the dependence of others on them (e.g., work, family, club); therefore, their absence will have less impact on those they leave behind and will not be so likely to require role substitutes. Second, because old people today tend to constitute most of the deaths (quite different from periods when major wars, plagues and epidemics, or simple lack of medical care distributed death almost randomly across the life span), many of us seem to look on death as the normal concomitant of age and are not especially shocked by it. Third, we know the old person is going to die soon anyway, so we are better prepared—perhaps *braced* would be a more appropriate term—for it when it happens. (If this seems to be a harsh statement, I believe that it reflects a harsh reality.) Fourth, many of us, old and young alike, feel that old people have already had the life which they were entitled to: to die at an old age does not involve being cheated. Fifth, our living style often brings us into contact with relatively few older people—the nonelderly remove themselves from the elderly both psychologically and physically. Sixth, old people have gone through the deaths of many others, and they themselves often indicate a greater readiness to die than people at other ages. And seventh, some old people have already deteriorated to the point that their future existence seems to hold limited value even for them; others have suffered physical, psychological, or social losses that may make further living less valuable. And there are undoubtedly additional reasons (Kalish, 1969, 1976).

I am not contending that these are all "good" reasons, but simply that they exist. Nor is it my intent to categorize all the elderly as deteriorated, since only a very small proportion are. But the more the losses and the deterioration exhibited by an older person (or a person of any age), the less tragic the death of that person is felt to be.

The Dying of the Middle Aged and Young

By reflecting on the reasons why the deaths of the elderly are perceived as less tragic, we can understand why the deaths of other age groups are more difficult to accept. Middle-aged people have substantial responsibilities and may have many people depending on them. Often the first question asked about a person who has just died (or, for that matter, who has just been divorced) relates to what is being done about the spouse and dependent children. Middle-aged people have a wide network of friends and associates and family members, normally much wider than the elderly. And they are seen as not yet having lived their allotted time.

In our society, the death of young adults is viewed as the most tragic of all (Kalish and Reynolds, 1976). They have not yet been able to make use of the lengthy schooling they undertook; their deaths are often sudden and unexpected; they are seen as having been deprived of their birthright. And since they are often younger than the rest of us, their death brings our own finitude painfully close to home.

In recent decades, a smaller number of pregnancies have resulted in a larger number of living children 20 years later. With infant and child mortality greatly reduced, the value of the individual child has probably increased and, with it, the pain of loss at the death of an infant or child. In earlier times, pregnancies and births were so common and so many died young, there seemed to have been a tendency to anticipate deaths of the very young in somewhat the same way that we now anticipate deaths of the very old. Infants or young children have a small network of social interactions, have no one dependent on them (except as someone to love and to give to, which is certainly a very significant role), and—if young enough—do not comprehend the process of dying. On the other hand, the love given to them, the vulnerability that they display, and the seeming meaninglessness of their death cause many people to view such an event as the most tragic of all.

PLANNING FOR DEATH

Economic and Legal Factors

It costs money to die; it costs money to be dead; it costs money to have been dead for a while. These crass truisms lead many families to plan for death as soon as there are family members to plan for, although others procrastinate in their planning, sometimes with the implicit feeling that to plan for death means they will die, while not planning means they will not die.

Financial advisors usually urge early and flexible planning. Even a very modest estate can be tied up in the courts for a lengthy period, depriving family members of the use of money at the very time that they need it most. Being uninsured or underinsured may leave survivors with immense financial problems, especially if the dead person had been the major breadwinner for a dependent spouse and minor children.

In this regard, anthropologist David Reynolds and I conducted a comprehensive interview survey of 434 adult residents of Los Angeles in 1970; our respondents were fairly equally divided among blacks, Mexican-Americans, Japanese-Americans, and Anglo-Americans, with older persons and persons of low and low-middle income overrepresented. Among the questions we asked were several related to having made out a will, having paid for a funeral, and having paid for a cemetery plot. Only a moderate proportion of these people (15 to 25 percent) had made such arrangements. This is somewhat surprising when we consider that the most frequently stated concern about dying is the welfare of the survivors. Yet in part because some taboo on death still exists, although certainly modified from a decade ago, and in part because of the embarrassment that family members feel in urging the breadwinner to make out a will, it would appear that many American family survivors find that they lack the protection of this document when death occurs.

The statistics for life insurance are more optimistic. In 1969, a national survey conducted for the Institute of Life Insurance (1972) found that at least one adult had some insurance in over 80 percent of all household units; this figure rose to over 90 percent when the adult was between 45 and 54 years of age. Even among those 65 years of age and older, two out of every three households had one or more persons carrying life insurance. (Not only were most men insured, but the great majority of women also carried some life insurance.) The total amount of life insurance in force in 1971 was $1.5 trillion! This was 2½ times as much as a decade earlier.

Although this appears to be an unbelievably large amount, it represents less than $22,000 per family and less than $26,000 per insured family. Even allowing for the distortions of an inflationary economy, the income that might be realized from these amounts would not do much to keep a family going for very long, while the need to take money from the capital for living expenses would quickly dilute that source of funds. Social security, burial insurance, and other sources of income, of course, provide significant supplements. Much criticism of social security as a retirement payment plan overlooks its importance as a life insurance supplement to surviving children and as a source of burial funds.

Although recent legislation reduces discrimination against women in obtaining credit, widows without recent work experience routinely learn that they do not inherit their husband's credit rating. If the women are elderly, the task is even more difficult. Minors, of course, are in still more tenuous circumstances.

Legal problems are even less likely to be anticipated in advance. Thus, in our Los Angeles survey, only slightly over one-fourth of the respondents had arranged for someone to handle their affairs. In many instances, there is the implicit assumption that a close family member will take care of the children or that other kin will provide for the widow (or, occasionally, the widower) regarding finances and legal responsibility. There is little, if any, documentation as to how often these assumptions work out well. Thomas Shaffer's helpful book (1970) does not offer an optimistic outlook.

The recent trend toward viewing death and dying more openly seems to have done little to enhance concern for the financial plight of survivors, at least not to the extent of encouraging more advanced planning for the economic and legal considerations that will weigh so heavily when dying and death do occur.

Sociological and Psychological Factors

Long before the dying process begins, the effects of eventual death influence relationships among family members. For some people, the taboo on death is so strong that they dare not refer to the possibility that someone else in the family, most especially the person to whom they are talking, will ever die. Many hold the feeling—recognized often as ridiculous even as it is maintained—that the other person cannot die so long as death is not mentioned. The discussion of death violates the taboo and might well be death-producing itself. Others base their avoidance of the topic on the feeling that such utterances would make their spouse or parent distinctly uncomfortable. And, of course, since such discussions often revolve around money, potential survivors may avoid the topic, lest they be perceived as a little too eager to guarantee themselves a portion of the estate.

In the Los Angeles study, just a little more than one-fourth of the respondents had ever talked "seriously . . . with anyone about your experiencing death someday" (Kalish and Reynolds, 1976). Of these, most described a family member as the other party in their most significant relevant conversation. No age or sex differences whatsoever were found in responses to the question. Considering the obvious import of the topic and the particular salience to the elderly, it does seem remarkable that so few of the respondents in any age, sex, or ethnic group had engaged in such a discussion.

The fact that personal death is not discussed in most families does not mean that its presence is not felt. In a content analysis of essays in which the writers projected themselves into a future state of dependency as a function of becoming old, over one-half of the women and over one-fourth of the men described themselves as being widow(er)ed (Kalish, 1971). Almost all of the participants were under 40 and most were unmarried, so this anticipation of widow(er)hood was even more unexpected, especially since the instructions spoke only of dependency and old age. It appears that young people, when forced to imagine their old age, think very much in terms of the loss of a spouse. The unanswered question is whether these same younger people would also anticipate such a loss were they not placed in such a contrived situation. My personal belief is that they would, although often in fleeting fantasies rather than concrete images or words.

In spite of the fact that a large majority of American families carry some life insurance, and of previously cited evidence that rehearsal for widowhood is quite common, the conscious thought that "I will die" or that "you whom I love, will die" often lacks the feel of authentic reality. Time seems to stretch far into the future, even though the same individual may have frequent nightmares about imminent death. At one level, death is very real; at another level, death is something that will occur only in an indefinite future.

Yet there is a magic, a mystique, attached to death that is undoubtedly stronger than that attached to any other familiar event in human existence. There is some evidence, albeit inconsistent, that certain ages are magic ages for given individuals. For example, a girl's mother dies when she is 9. The girl grows up, marries, and has her own children. When the oldest child becomes 9, i.e., recreates the circumstances under which the mother's death occurred, the present mother is more likely to display symptoms of serious emotional disturbance (Hilgard, 1953).

Can parents do anything that will enable their children to plan for and anticipate death with less fear, avoidance, and anxiety? Undoubtedly, they can, although Becker argues persuasively that " . . . the fear of death is natural and is present in everyone, that it is the basic fear that influences all others, a fear from which no one is immune, no matter how disguised it may be" (1973, p. 15). For Becker, young children direct their anger toward their parents, and this anger includes death wishes. The same magical power that causes food to be brought to them when they cry and produces a warm blanket when they demand it is perceived as bringing the possibility of magic-produced death to their parents when their anger is intense enough. Therefore, a comparable and reciprocal anger from the parents might well bring death to them, although the meaning of death is certainly unclear at early ages and the entire situation is repressed as children mature.

Perhaps the fear of death is an inevitable component of the human condition; perhaps its inevitability arises out of child-parent relationships; perhaps this fear can only be understood completely in terms of a social learning model. Whatever the case, little doubt exists that early learning in the family setting is a variable that can be modified. To some extent children develop their feelings regarding death from what they hear in their homes, from the tone of voice, the sentence broken off in the middle, the willingness to use the word *death* instead of euphemisms, attendance at a funeral. Children obviously pick up and respond to parental body language, decision making, overt and covert behavior. These parental behaviors can be modified, with the presumed result that the child's feelings, attitudes, and behavior will be altered in some rough accordance.

Death anxiety can obviously be communicated to children either directly by the parents or indirectly through the same environment affecting them both (i.e., a family in constant conflict might generate a high level of all kinds of anxieties due to a high level of tension, rather than communicating death anxiety directly to the children). What we do not know is whether such environments—or any environment—can be altered so that the subsequent fear of death dips to or near to a zero point, or whether there is an irreducible minimum, varying from person to person, beyond which the terror of death simply cannot be levelled, regardless of a warm and accepting home setting and no direct communication of death fear.

THE DYING PROCESS

Economic and Legal Factors

The financial costs of dying are horrendous. Most obvious are medical expenses: hospitalization, expensive drugs, extra nursing care, home care. We can also make a determination as to the future work-productivity potential of the individual who is dying and consider this as a financial loss. Then there is the emotional drain on the family that takes its toll in work that is missed or poorly done, in the disruption of work and family schedules of geographically scattered relatives who make the pilgrimage to the bedside or of those relatives who are close by and do the same. And there are other hidden and not-so-hidden financial costs.

Economics, law, and the family are involved with dying in another fashion. The cost of maintaining a dying person for an extended period can be overwhelmingly great. Although insurance and Medicare initially cover most costs, these may run out, leaving the individual or his or her family to provide the supplementary funds. A time sometimes comes when the health-care system can continue the existence of an individual indefinitely without meaningful cognitive powers. At present, this involves few enough people that the economics of the health-care system is not seriously affected, but the individual family unit can be utterly destroyed economically. Yet, in order to keep the family from pauperism, the physician may need to risk civil liability and even the chance of criminal liability (Manning, 1970) by terminating the care that keeps the patient existing.

The "living will" is becoming popular among persons who wish to make decisions concerning the conditions under which they want their lives terminated before they are too ill or too disoriented to partake in the decision making. The living will is legally binding only in California at present, but other states may soon follow suit. This document describes to health caretakers and family members the wishes of the ill, presumably terminally ill, person. But the wishes of the family may not coincide or, more likely, family members may disagree as to the best course of action.

A brother feels guilty over his real or exaggerated slights of the dying person and insists that his or her life be maintained, regardless of financial or personal drain; a daughter wants to try a painful, expensive, and high-risk operation she read about in a popular magazine; the eldest son, aware that his parents' funds are rapidly being depleted, and not eager to use his own, is easily reconciled with the stipulations of the living will.

How do people feel about the living will? Although our Los Angeles survey did not specifically ask about that document, it posed the question "Do you feel people should be allowed to die if they want to?" Nearly half of the respondents were in favor, with half of those giving as their primary rationale the fact that the person was expected to die anyway (Kalish and Reynolds, 1976). Half of those responding negatively did so because they felt only God has the right to take a life. The potential for a family schism over this issue is substantial, and there are psychological implications as well as financial and legal ones involved.

Psychological and Social Factors: Relationships with the Dying

Parsons and Lidz describe what they term *instrumental activism* as representing the general orientation of Western religions: "dedication to activity that can be expected on rational grounds to maximize human control over the *conditional* elements of the life situation" (1967). David Gutmann (1972) points out that young people utilize active mastery for coping with the world, while the elderly depend on magical mastery. Becker (1973) returns again and again to the theme of fear of death, relating it to loss of control, loss of power, awareness of one's vulnerability to death. And I would speculate that this increased awareness of our vulnerability to death has been the major cause of recent concern with death and dying. For many reasons, we have implicitly assumed that our science, technologies, and social activism would ameliorate our personal, social, and political problems. Instead, this very scientific bent has created problems of its own that are potentially more destructive than the difficulties it has cured. Therefore, we can no longer help being aware of the meaning of death, since we no longer believe in our own invulnerability.

We have simultaneously become more willing and more able to relate to dying people. No longer must we defend our own denial of death nor must we pretend to defend the denial of close family members by insisting that *he* or *she* (never *me*, always the other person) is better off not knowing of his or her terminal prognosis or upsetting herself or himself by discussing the condition with others. Individuals are increasingly perceived as competent, as being able to take responsibility for themselves and their problems, and as having the moral right to be aware of their condition even if it is emotionally upsetting. Further, there is the underlying assumption that most people are capable of dealing with their own difficulties when equipped with awareness and related to honestly, rather than being encumbered by uncertainty and related to with protective dishonesty.

Many tales of woe have chronicled the lack of open communication between dying persons and their family members. Glaser and Straus (1965) have made a strong case for the efficacy, for most individuals, of the open awareness context in which both the terminally ill person and members of the family know of the medical prognosis and can discuss its significance with each other. This stands in contrast to the mutual pretense context, in which both parties know of the impending death, but neither is certain of the extent of the knowledge of the other, and no relevant communication is possible. Share (1972) outlines the pros and cons of an open awareness context with children and concludes that the weight of professional opinion (as defined by those who write about the dying) and the weight of evidence (as defined by Share) are favorable to the open awareness situation. This situation has been widely discussed in academic journals and popular publications, and I will not pursue it here, except to point out its significance for family relationships.

Augustine and Kalish (1975) carry the matter a step further by hypothesizing that two of the three most important conditions that must be available for an "appropriate death" (i.e., for a person to die as much as possible the way he or she wants to—see Weisman, 1972) are open communication and warm personal relationships. They further point out that it is virtually impossible to have a warm personal relationship with a dying individual without being able to relate to that person in terms of his or her dying. I have referred to this as the "horse on the dining room table" syndrome. We are having a nice dinner together, while a horse sits in the middle of the dining room table; we all talk as if the horse weren't there, since for the host to mention the horse might upset the guests, while for the guests to refer to the horse would be embarrassing to the host. The horse, while ignored in conversation, is obviously constantly in the forefront of everyone's mind.

Returning to the concept of instrumental activism: our notions of the limitless potential of our culture's scientific, technological, and social activism run into serious conflict with the awareness that we will die. This affects not only the health caretakers but the individual and family members, who often feel that there is something "we should be able to *do!*" Up until recently, the answer was in terms of more technology. Now, increasingly cognizant of the limitations of technology, there appears to be a return to recognizing the importance of human relationships, and very likely the most significant of these are relationships with close family members.

That these family members do indeed attend to the dying person has been shown in a large and well-designed British study (Cartwright, Hockey, and Anderson, 1973) of 785 deaths in 12 areas. Each terminal person (according to extensive investigations subsequent to the death) had been helped by an average of three friends and relatives. For married persons, most of these helpers were members of the nuclear family (spouses and children); for those previously but no longer married, the proportion drops somewhat, but help received from a child-in-law rises substantially; help for single persons is roughly evenly drawn from relatives and from others; and the help from relatives is roughly evenly split between siblings and other relatives. The women relatives were most often responsible: "Wives and husbands generally bore the brunt of caring for the married, daughters for the widowed, sisters and other relatives for the single." And, since most wives outlived their husbands, women were the primary caretakers of the married. All considered, the wife was the most frequent helper and was also most likely to bear the major responsibility. When the primary caretaker was either a spouse or a sibling, the statistical probability was 50:50 that that caretaker was over age 65.

The extent to which this holds true in the United States and Canada is not known. Differences in income levels, geographical proximity, medical care systems, and value systems require that such generalization be made only cautiously. My own personal assumption is that the findings would not be much different if carried out in comparable communities in the United States or in Canada, but that hypothesis needs empirical testing.

The role of the primary caretaker of the dying person has received little attention. In some families, one individual assumes—or has thrust upon her or him—the major responsibility for care. According to the British study, the average period of time for this task was 5 months (Cartwright et al., 1973). However, the duration of the task is highly variable. Not infrequently, the primary caretaker becomes physically and psychologically exhausted during this period. Other family members are often relieved that the caretaking is being handled, and they may offer to help out either personally or financially to provide the primary caretaker with respite. There are forms of compensation for the job, nonetheless. The primary caretaker controls the information, the physical space, and the emotional contacts with the dying person. He or she (usually the latter) can decide who visits and when, who is privy to what knowledge, and what messages are carried. The primary caretaker may also anticipate some financial reward (and can become bitter if it is not forthcoming), although this is probably rarely a major motive; he or she will also expect to receive proper recognition from other family members of the important task being conducted (and again may become bitter if it is not forthcoming). After the death, this person may find adjustment the most difficult in terms of reëstablishing social activities, work career, or organizational involvement, but will probably have the least guilt and the fewest feelings of having unfinished business of anyone in the family.

Psychological and Social Factors: The Course of Dying

The effects of the dying process on family members vary as a function of innumerable factors: the nature of the terminal condition, personality of all involved persons, prior history of family relationships, the importance of the dying person to each individual family member, the ability of all concerned to establish the kind of communication that is most satisfying to everyone, and the rapidity with which death occurs.

The preferred death described by many people consists of having lived a long, healthy, and rewarding life and dying suddenly and painlessly of a condition that does not mutilate the physical body. In the Los Angeles study, half again as many respondents believed that a slow death was more tragic than a sudden death, although the figures changed to 50:50 among those 60 years of age and over (Kalish and Reynolds, 1976). If the person dying a sudden and unexpected death is very old, the effects on survivors would probably not differ much from any other kind of dying. The elderly have rehearsed their own deaths and have lived through the deaths of so many others that they claim to be (and I fully believe truly are) less afraid of dying and of death. Similarly, their close family members have probably anticipated their dying for some time and are relatively prepared for it. Older people, as I described earlier, are also more likely to have planned for their dying and their death.

When the nonelderly individual dies from sudden, unexpected causes, the situation is entirely altered. Both the practical and the psychological effects on the family are much greater. He or she is much less likely to have made plans for survivors, so that financial and legal matters are often in a state of confusion. More important psychologically, the survivors have had no time to deal with the death, no time to process and incorporate what is happening, no time for reminiscing, and no opportunity to work out unfinished business. (To switch abruptly from the academic back to the personal: The last time I saw my aunt, about 6 weeks before her death, I told her that I loved her, and she nodded and answered that she knew. It was very important to me that I said that, although she had no basis to doubt it. It was an appropriate act to close a 45-year relationship.)

I would assume that denial is greater for the survivors when the death is sudden and unexpected. "No, he couldn't be dead! Why, I just spoke to him 3 days ago and he was in perfect health!" Pine (1972) describes the way that close family members often recreate among themselves the events that led up to a death in an attempt to provide the dying with a social context, and probably also in an effort to "make sense" of the death. A sudden, unexpected death, standing by itself, is so jarring that people need to put it into historical and social perspective. Recall the day that President Kennedy was killed: Television and radio played and replayed and replayed everything that had happened, adding each new scrap of information as it came in, and then replayed it all again. And people throughout the country did the same thing for themselves.

Blauner (1968) carries the matter a step further, by suggesting that the virtually universal belief in ghosts in preindustrial societies came about because of the unfinished business between the quick and the dead. Family relationships with those who are dead, however, are not limited to the kind of ghosts that existed in preindustrial societies. The dead often reappear, either as seen or heard or felt, to loved ones, although the experience is often described in such terms as, "I saw him sitting in his favorite chair just as he always did after supper, although I know he wasn't really there" (Kalish and Reynolds, 1973; Parkes, 1972).

Further, the memory of the dead is often brought into family discussions, perhaps to prove a point or perhaps for the purpose of sharing. And the wishes of the dead are often honored. Nearly 80 percent of the Los Angeles interviewees responded in the affirmative to the question "Would you carry out your husband's/wife's last wishes even if they seemed to be senseless and caused some inconvenience?" (Kalish and Reynolds, 1976).

The impact of death on society, as Blauner (1968) points out, is closely related to how frequently it "strikes those who are most relevant for the functional activities and the moral outlook of the social order." This is similarly true for families. When death removes an individual whose family roles are still very important, her or his death is more socially disruptive than the loss of a less socially relevant person. The parent of young children or of teenage children normally performs a more important within-family role than the parent of middle-aged children or children themselves.

The Effects of Broken Attachments

Psychological disruption, as distinguished from social disruption, arises when the dying process severs emotional attachments between the terminally ill person and close family members. Common kinds of family responses have been described elsewhere (e.g., Parkes, 1972; Ross, 1969; Weisman, 1972). Among those most frequently observed is the cycle of anger and guilt. Family members feel anger toward the dying person for abandoning them, for the demands that her or his dying makes upon their emotional resources and their time and money and energies, and for other circumstances. Often the anger is repressed, since they are intellectually aware that the dying person's plight is hardly of her or his own choosing. Further, however they might justify to themselves that dying is "his or her own fault," they realize that death for most people is a severe penalty and that the losses suffered by the dying are in many ways much greater than their own losses. They may feel guilty because of their anger, and this guilt serves to intensify their anger which, in turn, intensifies their guilt.

The anticipated losses that face the family of the dying person are very real. Their emotional investment in the individual's presence, the satisfactions and warmth that they have received through their attachment to her or him, are soon to be ended. In order to cope with coming death, many close family members go through anticipatory bereavement, a kind of psychological rehearsal for the death that will come shortly. In this fashion, they work through a part of the distress of loss and are presumably better able to handle the death when it actually occurs.

The intensity of the sense of loss is largely a function of the intensity of the emotional attachments that have been built up over the years. Infants have had less opportunity to develop these attachments, and for the elderly, a process of emotional detachment has often been initiated. These two age groups also have fewer instrumental roles with those who will continue to live. Ross (1969) refers to the most appropriate final stage for the dying person as acceptance of his or her death, the result of disengaging from those in his or her milieu. In a very real sense, the individual's family members may well have withdrawn much of their affective involvement by the time of actual death, and the concept of acceptance might also be applied to them. At the same time, the need of the dying for warm, intimate human relationships precludes extensive detachment from being appropriately supportive. In some fashion that I must admit to not fully comprehending, an appropriate death must occur in a context in which good human relationships continue to the time of death, while these relationships simultaneously develop a kind of readiness to become detached that enables them to avoid being painfully destructive to the survivors. Anticipatory bereavement that extends over a long period may eventuate in a feeling of impatience, a feeling that the actual death seems unduly postponed and the dying process long drawn out.

Recent awareness of the importance of counseling both the dying and the family members has begun to attract a variety of professional groups to this task. In the San Francisco Bay area, a telephone service has been established that not only responds to questions of the dying and their family members for information but leads these persons to appropriate counselors. In San Diego, one group of funeral directors routinely offers the bereaved the services of mental health professionals who are attuned to their problems. Numerous other programs of a similar nature are now being developed elsewhere.

CONCLUDING COMMENTS

The effects of dying on the family are practical and personal, legal and economic, psychological and social, positive and negative, growth-producing and personally destructive, intense and modest, and present and future. They are rarely, if ever, absent, although physical and psychological distance can minimize them, and they diminish in time.

My aunt's death has affected my life only slightly. Neither my financial nor my legal status has changed at all; other than the cost and the effort of flying to Tucson, my day-to-day existence has not been altered. Although we were in fairly regular contact, physical distance prevented the development of a network of associations, so the loss did not sever an intimate relationship. There was no unfinished business, and I carry no guilt about my failures in the relationship since as nearly as I can discern, it was a successful and mutually rewarding relationship. She was old, her health had been failing for some months, and her death was expected.

However, since her death, I have thought about what will happen when I will need to face the death of someone who is physically closer, whose life is constantly intertwined with mine, with whom I do have unfinished business. The personal encounter with such a death, I know from my own experience, is a much different matter.

REFERENCES

Augustine, M. J., and Kalish, R. A. Religion, transcendence, and appropriate death. *Journal of Transpersonal Psychology,* 1975, **7**, 1–13.

Becker, E. *The denial of death.* New York: Free Press, 1973.

Blauner, R. Death and social structure. In B. Neugarten (Ed.), *Middle age and aging.* Chicago: University of Chicago Press, 1968. Pp. 531–540.

Cartwright, A., Hockey, L., and Anderson, J. L. *Life before death.* London: Routledge, 1973.

Diggory, J. C., and Rothman, D. Z. Values destroyed by death. *Journal of Abnormal and Social Psychology,* 1961, **30**, 11–17.

Geer, J. H. The development of a scale to measure fear. *Behavior Research and Therapy,* 1965, **3**, 45–53.

Glaser, B. G., and Strauss, A. L. *Awareness of dying.* Chicago: Aldine, 1965.

Gutmann, D. The premature gerontocracy: Themes of aging and death in youth culture. *Social Research,* 1972, **39,** 426–448.

Hilgard, J. F. Anniversary reactions in parents precipitated by children. *Psychiatry,* 1953, **16,** 73–80.

Institute of Life Insurance. *Life insurance fact book.* New York: Institute of Life Insurance, 1972.

Kalish, R. A. The effects of death upon the family. In L. Pearson (Ed.), *Death and dying.* Cleveland: Case Western Reserve University Press, 1969. Pp. 79–107.

Kalish, R. A. Sex and marital role differences in anticipation of age-produced dependency. *Journal of Genetic Psychology,* 1971, **119,** 53–62.

Kalish, R. A., and Reynolds, D. K. Phenomenological reality and post-death contact. *Journal for the Scientific Study of Religion,* 1973, **12,** 209–221.

Kalish, R. A. Death and dying in a social context. In R. Binstock and E. Shanas (Eds.), *Handbook of aging and the social sciences.* New York: Van Nostrand Reinhold, 1976.

Kalish, R. A., and Reynolds, D. K. *Death and ethnicity: A psychocultural investigation.* Los Angeles: University of Southern California Press, 1976.

Manning, B. Legal and policy issues in the allocation of death. In O. G. Brim, Jr., H. E. Freeman, S. Levine, and N. A. Scotch (Eds.), *The dying patient.* New York: Russell Sage, 1970. Pp. 253–274.

Moore, J. The death culture of Mexico and Mexican Americans. *Omega,* 1970, **1,** 271–291.

Parkes, C. M. *Bereavement.* New York: International Universities Press, 1972.

Parsons, T., and Lidz, V. Death in American society. In E. Shneidman (Ed.), *Essays in self-destruction.* New York: Science House, 1967. Pp. 133–170.

Pine, V. R. Death, dying, and social behavior. In B. Schoenberg, A. C. Carr, A. H. Kutscher, D. Peretz, and I. K. Goldberg (Eds.), *Anticipatory grief.* New York: Columbia University Press, 1972. Pp. 31–47.

Rahe, R. H., McKean, J. D., and Arthur, R. J. A longitudinal study of life-change and illness patterns. *Journal of Psychosomatic Research,* 1967, **10,** 355–366.

Ross, E. K. *On death and dying.* New York: Macmillan, 1969.

Shaffer, T. L. *Death, property, and lawyers.* New York: Dunellen, 1970.

Share, L. Family communication in the crisis of a child's fatal illness. *Omega,* 1972, **3,** 187–201.

Weisman, A. D. *On dying and denying.* New York: Behavioral Publications, 1972.

13

IMMEDIATE POST-DEATH ACTIVITIES IN THE UNITED STATES

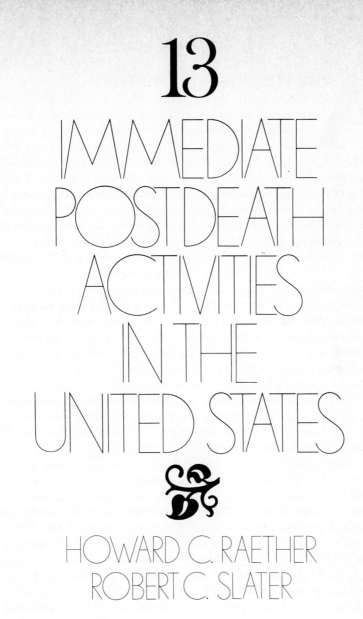

HOWARD C. RAETHER
ROBERT C. SLATER

THE FUNERAL—ITS HISTORY

American culture has inherent within it the long-established practice of the burial of its dead with attendant ceremonies. Our culture, however, did not invent the practice of burial of the dead, nor are the funeral rites and rituals that accompany it of American origin. Any sophisticated evaluation of immediate postdeath activities in the United States must begin with a tracing of the history of the practice of burial of the dead. It has been said by sociologists, anthropologists, and historians alike that humanity is an animal that buries its dead with dignity. They go on to exemplify from many cultures the practices and procedures to support this thesis. It is not our intention to give an in-depth history of funerary practices throughout the centuries. However, it becomes necessary to examine the past in order to more adequately evaluate the present and project the future.

The source that one would choose to document early funeral and burial practices will determine the date of the beginning of these practices.

If one accepts the Bible as authoritative, in the fiftieth chapter of the first book of the Bible—Genesis—there is evidence that the dead were prepared for burial. In the last verse of this chapter, the Oxford Text of the New English Bible uses both the words *embalm* and *coffin.*

If one chooses to use recorded history as the authority, one would turn to *The Persian Wars* by Herodotus (c. 484–424 B. C.) and read within his writings an extensive commentary about the preparations of the dead, particularly for anatomical study.

If one chooses rather to delve deeply into anthropology, one will probably turn to the Egyptian culture, which predates both of these references, and seek out the documentation of the Egyptian practice of mummification of the dead. It is interesting to note that if one uses the Egyptian source as a reference, the functionary was called a priest-doctor, implying that burial of the dead took on both a religious as well as a sanitary or health aspect.

As we progress in a brief historical overview, it is revealed that in the early centuries after the death of Christ much of the preparation and care of dead bodies that was a part of the funerary practices was performed by anatomists, doctors, or paramedical practitioners. There was an intense interest in the temporary preservation of the body in order to study further its functions and its relationship to the overall physical well-being of humanity.

In the middle of the seventeenth century, with the advance of anatomical and physiological study, particularly that pertaining to the circulatory systems of the human body, the practice of temporarily preserving the dead became much more prominent. In the devastating bubonic plague that attacked continental Europe, we find evidence that preparation and care of the dead was practiced in order to curtail the spread of the plague from the dead bodies.

In the nineteenth century (c. 1800–1850), some of the sophisticated practices used to preserve the dead body were brought to the North American continent. With the advent of the Civil War and the movement of men away from their families and homes, funerary practices which are still used in this decade were developed. A primary motivation for their development was that the bodies of the fallen dead of the Civil War might be returned to their homes for funeralization and burial.

In the late nineteenth century and early twentieth century, technology advanced to the present "state of the art" of caring for the dead, while serving the living and giving dignity to humanity.

This is a brief overview of the development of funeralization that has accompanied humanity's concern at the time of separation of the dead from the living.

It is important to realize that from these actual processes involved in the preservation of the dead a functionary emerged who was concerned not only with the preservation of the dead body but also with funeralization for the dead and the needs of those who survived.

Sociologists indicate that the funeral functionary in early history was granted the privilege of the "laying on of hands" that was extended to the doctor, the religious functionary, and the artist. In these instances the human body was exposed to the care and keeping as well as ministrations of such functionaries. It is interesting to note that funeral practitioners have always enjoyed the privilege of taking unto themselves the care and shelter of the remains of the human dead during the funeral process. This privilege has been sanctioned and approved by the community in which the funeral practitioner serves and the nation that is made up of such communities.

As we examine funeralization today, we have every reason to believe that it has reached an optimum form in that it permits the survivors of the deceased to work through their grief through a socially approved pattern of behavior. In many instances this behavior is a dramatization or acting out of the deep and intense feelings that survivors and mourners possess. From the standpoint of psychological and psychiatric evaluation, the very process becomes therapeutic. Much of the literature in the past decade relative to the subject of dying, death, grief, and bereavement has pointed out the psychological impact of grief, and the need to work toward its resolution.

The emphasis on immediate and sometimes anniversary rituals has shifted from those with a preoccupation with death to those motivated by a genuine concern for life and the living, for safeguarding the physical as well as the emotional and mental health of the survivors.

This is one of the reasons for acceptance by American culture of the role of the funeral service practitioner, including the providing of staff, facilities, equipment, and merchandise to meet needs, desires, and often demands following a death. There are few who personally care for their own dead, whether the postdeath activity is a funeral, a memorial service without the presence of the body, or a direct disposition as soon after death as possible. Today, most deaths are followed by a funeral period with a funeral-service licensee retained to coordinate all of the details associated therewith.

The modern funeral home has been established as an appropriate place for making arrangements for the funeral—for the "in-state" period during which a visitation, wake, or shiva is conducted—and in which funeral rites may be performed in whole or in part. The modern funeral home is designed and equipped to relieve the burden of the sorrow of death in comfortable and convenient surroundings.

Responses to Death

The response to death in contemporary America is important. Furthermore, many responses and their aftermath are predicated on new insights into dying, death, and bereavement.

For the great majority, the pattern of response to death is as follows:

1. Shock, because of the severing of attachments, personal and community, accompanied by a sense of frustration and loss
2. A religious service, if the deceased and/or his or her survivor had or have a religious belief, with the clergyman as an officiant
3. A humanist or secular service, if the deceased and/or his or her survivors find a religious service dysfunctional
4. Caretaking on the part of the funeral service licensee to whom the body of the dead person is entrusted, and also care giving in meeting certain of the needs of the mourners

Modifications and/or intensifications of these responses exist based on:

1. The ethnicity of the group to which one belongs.
2. The attitude toward dying which favors "death with dignity," i.e., favors the release of supportive measures when the person is being kept alive but is not really living, or favors *euthanasia* as the overt act of "mercy" killing.
3. The mobility of population and community attachments, which results in fewer people directly affected or highly involved.
4. The segregation of the aged and concomitant "anticipatory grief"—out of sight, out of mind; out of mind, out of heart.

5. Where death occurs. About 70 percent of all deaths occur in medical institutions, with the percentage in excess of 90 percent in some metropolitan areas.

6. The impact of youth, many of whom are concerned with meeting human fulfillment of wants and needs.

7. The Uniform Anatomical Gift Act existing in some form in every state, which gives a person the right to determine what should be done with his or her body following death.

THE FUNERAL—ITS FACETS

It is difficult to establish an all-inclusive definition of the funeral. This is especially true when you try to determine from which discipline and perspective the definition should be established.

Dr. William M. Lamers, Jr. (1969), a West Coast psychiatrist, has developed a definition of the funeral which is widely used and quoted. He says that a funeral is an organized, purposeful, time-limited, flexible, group-centered response to death. Coming from the perspective of a psychiatrist, this becomes an adequate definition. Psychologists and pastoral counselors tend to define the funeral on the basis of the needs that a family in bereavement are experiencing. A combination of many of these definitions would indicate that a funeral becomes that experience in which a person can face the reality of what has happened, let memory become a part of the process of grieving and, in the experience, express honest feelings, accept the community support that is freely proffered, and attempt to place the death in a context of meaning acceptable to the individual experiencing the trauma of the separation.

It is the feeling of the authors that each of these definitions is important and certainly not mutually exclusive. We would add, however, that the funeral cannot be defined in a single sentence but perhaps can be defined in terms of the phases or experiences that the bereaved family goes through in their process of bereavement. We would suggest that there are five such phases.

Removal

The first would be removal or the separation of the dead from the living. In today's practice of health-care delivery, it is not too infrequent to find this phase of the funeral process missing. With a high percentage of deaths occurring in hospitals, extended care facilities, and senior citizen centers, members of the immediate family may not be present at the time the actual death occurs. This is in direct contrast to the situation of 3 or more decades ago when the family was a multigenerational unit, and all of life's great experiences—namely, birth, marriage, and death—were experienced within the context of the family home. However, there is for all people that moment of the separation of the dead from the living, whether it be an experiential moment or one which is based upon the last contact with the deceased while the person was still alive. Today's funeral practice supports the age-old custom of removing the dead from the living for a period of preparation and arrangement.

The Visitation Period

The second phase of the funeral which becomes a part of its definition is what is commonly referred to as the visitation period. This may be simply a period of time for social intercourse, or it may also take on a religious function. Again this practice today is most commonly done in the funeral home. Exceptions to this would be those few remaining instances in which the deceased is placed in state in the family home or residence. Another variation would be one in which the in-state period would be in a church or religious edifice or, for persons of important political impact, in governmental buildings. A few others may choose to have an "open house" format prior to or after the disposition of the body. Wherever the visitation with the body present is held, its purpose is to meet the need of the reality of what has happened and to provide a climate for mourning.

It is at this point that the definitions of the sociologists and psychiatrists take on added meaning when they speak of the need of facing the reality of what has happened. Dr. Eric Lindemann, the psychiatrist who is credited with some of the current development of the symptomatology of grief, spoke of this as being the point from which each person must start to reorder and readjust his or her life following the traumatic separation caused by death (Lindemann, 1944). It is a time when the community can come to the family and with verbal and nonverbal expressions convey to them their empathy, sympathy, and support. Within the religious context of the Roman Catholic, it is now referred to as the scripture service, and for the person of Jewish faith it is a part of the practice of shiva. For all people it is that moment in the period of bereavement when in an atmosphere which permits and is conducive to honest and open expression of feelings they can take the first firm step of reordering their lives without the presence of the person who is now dead.

The length of the visitation varies depending upon ethnic, parochial, and provincial customs. In many ethnic groups, there are at least 2 nights of visitation—the first night often being designated for members of the family and the second night being designated for members of the community. Perhaps the modal practice is for one night of visitation immediately preceding the day of the funeral ceremony. In some parts of the United States, the practice of visitation is limited to a few hours before the actual ceremony, with no formal visitation occurring the day or night before the funeral. From those well qualified to evaluate the psychological value of the visitation, the majority declare that it is inherent in the process of providing a therapeutic value to funeralization (Lindemann, 1944).

The Funeral Rite

It is important to see the funeral as part of a total process. The authors see funeralization as those activities that occur from the moment of death to the final resolution of grief. The funeral rite is that specific time period when rites and rituals are invoked to meet the needs of those who mourn. Some tend to think of the funeral in America as that brief period of time, ordinarily no more than 30 to 60 minutes in duration, when an officiant, reader, or leader will conduct a ceremony that will declare that a death has occurred but, equally important, will give testimony to the life that has been lived. Regardless of how people conceive of a funeral, we would look at it from two perspectives and, finally, from the viewpoint of alternates to the funeral.

Approximately 75 percent of the funeral has a religious connotation. This means that there will be a period of worship during which a formalized liturgy or a less structured order of worship will be conducted by a religious officiant. The music, the readings, and the prayers used will be those that are considered "traditional" at the time of the funeral. However, the religious service may also take on a context that is now being referred to as "contemporary": the formalized, structured, religious form of worship will give way to a less structured content and involve a great deal of participation by those in attendance in terms of singing, the use of litanies especially prepared for the occasion, the confession of creeds and statements of belief, as well as corporate and responsive prayers. The music will become more contemporary in lieu of some of the older hymns of faith that may be particularly indigenous to whatever religious discipline is being followed for the funeral. Both of these services are religious in context, rely on the concepts of humanity and creator, finite life and infinite life, and will center on comfort and consolation on the basis of resurrection and hope of an afterlife.

In contrast to the religious service, an alternate order of service is being referred to as the humanist or secular funeral. In this instance the readings, music, and verbalization will be devoid of religious content. The leader or officiant will usually be a close friend of the family chosen for her or his knowledge of the family and her or his ability to speak in public. Such persons may be teachers, lawyers, judges, political officials, or in some instances even the funeral director that has been called to serve the family. This service takes on meaning and significance for the person for whom religion is dysfunctional. Therefore, while a clergyman may offici- ate, this is usually not the case.

It is interesting to note that it is not infrequent that a family will have two services for the deceased from the standpoint of the actual formal funeral service. One will be of religious content and one will be humanistic in form, thus meeting the needs of the various members of the family, which may not be compatible.

Even these alternates to the funeral find within them a context or facet of what most regard as funeralization. Some persons may request a direct disposition service. By definition, this usually involves removal of the body from the place of death, no embalming, and cremation or burial without any formal rites or ceremony. There is also the securing and filing of necessary forms and permits. In some instances, particularly where cre- mation is practiced, there may be a disposition of the ashes by scattering them in, on, or above a specifically requested location. For some persons this may take on the aspect of a funeral.

Another alternate to the funeral is that of body donation. There are less than 7000 body donations annually. Most medical and teaching insti- tutions that become the prospective donee of a dead human body will grant permission for a funeral with the body prior to its delivery to the institution. Families should be counseled as to the final disposition of the residue of the body. Many who are involved in a body donation request that the remains of the body be returned to them for some form of disposi- tion following utilization of the body by the donee institution. This may be the residue of the body or the cremated remains of the residue.

Another form of service that is an alternate to the funeral that was referred to earlier is that of the memorial service. Postdeath services with- out the body present, which is ordinarily the acceptable definition of a memorial service, have existed for many years. Most times in the past the body was absent because there was no body available inasmuch as it was not recovered following death. However, more recently, memorial services without the body present are being held even though the body is available. Some will choose this type of service because they feel it is more spiritual since emphasis is not on the body, and this in turn makes the service more Christian and less pagan. Others will indicate that it makes the service less emotional. Still others will choose it because the focus is on life, or it is more convenient or economical. While the memorial service—that is, a funeral without the body present—may meet the needs of some individu- als, it should be decided on carefully and not based on avoidance of the reality of what has happened or on the fact that it is more convenient. Recognizing the reality of the death is important and is the beginning of the resolution of grief. Convenience is not a valid reason for taking any action that involves deep personal, emotional reaction.

It is seen then that the funeral, as a specific aspect of the broader act of funeralization, exists today in our culture in many types and forms. It is flexible and can be adapted to meet the needs of each and every individual. In this respect, it is important to choose a funeral that will meet the significant needs of the bereaved rather than those which address themselves to superficial wants or desires.

The Procession

As we look at the facet of the funeral process known as the procession, we find that throughout recorded time humanity has made special acknowledgment of the movement from the place of death and/or the place of the final service to the place of final disposition. Some of the great works of art depict humanity's "last journey" as a part of the burial rite. Psychologically, the procession adds to the impact of the movement which occurs as a person moves from the place of death to taking those firm steps of resolution and living a life without the presence of the deceased. Few, if any, cultures have no counterpart to the procession. The only instance of this appears to be when the dead are left at the place where they died and the living move away, leaving the last place of abode as the place of final disposition of the dead. Even here we have the procession away from the place of death without the deceased.

Recent criticism has been leveled at the funeral procession in a mobile, modern, highly mechanized society such as our culture enjoys. However, such criticism is unrealistic, if not illogical, in a culture that still finds time and place for all of the other parades associated with life's great events—patriotic, religious, and ethnic celebrations, homecomings, athletic events and the like. Therefore, this facet of the funeral is still one of great significance for those most directly involved. As is indicated, the procession serves a dual purpose. Moving *to* the place of final disposition helps one to accept the finality of what has occurred, and moving *from* the place of final disposition helps one get back into the normal mainstream of life.

The Committal

The final phase of the funeral process that is most common is the act of committing the body to its place of final disposition. Psychologists have agreed that this simple act, like none of the others, emphasizes and under-girds the finality of what is experienced. For the religious person, it is a return to the creator from which the substance of the body has come. For the humanist, it is evidence of the cyclical nature of life that begins and ends and is recycled into another beginning. It is also of psychological import because it is that milestone from which one turns to begin a new life without the presence of the person who was deeply loved and whose life had been an intimate part of the lives of those who survived. Pastoral counselor-psychologist Paul Irion (1966) has made the statement that the committal that does not commit in essence is not a committal at all. Therefore, the committal should be at the place of final disposition and should involve an act of committal.

The authors feel that these five phases of the funeral process give the reader an overview of the facets of the funeral as it is experienced in our American culture.

THE FUNERAL—PROS AND CONS

As with any practice which evokes strong emotions, people develop positive and negative attitudes. This is a natural process. What is important is that a person expose his or her attitudes to careful evaluation and rational thinking. We have indicated in this section some of the areas where there are deviations or alternates to the funeral. We would like now to examine these in more detail and also to present some facets of funeral practice that tend to polarize people's attitudes.

Direct Disposition

The definition of this postdeath activity given previously is self-explanatory. Not much more can be said than that there are deaths which are followed by direct disposition. Most of the time this is by cremation. The disposition of the cremated remains is determined by the family. The cremated remains can be placed in a receptacle for the next of kin to keep or which they may bury or place in a columbarium. Or, the next of kin, where not prohibited by law, can scatter the ashes or engage someone else, which is most often the case, to scatter the ashes for them at a particular place, often at sea. This must be done within the law, both state and federal, where applicable.

Although this service is most often provided by funeral service licensees, there are some companies established solely for the direct disposition of the dead without any attendant rites or ceremonies.

The Body Present and Viewed

The primary distinction between the funeral and the memorial service and direct disposition is the presence of the body. Insofar as the presence of the body is inherent in the funeral, an examination of the reasons for the support of what most people have done and do is in order.

Those who in any way are associated with individuals immediately following a death and throughout the first days therafter hear many statements made by the mourners. The most common statement is the denial of that which has taken place. This denial is often verbalized in the expression, "I can't believe that he (or she) is dead." Naturally, feelings and expressions vary with the kind and nature of the death. Sudden death, such as that caused by a heart attack, an accident, or suicide, perhaps evokes the most emphatic, if not abnormal, expressions once the numbness leaves the survivor after being notified of the death.

Next in the order of intensity of expression are those which follow a short illness or surgery or hospitalization in which it seemed as though the individual was recovering.

Perhaps those who are least prone to openly express themselves are those who have had someone die of a lengthy illness. The authorities say that survivors of persons who have died of a lingering illness or of persons who have lived their 3 score years and 10 have gone through anticipatory grief and in the process may have done during the illness what others do following death. However, there is the pain which comes when death does occur. Also there are those members of a new group which included the deceased. To them the loss is pronounced. In fact, it may not have been anticipated because to anticipate the loss of others is to anticipate the loss of self. Even when death has brought release and relief, many times there is hostility, ambivalence, despair, and depression and often denial that the body which once was a person that loved and was loved in return is no longer alive.

When someone dies, a life on earth has ended. What remains is not that living person, but the body of a man, woman, or child. And remembrance of someone most of the time is in terms of physical being—their body.

That is why it is difficult for many survivors to disassociate themselves immediately from the lifeless body. The finite mind requires evidence that an earthly existence has ended. With the body present, opportunity is also provided for recall and reminiscence, for the sharing of experiences with others who have related to the life that was lived by the person now dead.

With the body present, the dead person can be viewed. This is perhaps of greater importance today than ever before. Most people die away from home, often in distant medical institutions. There are more deaths which follow a devastating lingering illness. There are more people whose lives end under tragic circumstances.

Several helpful purposes are served by the custom of viewing:

Realization Viewing the dead body makes those who survive more aware of the reality of sudden, accidental, or lingering death. Seeing helps us to believe. Often much time, effort, and money are expended to recover a missing body for the purpose of confirming the fact that the death has occurred.

Recall Before a long, lingering death, the face of someone loved may be lined with the effects of pain or malignancy. With accidents and violence, the entire body may be disfigured.

Proper preparation and, when necessary, restoration help to modify and remove the marks of violence or the ravages of disease. Preparation, restoration, and the use of cosmetics are not meant to make the dead look alive. They provide an acceptable image for recalling the deceased.

Viewing is therapeutic for many people regardless of age. It is especially helpful for a child. Instead of fantasizing in his or her vivid imagination, with the body present, he or she is able to comprehend the real meaning of death.

Expression In many circumstances, such as economic distress, poor health, or domestic difficulties, comfort is given to those involved. In most instances, opportunities present themselves for such expression days, weeks, and even months later.

Death is different. Time is an immediate factor. Many find it difficult to express themselves. They may talk about every subject but the reason why they are making a sympathy or condolence call. The presence of the body during the visitation or wake provides an immediate and proper climate for mourning. With the body present, it is natural to talk about the deceased.

If tears are shed, they flow less self-consciously for both survivors and those who call. If there is a religious service, the body present and viewed before the ceremony helps the sorrows of one become the sorrows of all.

A summary of this section could be the statement of a student, Jan Brugler, at the Indian Lake, Ohio, high school, responding to how she felt about death. The question came up during a course, Perspectives on Death, and was reported in a feature article in a popular magazine for young persons, *TEEN*. Her words were brief but, as the writer of the article indicates, Jan said it all when she remarked, "You must express your grief at the death of a loved one, and then you must go on. The eyes of the dead must be gently closed, and the eyes of the living must be gently opened" (McCoy, 1973, p. 66).

For most people the funeral with the body present does what this high school student wisely said must be done.

Prearrangement of Funerals

The prearranging and prefinancing of funerals is on the increase. The following suggestions should be kept in mind when prearranging and prefinancing a funeral:

1. The possible effect on survivors should be considered whether the funeral is just prearranged or prearranged and prefinanced. It is difficult for anyone to know the time, place, or circumstance of his or her death. Therefore, survivors should be able to alter instructions or recommendations which would prove difficult, ill-advised, or guilt-producing for them.

2. A realistic approach should be taken to the logic and economics of planning now what might not take place for many years.

3. Keep in mind that the selection of a funeral director or a funeral firm as well as of burial merchandise for use at a future, indeterminable time must be, of necessity, on a tentative basis.

4. Monies paid in advance of need for funeral services and merchandise, including burial vaults, are governed by law in most states. If there are no such laws in the state in which the prefinancing is made, it is recommended that the prepaid funeral agreement include the provision for a trust fund, with the person making the payment maintaining control of the account. The fund should include all monies paid in advance of need for services and merchandise, including burial vaults. The agreement should also entitle the person in control of the trust to the interest earned, with the option of applying it to the principal to offset any increased inflationary costs. Such person making the payment should retain the right to terminate the contract at any time without forfeiture of any of the funds paid or earnings accrued.

In any event, the inherent uncertainties of a prefinanced funeral agreement, even an informal one, make it highly desirable to seek expert, professional counseling.

THE FUNERAL—ITS FUTURE

Professor Paul E. Irion (1966) questioned some facets of the American funeral in his *The Funeral: Vestige or Value?* He writes:

The funeral can, however, be a means by which the attitudes of the culture toward death and mourning are reshaped. Ritual is not merely a passive reflector of cultural values; it also can participate in the structuring of these values. It is not impossible for the funeral to be restored to its basic purposes and functions and to exert a potent influence upon American thought and behavior. It can be a force in stemming the neurotic flight from reality of our time by affording the support that is necessary for the individual to confront death and loss realistically. It can undergird acceptance and defiance of death rather than the denying of death. It can resist the radical separation of death from life and deepen life's meaning by acknowledging the dramatic encounter with the reality of death [p. 59].

The *Archives of General Psychiatry* (1971) reports on the findings of a study by Eugene S. Paykel and Brigette A. Prusoff of Yale University School of Medicine and E. H. Uhlenhuth of the Chicago Pritzker School of Medicine. These psychiatrists judged the degree to which 61 life events were upsetting. The first five were (1) death of a child, (2) death of a spouse, (3) jail sentence, (4) death of a close family member (parent, sibling), and (5) unfaithful spouse.

The findings substantiate what many have emphasized for years—that for most people the death of someone loved is a traumatic event, a major life crisis. Funerals provide for the final disposition of the body of the deceased and serve the survivors in the process.

For many years those with expertise and competence based on death-related studies have maintained that dying is a process with death the terminal event. There are some who look at this differently. They maintain that death is a proces of which dying is a part.

IN CONCLUSION

Most cultures dispose of their dead with ceremony. This ceremony, no matter how primitive or how sophisticated, includes some form of funeralization in its postdeath activity. The funeral has become for most people a way of working through strong feelings and emotions. For this reason, the funeral has an inherent value and should not be seen merely as a vestige of history that can be cast off as irrelevant or dysfunctional.

The funeral as a postdeath activity finds expression in three fundamental approaches or characteristics—psychological, theological (philosophical), and sociological. A cursory examination of these characteristics will give support to the relevancy of the funeral as the first firm step toward the resolution of grief caused by the separation crisis of death.

Firstly, the literature of the past 3 decades is replete with studies of the psychology of grief, the first of which dates back as far as some of Freud's early writings on melancholia. Grief is an emotion; and as such, it will be expressed. A person chooses only its manner of expression by either openly confronting it or repressing it. As with all emotions, the acceptable procedure in working them through is to place the persons experiencing the emotion into an atmosphere of acceptability. Our culture has developed the funeral as that time and place where each person is permitted to work through his or her strong feelings of grief. Here the reality and finality of the death which has occurred can be the focus of readjustment to the loss. For all persons involved the funeral is a psychological experience, differing only in the degree to which it affects each individual.

Secondly, the funeral is based on a theological or philosophical experience. To some, these may be perceived as synonymous, but to others, they present an either/or proposition. What is relevant is that each contains within it a concept of life and death. Theologically, it will involve concepts and interpretations of birth and death as seen in the context of life and afterlife. Philosophically, it is more apt to encompass the concept of biological life and death. Important to the issue is that in either case it places the death in a context of meaning for the survivors and enables the funeral to become a meaningful postdeath activity.

Thirdly, the funeral should be viewed in its sociological context. The funeral, like all other ceremonies, is a people- (group-) centered activity. During most times of emotional stress, a person will find great support in interacting with other persons. This interaction is supportive at both verbal and nonverbal levels. Similarly, it is supportive to mourners to know that others care enough to want to share this experience with them. It is also supportive in that the presence of others who have gone through a grief experience demonstrates that the grief can be resolved and necessary adjustments made. This concept is paraphrased in a lyric from a recent musical, "People who need people are the luckiest people of all." If there was no one with whom to share one's grief, the funeral most likely would become dysfunctional.

Seen in this light—psychological, theological (philosophical), and sociological—the funeral as a postdeath activity takes on added form and function. Funeralization through the ages has served each culture well. It can continue to do so if it remains *sensitive, perceptive* and *adaptive* to the needs of people. The funeral is an organized, purposeful, time-limited, flexible, group-centered response to death. It is a meaningful and significant postdeath activity that serves the needs of grieving persons well.

REFERENCES

Habenstein, R. W., and Lamers, W. M., Sr. *Funeral customs the world over.* Milwaukee: Bulfin Printers, 1960–1961.

Irion, P. E. *The funeral: Vestige or value?* Nashville: Parthenon Press, 1966.

Lamers, W. M., Jr. Funerals are good for people—M. D.'s included. *Medical Economics,* **46** (June 23, 1969), 104–107.

Lindemann, E. Symptomatology and management of acute grief. *American Journal of Psychiatry,* 1944, **101,** 144–148.

McCoy, K. Death: Hot controversy/cold facts. *Teen,* June 1973, pp. 62–66.

Paykel, E. S., Prusoff, B. A., and Uhlenhuth, E. H. Scaling of life events. *Archives of General Psychiatry,* 1971, **25,** 340–347.

Raether, H. C., and Slater, R. C. *The Funeral, Facing Death As An Experience of Life.* Milwaukee: National Funeral Directors Association, 1974.

Slater, R. C. *Funeral Service: Meeting Needs . . . Serving People.* Milwaukee: National Funeral Directors Association, 1974.

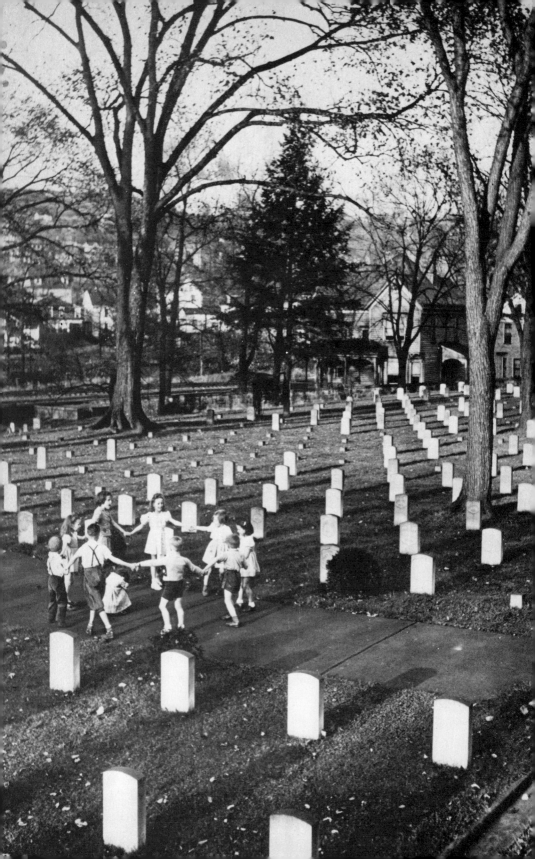

PART
FIVE

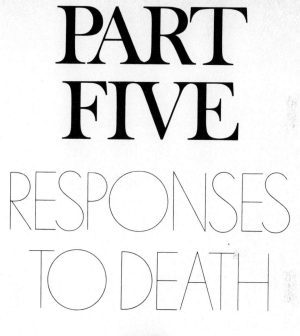

RESPONSES
TO DEATH

14

DEATH EDUCATION

DANIEL LEVITON

Until recently, death education was proscribed because of its potentially painful subject matter. Slowly but surely, however, education about death is being accepted as a legitimate need for the living. Yet we possess minimal understanding of the effects of death education on people. Such questions as "Who should do the educating?" "What are the guidelines for selecting death educators?" "Which are the target populations?" and "What should be the goals and content of courses in the area?" still require more informed answers.

REFLECTIONS ON THE HISTORY AND DEVELOPMENT OF DEATH EDUCATION

One day a bright graduate student will seek the motives which led early death educators to embark upon their venture. Some were involved in teaching about human sexuality and saw parallels in the study of death. Others became aware of the abysmal training given to physicians and nurses as they watched dying patients and their families endure needless isolation, ostracism, and suffering. Indeed, some may have been affected as their own loved ones endured a dying process. Still others, perhaps, striving for their fair share of what Robert J. Lifton calls "symbolic immortality" (1967) saw their involvement with death as an opportunity to be remembered by future generations. But whatever the personal motives, most would agree that Herman Feifel's *The Meaning of Death* (1959) was a prime mover in legitimizing the study of and teaching about death. For in that work, the message was loud and clear: the study of death and dying was a valid and necessary area for scientific inquiry, especially for the behavioral scientist. It emphasized that death was more than merely an isolated, personal event; that awareness of personal death, and knowledge of vulnerability and the constraints of time, affected not only individual behavior but social conduct as well. The book did more than help individuals reflect upon a personal cosmology and eschatology; it provided the pioneering death educator with a *subject matter* basis for teaching. Here was a convenient source which presented information and considered reflections from philosophical, artistic, theological, and, more importantly, theoretical and scientific bases.

The 1960s witnessed the first systematic attempts to introduce death education in the college setting. Any list of those who contributed to the literature and taught *formal* courses up to and including 1971 would have to include Edgar Jackson, Richard Kalish, Robert Kastenbaum, Herman Feifel, Robert Fulton, Edwin Shneidman, Alan Berman, Herbert Anderson, Betty Green and Donald Irish, Francis Green, John Black, Francis

254

Scott, James Carse, James Farmer, Jacques Choron, and Douglas White. Others like Avery Weisman, Herman Feifel, Robert J. Lifton, Kurt Eissler, Elisabeth Kubler-Ross, and Lawrence LeShan integrated their medical colleagues and students into a learning relationship with dying patients.

If Feifel's book heralded the renaissance of serious acknowledgement of the existence of death and its pervasive effects on life, it was not the first to suggest the need for death education. The honor, seemingly, goes to T. O. Elliot who wrote a chapter, "Bereavement: Inevitable But Not Insurmountable," published in 1955. At that time, Elliot wrote: "If good sex education is important, delicate and subtle, so is proper 'death education.' "

That valid sex and death education are important to healthy physical and mental development is a consistent theme sounded by proponents of death education. Penniston, in an article published in 1962, "The Importance of Death Education in Family Life," serves as an example:

> We have surrounded it [death] with taboos and we are unable to speak about it easily. The result is, just as it was with sex, that there is a good deal of misinformation which needs to be corrected especially in regard to the grief process and to understanding what the experience of bereavement is really like. As with sex, it is a subject which ought to be sensibly discussed before we become emotionally involved with it as a problem. Hence, the title of this paper [p. 15].

Wahl (1959), too, uses the analogy of sex education; moreover, he implies that death education can be therapeutic. He writes:

> Modern parents, thanks to Freud and to the generation of educators sparked by his genius, are now able, for the most part, to approach the problem of the child's sexuality in a rational and sensible manner, and as a result *there has been a steady diminution during the last fifty years of neurotic symptom formation such as conversion hysteria, whose main etiology is massive sexual repression* (my emphasis).
>
> I suggest, however, that there is a second half to the riddle of the Sphinx to which we have not addressed ourselves. I refer to the complement of 'Whence came I' viz., 'Whither go I?' or in the child's language, 'What is it to be dead?' Again, clinical experience abundantly proves that children have insatiable curiosity not only about 'where people came from' but also about 'where people go to.' In his efforts to find an answer to this conundrum, he is met today, as his questions about sexuality would have been met in the 1890's, with evasion and subterfuge [p. 26].

Was it the times, the *Zeitgeist,* which were appropriate for the emergence and high interest in taboo topics such as sex and death? I think so. As a result of an interminable war yet to end, increased technology, and the depersonalization expressed in the perceived inability to control one's own life, the old forbidden unmentionable death was cast into the sunlight for scrutiny. From the mid-1960s onward death education accelerated in the United States.

While a variety of symposia and workshops on death and dying were organized after the publication of Feifel's book, the first significant symposium on death education was held at Hamline University, St. Paul, Minnesota, in 1970. Organized by two sociologists, Betty Green and Donald Irish, that two-day conference attracted over 2000 people from all walks of life. Subsequently, the proceedings of the conference were published in 1971 and served to stimulate interest in the field. The interest in death education was further fanned by the appearance of articles by D. Leviton (1969) and R. M. Somerville (1971) devoted exclusively to the issue, and by the best selling book, *On Death and Dying,* by Kubler-Ross (1969).

In March 1966, the first newsletter on death and dying appeared, edited by two psychologists, Richard Kalish and Robert Kastenbaum. In 1970, that newsletter evolved into *Omega: An International Journal for the Psychological Study of Dying, Death, Bereavement, Suicide and Other Lethal Behaviors,* with Richard Kalish as editor and the sociologist Robert Fulton as associate editor. The title was later shortened to *Omega.*

The appearance of *Omega* was significant and vital. As a scientific journal, it not only provided expression for high quality scholarly efforts but also stimulated a sense of camaraderie among those working in the thanatological domain.

The number and types of requests for death education curriculum materials cover all grade levels from elementary school through high school and college, and such professional schools as law, medicine, nursing, and theology. Death education is a topic of interest in adult education circles and in in-service training programs for nurses, police officers, physicians,[1] and self-help groups (such as Parents Without Partners, widow-to-widow programs, and memorial societies). In truth, we do not know with any great exactitude the number of death education courses existing today. David Berg, a former teacher of death education at Northern Illinois

---

[1] At this time formal school and university death education outside the United States seems to exist only in medical education. At the International Conference for Leaders on Death and Dying, November 1974, representatives from Sweden, Canada, West Germany, and Great Britain reported no significant effort to develop death education in their public school or university sectors.

University's Laboratory School and coauthor of a teaching unit on death,[2] estimates that some 200 high schools, mainly public, use his program alone. An article in *The New York Times* on July 21, 1974, stated that there were more than 165 college level courses on death and dying. Robert Fulton, director of the Center for Death Education and Research,[3] in a personal conversation in 1974 indicated that over 1100 courses existed above high school level. In a 1975 survey, Liston found that 41 medical schools had formal training programs to help their students interact more meaningfully with terminally ill parents and their families. Similar education is also being provided in numerous nursing schools. In this context, a course for Montgomery County (Maryland) policemen was instituted in 1974 under the aegis of the Department of Health Education, University of Maryland. And so it goes and grows. But what does it mean? What can death education achieve?

CONTRIBUTIONS OF DEATH EDUCATION

When I first began teaching, my naïve assumption was that death education would resolve existing fears or anxieties concerning death, and predispositions toward suicide. All participants would look forward to accomplishing the "healthiest" death, that is, *acceptance* of death. Initial research investigations indicated that the course did indeed reduce fear of death in some of the students. Others, however, evidenced an increase in fear of death. Still others showed no change. Similar results have been reported by other death educators (Feifel and Branscomb, 1973). One possible explanation of these varying effects is the use of measuring instruments which tap different levels of awareness.

What of suicide? One would think that a course on death education would significantly reduce suicidal intent. My precourse tests indicated that 3 percent of 230 students taking a 1974 course were contemplating suicide then and there. After one semester of inspired and scholarly lectures and discussions, I found no change! "What in the hell," I asked myself, "was the course accomplishing?" The answers were there in both the objective and subjective data. Some students had changed from suicidal to nonsuicidal, or vice versa. Others held on to their precourse outlook. My expectations had simply been unrealistic, almost romantic.

Yet the course did have some significant effect. Almost unanimously

---

[2] For information, write to Perspectives on Death, P. O. Box 213, DeKalb, Illinois.

[3] Address: Center for Death Education and Research, 1167 Social Sciences Building, University of Minnesota, Minneapolis, Minn. 55455.

the students responded that the course had helped them catalyze and synthesize attitudes and thoughts concerning death in a more positive manner. Death was now seen as something necessary and less horrible than originally preceived. Many now felt confident enough to demand direct answers from physicians and other health-care givers concerning their dying and that of others, and more comfortable in interacting with a dying person. Further, discussion of the topic of death was no longer taboo. Interestingly, there was an increase in preference for an educator rather than parent to teach children about death. Additionally, almost all saw a need for death education to begin early in childhood and to continue on a developmental basis. Finally, most felt they would now be more sensitive to the needs of their children in the area.

Incoming findings tentatively suggest a set of realistic goals for death education:

1. Gently remove the taboo aspect of death language so students can read and discourse upon death rationally without becoming anxious.

2. Promote comfortable and intelligent interaction with the dying as human beings who are living until they are dead.

3. Educate children about death so they grow up with a minimum of death-related anxieties. Anxieties are too often based upon irrationality and myth rather than fact.

4. Assist the individual in developing a personal eschatology by specifying the relationship between life and death.

5. Perceive the health-care giver as a professional and human being, neither omnipotent nor omniscient, who has an obligation to give competent and humane service, attention, and information without mendacity to the dying and their families.

6. Understand the dynamics of grief and the reactions of differing age groups to the death of a "significant other."

7. Understand and be able to interact with the suicidal person.

8. Understand the role of those involved in what Kastenbaum and Aisenberg (1972) call the "death system" and the assets and liabilities of that system.

9. Educate consumers to the commercial death market.

10. Recognize that war and other holocausts are related to feelings of personal immortality and omnipotence. War might be avoided if we realize that it may be ourselves or our children who would be killed or mutilated as well as an amorphous "enemy."

11. Recognize the variations involved in aspects of death both within and between cultures. Death means different things to different people.

12. Know the false idols and mythology existing in the growing field

of thanatology, the salient heuristic questions, and the great need for research.

Obviously, specific goals will vary according to the target population. For example, physicians and nurses might focus on the goals of learning to deal intelligently and humanely with dying patients and their families, and to recognize that they themselves will need support as a result of making an emotional investment in their dying patients.

As already indicated, we find that students react in different ways to a course on death. Many feel that it is therapeutic. Some, however, find their anxieties being exacerbated by the course. One young man came in following a class to discuss his increasing fear of ceasing-to-be, of nothingness and annihilation, as the course progressed. I suggested he read the works of Ernest Becker, Peter Koestenbaum, Norman O. Brown, and Jacques Choron. Subsequently, he consented to see a thanatologically oriented psychotherapist. Unfortunately, this was of no avail. I agreed with him that he would be wise to drop the course. We must realize that the death educator can provide no *answer* concerning status after death. He or she can provide no guarantee of a heaven or a sublime afterlife, or a hell for that matter.

What the death educator can do is work toward an easy dying. We can inform about the importance of pain reduction for the dying person. Pain is a priority issue for the dying. We can teach that style of dying is individualistic. Must we suffer the dying to minister to the living's need to avoid reality? We can help the dying die an "appropriate death" to use Avery Weisman's terminology (1972). We can also help students learn that the dying do not have to go through five stages of death ending in "acceptance." One is not "unhealthy" or "abnormal" if he or she dies "denying."

A word about false, unproven idols. Elisabeth Kubler-Ross has probably done more to make the public aware of the needs of the dying than any person working in the field today. She hypothesized that the dying person goes through five psychological stages prior to death (1969). Further, she explicitly stated that the stages should be tested under more rigorous conditions. What has happened? We find not only novices but experienced death educators and thanatologists accepting the five stages as invariant, as gospel. Health-care givers find themselves being forced to think in terms of whether they were "unsuccessful" in meeting the ultimate goal, the big number 5—"acceptance" of death.

In this regard, Richard Schultz and David Aderman, reviewing research on the process of dying, found that a "stages of dying" concept was unsupported. They report that data "show the process of dying to be less rigid and even stageless. There is some consensus among all researchers that terminal patients are depressed shortly before they die, but there is no consistent evidence that other affect dimensions characterize the dying patient" (Schulz and Aderman, 1974, p. 137). It would be wise if educators and researchers simply viewed any "stages of death" scheme as simply theoretical until proven by more rigorous scientific procedures.

RESEARCH IN DEATH EDUCATION

The need for research to determine more fully the effects of death education courses is obvious. We need to know what is happening to our students, under what conditions, and for how long. Most of the research accomplished thus far in the field of death education has been essentially descriptive, although a few investigators have used sophisticated experimental design. Unfortunately, deficiencies in sample selection and size, inappropriate testing procedures, and failure to consider external and internal sources of validity mar most of the studies reported thus far (Campbell and Stanley, 1963). Additionally, replication studies need to be carried out to determine the representativeness of present findings. Nonetheless, there is strong evidence that courses in death education generally have a positive effect on participants with regard to attitudes about dying, death, and grief.

THE DEATH EDUCATOR

To the best of my knowledge, no data exist which define criteria for selecting the competent death educator. Some criteria, however, have been suggested as possible guidelines. Leviton (1971), for example, adapting recommendations for sex educators by Warren R. Johnson (1973), suggests the following:

1. The teacher must have come to terms with his or her own death feelings and be aware of their influence on his or her total personality functioning.

2. Plainly, the teacher needs to know the appropriate subject matter he or she is to teach.

3. The teacher of death education needs to be able to use the language of death easily and naturally, especially in the presence of the young.

4. He or she needs to be familiar with the sequence of psychothanatological developmental events throughout life, and to have a sympathetic understanding of common problems associated with them.

5. The teacher needs an acute awareness of the enormous social changes that are in progress and of their impact on our patterns of attitudes, practices, laws, and institutions concerning death.

Theodore Dougherty (1974) elaborated upon the above criteria and found them "having definite validity for assessing the minister as a death educator. To be an effective teacher about death, the minister would do well to take these beginning standards seriously" (p. 85).

Sex education, death education's older sister, has now developed to the point where professional organizations such as the American Association for Sex Educators and Counselors (AASEC) have formulated standards for the accreditation of sex educators (Johnson and Belzer, 1973). Undoubtedly, death educators soon will be organizing their own professional and scientific associations to disseminate information and suggest standards.[4]

CHARACTERISTICS OF THE STUDENT TAKING DEATH EDUCATION COURSES

The one commonality which can be attributed to students attending death education courses is that they are diverse. Diverse in their attitudes concerning death, knowledge about death, fears, and previous experience with death.

In this respect, the death educator must be sensitive to the suicidal student registering for his course. Indeed, in one of my recent death education courses, 8 of 230 students admitted to a previous suicide attempt; 15 responded they were contemplating suicide at the beginning of the course, 8 of whom still reported contemplating suicide at the course's end. One student, it later turned out, enrolled in every death-related course offered on campus (for example, Crisis Intervention, Death Education, and Self-Destructive Behaviors) and, after a semester interval, eventually suicided. It was as though he was working through his ambivalence over whether to live or die. After determining to suicide, it seems that he systematically set about to gather information which would ensure success, that is, he devel-

---

[4] Ars Moriendi, a Task Force of the Society for Health and Human Values, 3601 Locust Walk, Philadelphia, Pa., 19104, under the direction of Kenneth Spilman and John Fryer, held a week-long international conference for leaders in death and dying during November 1974 to discuss this issue among others. Another working group organized to deal with death education and with meeting the needs of health care givers is The Forum for Death Education and Counseling. Along with sponsoring conferences, a newsletter, and resource materials, The Forum has developed a code of ethics for death educators and counselors. Its address is P.O. Box 1226, Arlington, Virginia, 22210.

oped a highly lethal plan of action. Eventually, he shot himself. Whether the probability of suicide is different for those enrolled in other courses remains to be determined.

One can argue that students commit suicide who are not enrolled in a death education course, or that the course may very well serve to prevent the suicide of those who may be ambivalent in their desire to suicide or to live. In any case, the death educator stands the *risk of being accused* of stimulating students to suicide by the very nature of the course.

In the hope of establishing rapport with students, especially those anguishing with the idea of suicide, I try to answer their "call for help" in several ways. During the first lecture, students are informed that my data indicate that approximately 3 percent of the class are contemplating suicide at that moment. They are given my home and office phone numbers and addresses. They are requested to telephone or visit me and/or my graduate assistant at any time. If we administer a research protocol before and after the course, the question "Are you contemplating suicide now?" is included. Another method is to use one's eyes during class. Even in an auditorium of 300 or more students, a truly depressed or emotionally upset student can be identified and a conference arranged.

When asked why they enrolled in the course, about half of a 1972 class gave pragmatic responses: they were curious about the subject matter, it filled an elective need, or it fitted an available time slot. Thirty-six percent took the course to overcome personal fear of death, and 11 percent reported enrolling with the hope of overcoming their fear of the death of others. Interestingly, 11 percent reported feeling guilty over the death of another, while 10 percent reported worry over the eventual death of another.

Others enrolled to enhance their communication about death and to become better educated about death. Twenty three percent wished to learn to help others overcome their fear of death as part of their professional training (nursing, medicine, psychology, law enforcement). Only 9 percent mentioned taking the course to prepare for their own eventual death. Between 2 and 3 percent were motivated to enroll because of their experiential contact with death. Six students experienced the so-called "death-trip" while using psychedelic drugs, and reported having a "close call" with death.

Thus, the death education student comes to class representing a variety of experiences and attitudes. Two extreme cases make the point: One Vietnam veteran in combat received a telegram informing him of the death of his recently born son. On the same day his buddy had been decimated by a booby trap only a short distance away. Today, he suffers recurrent nightmares representing the symbolic or real death of children and others. His feelings of guilt and despair are heart-rending to the listener. Too many of these men have returned from a montage of wars to too little understanding of their confrontation with death (Lifton, 1967, 1973).

The other extreme is represented by a young woman who enrolled because, according to her own testimony, "I know absolutely nothing about death yet live in utter fear of it." She had never witnessed the death of grandparents, parent, friend, or pet. For her death and dying were the mysteries *par excellence,* exacerbated by their remote yet ubiquitous qualities.

To reiterate, while subjective assessments are helpful, we still need to run systematic research to determine the characteristics of students who come for death education and its impact on them.

VARIATION IN DEATH EDUCATION COURSES

Just as variation is evident among students enrolled in death education, the courses themselves show variation. On an a priori basis, sources of variation include at least six factors: (1) *target audience:* elementary, high school, college and university students, professional school personnel, special groups (handicapped children, the elderly, the terminally ill, police officers, firefighters, military personnel); (2) *target domain:* course which is "feelings"-oriented (affective), intellect-process–oriented (cognitive), or interaction-with-the-dying–oriented (activity); (3) *number of students;* (4) *endorsing discipline:* health education, psychology, literature, sociology, art; (5) *methodology:* lecture, small group discussion, role playing, use of films, interaction with the dying person, literature; and (6) *goals:* therapy, knowledge, social reform, professional preparation, global concerns (such as elimination of war and other destructive behaviors prevalent among people).

I have selected six courses to give some idea of existing variations. Obviously, some excellent courses are not listed simply due to lack of space or my unfamiliarity with them. Parenthetically, it is helpful to know that *Omega,* the journal of death and dying sponsored by Ars Moriendi, devoted one of its 1975 issues to death education (see Volume 6, Number 3).

Table 14-1 shows that specific courses have been designed for both general and specialized audiences. Most of the courses are devoted exclusively to thanatology. Exceptions are those designed for elementary school children when death is discussed during the "teachable moment" or when appropriate (Leviton and Forman, 1974). Such opportunities are commonplace as children develop throughout the life process—a process characterized by adapting to the death of plants, seasons, pets, and humans. Only one course (Barton, Flexner, Van Eys, and Scott, 1972) seemed to make a concerted effort to include "activity" as a target domain (defined

TABLE 14-1 SELECTED DEATH EDUCATION COURSES

Instructor and Location (Reference)	Audience	Domain	No. of Students	Sponsoring Discipline	Methodology	Goals
Anderson & Migliore (1972), Princeton Theological Seminary	Theologians	Affect, knowledge	80	Theology	Lecture, discussion, readings	Professional preparation
Scott (1971), University of Oregon	College students	Primarily affect	30–36	Gerontology	Role playing, films, readings, discussion, "sensitivity weekend"	Sensitive to death
Barton et al. (1972), Vanderbilt School of Medicine	Medical students	Affect, knowledge, activity	6–10	Medicine	Readings, discussion, interaction with dying person, role playing, lecture	Professional preparation
Leviton & Forman (1974), Kenmoor Elementary School, Prince Georges County, Md.	Kindergarten students	Affect, knowledge	25	Elementary education	Discussion, sharing experiences, role playing	Appropriate understanding of death & dying
Bertman (1974), Equinox Institute Brookline, Mass.	Elementary, secondary school students	Affect, knowledge	No indication	Outside agency	Discussion, readings, music, films	Appropriate understanding of death & dying
Leviton (1971) College Park, Maryland	College students	Affect, knowledge	300–400	Health education	Lecture, discussion, role playing, films	Improve human interaction and quality of civilization and life; understanding of death & dying

as "overt interaction with the dying person"). In this vein, Kubler-Ross's work (1969) exemplifies the "activity" approach of students and their teachers with the dying person. I make every effort to have a dying person speak to my smaller graduate level classes. However, I do feel some hesitancy in having such an individual speak to my large class unless he or she is extremely motivated to do so. Perhaps I am overly concerned about "using the dying person for showmanship and bizarre effects," that is, exploitation of the dying person. Obviously, there is a difference between structuring a situation where students *learn* from the dying and participating in his or her exploitation.

Sample Courses

In order to give the reader a better idea of differing approaches to death education, I shall briefly describe three courses.

The first is entitled Confrontations of Death, which utilizes small groups and a "task-oriented T-group" orientation. It was developed by Frances G. Scott and her colleagues at the University of Oregon (Scott and Brewer, 1971). Topics include: preliminary considerations of life and death (exercise—students write their philosophy of life and death), philosophical considerations of the meaning of life and death (film—*Ikiru*), the theme of death in poetry (selected readings in texts), the theme of death as presented in classical and contemporary music (selected classical and contemporary music), doctors and hospitals (guest lecturer—a physician, followed by a T-group interaction), and the process of dying (death-related videotapes and T-group discussion follow). The sixth week is highlighted by a weekend retreat entitled "A Sensitivity Group Week-End Group Experience," (which is described in Scott and Brewer's text). At the end of the seventh week, students are again asked to write on their philosophy of life and death and also to discuss their weekend experience. The number of participating students is limited in order to facilitate discussion, and classes usually take place in the university setting.

A second approach is that of Sandra Bertman (1974), who is unique because she has taught death education to a variety of groups ranging from children to adults. The following is a description of her course, Perspectives on Death, which is designed for adult education classes but is easily adaptable to high school, college, and professional classes. By way of introducing her course she writes:

> American people have been characterized as death-denying, implying bewilderment when dealing with the death and loss experiences amongst us. In an effort to become more comfortable with the subject of death, grief, and bereavement, we shall explore attitudes and feel-

ings expressed in the written and visual arts; most especially poetry and film. Materials ranging in tone from Tolstoy to Twain to Brel and the Beatles shall provide the points of departure for reflecting on such concerns as isolation, depersonalization and lack of communication, ritualization; repercussions (creative and non) that accompany loss; growing old; *carpe diem,* a meaningful death; and talking about death with children [p. 356].

Her 10-week course includes the topics: the scope and meaning of death (film—*How Could I Not Be Among You?;* read Tolstoy's *The Death of Ivan Ilych*), the sudden death (film—*All the Way Home;* read Agee's *A Death in the Family*), the hospital (read Kubler-Ross's *On Death and Dying*), who owns my life? (videotape—*Whose Life Is It Anyway?*), will you still need me; will you still feed me? (film—*Home for Life*), suicide (film—*The Slender Thread*), the funeral (film—*The Loved One*), grief and bereavement (attitudes toward death as reflected in music and song: spirituals, rock 'n roll and folk music), death rituals in primitive cultures and mythology (films— *Dead Birds* and *Day of the Dead*), treatment of death in the visual arts (film—*La Jetée*).

The topic of death can be handled both formally and informally. The trained teacher working at any level is able to use the teachable moment to explore death-related questions raised by students. A death in the family of a child of elementary school age can provide the stimulus for expressions of feelings and learning about grief and death in the classroom. One knowledgeable elementary school teacher did just that. She used a child's experience with the recent death of a sibling to initiate death education. She legitimized the students' psychological and physiological reactions to death, so well documented and described recently by Parkes (1972). Using Bertman (1972) as a source, she fashioned an informal curriculum which allowed students to see the pervasive influence of death upon behavior and culture. Her most difficult task was in dealing not with her children but with the school principal. Upon hearing what she was doing, he demanded that she stop her activities lest she "corrupt" her students. Luckily, she was able to rationally demonstrate to him the therapeutic value of death education over time and gained his support. Children are often more receptive to death education than either colleagues or supervisors. If death education is to succeed, its curriculum must be accepted by the community.[5]

---

[5] My own clinical work with elderly persons, and in the death education area, has been labelled "obscene and perverse" by a local county organization to "stamp out obscenity." Pressure has been brought to bear on the administration of the University of Maryland who, to date, have remained most supportive.

Already there is evidence that those same forces that attacked sex education as "subversive" and "perverted" see death education as a similar sinister force.

A third approach is one I use on the university level for rather large classes of 300 to 400 persons. The course has served as a model for undergraduate classes, nursing students, and police officers (Leviton, 1969, 1971). Recognizing the "taboo" nature of the language of death, its approach is "hierarchical." Topics, initially, are of an impersonal, objective nature, and then evolve into more personal and affect-arousing aspects. During the first half of the course, subjects include the language of death, definitions and taxonomies, philosophies of death, anthropological views, social factors affecting death and dying, legal-historical view of death, theories of death, and Judeo-Christian views of death. By this time, it is assumed that the student is adequately acclimated to death language to rationally carry on a dialogue without emotional upset. Topics during the second half include developmental views of death (from children, adolescents, and young adults to the middle-aged, aged, and dying), bereavement, grief, and mourning, sudden infant-death syndrome, widowhood, funeral industry, consumer's view of the funeral industry, interacting with the dying person and his family, other types of intervention and therapy with the dying and family (for example, psychoactive-assisted psychotherapy, the Adults' Health and Developmental Program), nature of suicide, sexuality and suicide, crisis-intervention fundamentals, and ethical issues (for example, euthanasia, war).

Texts which have been well received over the years include Alvarez, *The Savage God;* Feifel (ed.), *The Meaning of Death;* Kastenbaum and Aisenberg, *The Psychology of Death;* Elliot, *Twentieth Century Book of the Dead;* Perlin (ed.), *A Handbook for the Study of Suicide;* Kubler-Ross, *On Death and Dying;* Weisman, *On Death and Denying;* and Shneidman, *The Deaths of Man* and *Death: Current Perspectives.*

Two objectives tests are given each semester to determine students' grasp of the subject matter. They are also asked to write a short, 3-page, "I-oriented" essay describing their personal reaction to death. Its purpose is to allow the student to gently face the thought of death while considering his or her own psychothanatological strength. Films are shown on an optional basis. One film, *Death* (produced by Filmmakers Library), follows the dying of two men from cancer at Calvary Hospital. It is an extremely powerful film requiring the emotional preparation of the class before and during the viewing. Another film *The Autopsy and Reconstruction* (produced by the University of Iowa), is usually attended by one-third to one-half of the class, and is generally well received. Parenthetically, I have found that much of the initial emotional upset resulting from this film can be alleviated if the instructor talks through the first part of the film, especially during the showing of the first incision. The use of humor is highly recommended.

Audiovisual Bibliographies

A plethora of audiovisual aides is beginning to invade the market similar to that which occurred in the fields of sex and drug education. To date, most of the films designed specifically for classroom education (grades 1 to 12) are mediocre, patronizing, and unrealistic in my opinion. Clarence W. Collins has prepared a helpful bibliography of approximately 30 films on the topic of death.[6] Unfortunately the list is not annotated.

Other audiovisual bibliographies germane to death education can be obtained from:

The Center for Death Education Research
1167 Social Sciences Bldg.
University of Minnesota
Minneapolis, Minn. 55455

The Institute of Society, Ethics and the Life Sciences
623 Warburton Ave.
Hastings-on-Hudson, New York 10706

CONCLUSION

It is probable that death education, like sex education, is here to stay. Organizations such as The Forum for Death Education and Counseling, Ars Moriendi in Philadelphia, Equinox Institute in Brookline, Massachusetts, Foundation of Thanatology, Continental Association of Funeral and Memorial Societies in Washington, D.C., and National Funeral Directors Association in Milwaukee, among others, are joining together with interested scholars to provide valid death education. Toward this end, two caveats should be voiced.

The first concerns the training of teachers. It was once assumed that any married person could teach sex education. Unfortunately, the subject matter is often too diverse and profuse for the lay person. Too often his or her armamentarium of knowledge is based upon myth and stereotype. Once, at a parent-teacher's symposium on sex education, I was asked if I

---

[6] c/o Horizons, The Riverside Church, 490 Riverside Dr., New York, N.Y. 10027

categorically would approve of formal sex education for my daughter. My reply was "Absolutely not!" I would want to know what the teacher knows about the subject area, whether he or she considers himself or herself to have the last word on sexual morality, and so forth. I take the same attitude toward death education. In addition to knowledgeability and balanced good will, understanding and empathy for students and an ability to communicate are important characteristics of teachers. For the teachers of my child, I would prefer the five criteria listed earlier in this chapter.

My second caveat concerns the misuse of death education. I worry over the possibility of death education becoming a means to condition people to kill and/or die for ignoble causes. "To die for the glory of the State" is all too common a rallying cry throughout history. Kamikazi pilots, My Lai, and the suicidal and destructive preoccupations of the Dadaists in the early twentieth century, all give indications and warning that people can be rather easily persuaded to forsake life.

Again, the hope is that death education will contribute to a greater empathy and humane concern for one's fellow humanity. If the universal denial of death postulated by Freud (1961) can be somewhat lessened to the extent that we come to know that life is fragile, that death can occur at any moment, then perhaps life will become more valued. Erich Fromm (1964) suggests the need to become more *biophiliac* as opposed to *necrophiliac,* that is, more life-loving than death-loving. Such a framework prompts us to ask three interrelated questions: (1) Can the study of death affect the quality of life? (2) How can our psychosocial environment be guided to best assure the attainment of an improved quality of life and dying? and (3) Can we be educated to achieve these goals? Feifel (1971) is aware of the close relationship between an understanding of death and the improvement of civilization. He writes,

> Death comes not to the dead but to the living. To deny or ignore it is to distort life's pattern. We dread death because we refuse to understand it. As Paz, the Mexican author and diplomat, has insightfully stated, "a civilization that denies death ends by denying life." Death makes an authentic statement about life's actuality and meaning. It helps clarify and intensify our image of man and his world. Herein lies the summons to advance our comprehension of how death can serve life. To die—that is the human condition; to live decently and to die well—this is man's privilege [p. 12].

All of us need to make our contribution to answering the salient question concerning the quality of life and death. Certainly such health-care givers as the physician and nurse should be among the leaders. It is true that many of them have done pioneering work in educating their professions so that dying is made easier for patient and family. Yet their numbers are all too few.

A nurse attending one of my courses summed up her resentment when she said in class, "Where are the doctors when we need to talk, to explain things to the patient; to hold his hand, to provide the shoulder for his wife to cry upon? Where is the physician? They leave the job to us while they take off. They're more at home reading charts and printouts than helping a dying person overcome his apprehensions, doubts, and fears."

Progress is being made, however. The plethora of influential books, the new breed of humanistically oriented physicians, nurses, and police officers, among others, suggests hope. Yet progress is too slow if it is you or yours who is dying.

But the scope of death education is larger and more global than simply client-caregiver relationships. Would national and world political leaders deal more effectively in striving for peace, in the eradication of famine, pestilence, and disease, if they were forced to face the meaning of death for themselves or their children? As Lifton (1967) has ably demonstrated, those who come into repeated contact with death develop a defense posture called "psychological closure." One becomes benumbed to the starving child times 2, 4, 100, 200, 2000, 200,000. But if one's own child is starving, who would not steal or perhaps kill to obtain food? Feifel has said on many occasions that death is for all seasons and for all people. If death is egalitarian, then death education can strive to democratize us all in a reverence for life—and in striving for world harmony—or at least warn us of the dangers should our denials obscure intellect and reason.

The subject matter of death exists and is now readily available. Those interested can consult journals devoted exclusively to thanatology and suicidology such as *Omega, Journal of Life-Threatening Behaviors* (now *Journal of Suicide*), and the *Journal of Thanatology*. Bibliographies on death, dying, and suicide are available (for example, Kalish, 1965; Vernick). Both general and specialized sources are there for the serious scholar and educator.

Death education has come of age to receive its confirmation. Whether the child prodigy is father to the Promethean man, whether death education becomes a worthwhile, mature entity and a moving force contributing to the improvement of the human condition remains to be seen.

REFERENCES

Alvarez, A. *The savage god.* New York: Random House, 1972.

Anderson, H. Panel presentation on the teaching of death. Paper presented at the meeting of the American Psychological Association, Honolulu, September 1972.

Barton, D., Flexner, J., Van Eys, J., and Scott, C. Death and dying: A course for medical students. *Journal of Medical Education,* 1972, **47,** 945–951.

Bertman, S. L. Death education in the face of a taboo. In E. A. Grollman (Ed.), *Concerning death: A practical guide for the living.* Boston: Beacon Press, 1974.

Campbell, D. T., and Stanley, J. C. *Experimental and quasi-experimental designs for research.* Chicago: Rand McNally, 1963.

Death education 1975. *Omega,* 1975, **6,** 179–287.

Dougherty, T. E. *An appraisal of a death education process in clinical pastoral education.* (Unpublished doctoral dissertation, The Southern Baptist Theological Seminary), 1974.

Elliot, G. *Twentieth century book of the dead.* New York: Scribner, 1972.

Elliot, T. O. Bereavement: Inevitable, but not insurmountable. In H. Becker and R. Hill (Eds.), *Family marriage and parenthood.* (2nd ed.). Cambridge, Mass.: Heath, 1971.

Feifel, H. (Ed.) *The meaning of death.* New York: McGraw-Hill, 1959.

Feifel, H. The meaning of death in American society: Implications for education. In B. R. Green and D. P. Irish (Eds.), *Death education: Preparation for living.* Cambridge, Mass.: Schenkman, 1971.

Feifel, H., and Branscomb, A. B. Who's afraid of death? *Journal of Abnormal Psychology,* 1973, **81,** 282–288.

Freud, S. *Beyond the pleasure principle,* New York: Liveright, 1961.

Fromm, E. *The Heart of man: Its genius for good and evil.* New York: Harper and Row, 1964.

Green, B. R., and Irish, D. P. (Eds.) *Death education: Preparation for living.* Cambridge, Mass.: Schenkman, 1971.

Johnson, W., and Belzer, E. *Human sexual behavior and sex education.* (3rd ed.). Philadelphia: Lea & Febiger, 1973.

Kalish, R. A. Death and bereavement: An annotated social science bibliography through 1964. *SK & F Psychiatric Reporter,* (Smith Kline and French Laboratories, 1500 Spring Garden Street, Philadelphia, Pa 19191), March-April 1965, pp. 1–38.

Kastenbaum, R., and Aisenberg, R. *The psychology of death.* New York: Springer, 1972.

Kubler-Ross, E. *On death and dying.* New York: Macmillan, 1969.

Leviton, D. Education for death. *Journal of Health, Physical Education, Recreation,* 1969, **40,** 46–51. (a)

Leviton, D. The need for education on death and suicide. *Journal of School Health,* 1969, **39,** 270–274. (b)

Leviton, D. A course on death education and suicide prevention: Implications for health education. *Journal of American College Health Association,* 1971, **19**, 217–220. (a)

Leviton, D. Death bereavement and suicide education. In D. A. Reed (Ed.), *New directions in health education.* New York: Macmillan, 1971. (b)

Leviton, D. The role of the schools in providing death education. In B. R. Green and D. P. Irish (Eds.), *Death education: Preparation for living.* Cambridge, Mass.: Schenkman, 1971. (c)

Leviton, D., and Forman, E. C. Death education for children and youth. *Journal of Clinical Child Psychology,* 1974, **3**, 8–10.

Lifton, R. J. *Death in life: Survivors of Hiroshima.* New York: Vintage Books, 1967.

Lifton, R. J. *Home from the war.* New York: Simon and Schuster, 1973.

Liston, E. H. Education on death and dying: A neglected area in the medical curriculum. *Omega,* 1975, **6**, 193–198.

Parkes, C. M. *Bereavement: Studies of grief in adult life.* New York: International Universities Press, 1972.

Penniston, D. H. The importance of death education in family life. *The Family Coordinator,* 1962, **11**, 15–18.

Perlin, S. (Ed.) *A handbook for the study of suicide.* New York: Oxford, 1975.

Schulz, R., and Aderman, D. Clinical research and the stages of dying. *Omega,* 1974, **5**, 137–143.

Scott, F. G. and Brewer, R. M. (Eds.) *Confrontations of death.* Corvallis, Oregon: Continuing Education Pubications, 1971.

Shneidman, E. *The deaths of man.* New York: Penguin, 1974.

Shneidman, E. *Death: Current perspectives.* Palo Alto, Calif.: Mayfield, 1976.

Sommerville, R. M. Death education as part of family life education: Using imaginative literature or insights into family crises. *The Family Coordinator,* 1971, **20**, 209–224.

Vernick, J. J. *Selected bibliography on death and dying.* Superintendent of Documents, U. S. Government Printing Office , 1971.

Wahl, C. C. The fear of death. In H. Feifel (Ed.), *The meaning of death.* New York: McGraw-Hill, 1959.

Weisman, A. D. *On dying and denying: A psychiatric study of terminality.* New York: Behavioral Publications, 1972.

15

THE SENSE OF IMMORTALITY: ON DEATH AND THE CONTINUITY OF LIFE

ROBERT J. LIFTON

Serious concern with the way in which people confront death leads one to question the nature of death and the nature of life in the face of death. In my work in Hiroshima I found that studying an extreme situation such as that facing the survivors of the atomic bomb can lead to insights about every-day death, about ordinary people facing what Kurt Vonnegut has called "plain old death." I feel that our psychological ideas about death have been so stereotyped, so limited, so extraordinarily impoverished, that any exposure to a holocaust like Hiroshima, or My Lai, or in fact the entire American involvement in Indochina, forces us to develop new ideas and hypotheses that begin to account for some of the reactions that we observe. I want to suggest a few such principles that are both psychological and historical.[1]

My basic premise is that we understand humanity through paradigms or models. The choice of the paradigm or model becomes extremely important because it determines what might be called the *controlling image* or central theme of our psychological theory. Human culture is sufficiently rich that a great variety of paradigms are available to serve as controlling images, including those of *power, being, instinct and defense, social class, collective unconscious, interpersonal relations,* etc. These paradigms are by no means of equal merit, but each can be used to illuminate some aspect of human experience.

At the end of my study of Hiroshima, *Death in Life,* I stated that sexuality and moralism had been the central themes confronted by Freud in developing psychoanalysis, but that now unlimited technological violence and absurd death have become more pressing themes for the contemporary person (Lifton, 1968). During the Victorian era, when Freud was evolving his ideas, there was an overwhelming repression of sexuality but a relatively greater openness to the reality of human death. The extent of sexual repression is revealed by the Victorian custom of putting doilies on table legs because these were thought to be suggestive of the human anatomy. There has been a historical shift, and the contemporary situation is one in which we are less overwhelmed by sexual difficulties but more overwhelmed by difficulties connected with death. One can characterize the shift as covering the legs of tables with doilies to wearing hot-pants, and the change from the grim reaper as public celebrity to the Forest Lawn syndrome. The fact that Freud's model of libido and repression of instinctual sexual impulses was put forth during the late Victorian era, at a time when society was struggling with these issues, does not

---

[1] *Note:* This chapter is the text of the Twentieth Annual Karen Horney Lecture presented in New York City, 1973, and reprinted from *The American Journal of Psychoanalysis,* 1973, **33**, 3–15.

invalidate the generalizability of his ideas: their power lies precisely in that generalizability. But it does raise the important point—not only for Freud but for our own work now—of the influence of historical forces on the psychological theories we choose to develop. If we now begin to build psychological theory around death it is because death imposes itself upon us in such unmanageable ways.

In my own psychological work on extreme historical situations involving ultimate violence and massive death, I have preferred to speak of a process of psychic numbing rather than repression. Repression occurs when an idea or experience is forgotten, excluded from consciousness, or relegated to the realm of the unconscious. Repressed childhood memories and repressed instinctual impulses are illustrations of this process. Repression is part of a model or controlling image characterized by drives and defenses and refers to the compensatory effort of the organism to cope with innate or instinctual forces that dominate emotional life. The original idea was to analyze these forces and thereby bring the patient to cure.

Psychoanalysis has been changed significantly by the development of ego psychology, by various neo-Freudian modifications, and by many new influences including ethology. But I think that psychoanalytic theory is still bedeviled by its traditional imagery of instinct, repression, and defense. This imagery yields limited and distorted insight when one approaches the subject of death and the relationship of death to larger contemporary experience. The concept of psychic numbing, in contrast, suggests the cessation of what I call the formative process, the impairment of humanity's essential mental function of symbol-formation or symbolization. This point of view is strongly influenced by the symbolic philosophy of Cassirer (1946, 1953–1957) and Langer (1942, 1953, 1962, 1967). Psychic numbing is a form of desensitization; it refers to an incapacity to feel or to confront certain kinds of experience, due to the blocking or absence of inner forms or imagery that can connect with such experience.

The importance of this kind of phenomenon was impressed upon me very profoundly by my work in Hiroshima. It would appear that the technology of destruction has had a strong impact on the spread of psychic numbing. But my assumption is that psychic numbing is central in everyday experience as well, and may be identified whenever there is interference in the *formative* mental function, the process of creating viable inner forms. The *psychoformative* perspective would stress that a human being can never simply *receive* a bit of information nakedly. The process of perception is vitally bound up with the process of inner recreation, in which one utilizes whatever forms are available in individual psychic existence.

Within this psychoformative perspective the central paradigm I wish to develop is that of *death and the continuity of life*. In elaborating this paradigm I will speak first of a theory of symbolic immortality, then of an accompanying theory of evolving death imagery, and finally discuss the application of this paradigm to clinical work and psychopathology.

I want to emphasize at the beginning that this approach to psychology and history is impelled by a sense of urgency about our present historical predicament, and by a strong desire to evolve psychohistorical theory adequate to the dangerous times in which we live. In this approach it is necessary to make our own subjectivity as investigators clear and conscious, to try to understand it and use it as part of the conceptual process. I have elsewhere suggested possibilities for going even further and making our forms of advocacy clear, forthright, and, again, part of the conceptual process (Lifton, 1972). In presenting this paradigm of death and the continuity of life I also assume a sense of urgency in our intellectual and professional lives. A crisis exists in the psychiatric profession, and in other professions as well, that has to do with despair about the adequacy of traditional ideas for coping with new data impinging from all sides.

In his book, *The Structure of Scientific Revolutions,* Thomas Kuhn (1962) describes a sequence that occurs in the development of scientific thought when the data can no longer be explained by prevailing theories. Kuhn observed that when this happens the usual reaction among scientists is to cling to the old theories all the more persistently. At a certain point the incongruity between the theory and data becomes so glaring—and the anxiety of those defending the theory so great—that the whole system collapses and the paradigm changes. I think we are at a point something like that now, and that a new depth-psychological paradigm is required. Ironically, the paradigm of death and the continuity of life is actually humanity's oldest and most fundamental paradigm.

Psychiatrists and psychoanalysts have for the most part left the question of death to philosophers. Freud's theory (1957) legitimized this neglect when he said:

> It is indeed impossible to imagine our own death: and whenever we attempt to do so we can perceive that we are in fact still present as spectators. Hence the psychoanalytic school could venture on the assertion that at bottom no one believes in his own death, or, to put the same thing in another way, that in his unconscious, every one of us is convinced of his own immortality.

Freud viewed all interest in immortality as compensatory, as a denial of death and a refusal to face it unflinchingly. Freud insisted that we look at death squarely, that we cannot psychologically afford the consequences of denial. But Freud had no place in his system for the *symbolic* significance of the idea of immortality as an expression of continuity. For this reason I call Freud's approach *rationalist-iconoclastic.*

Jung's approach was very different; he took the mythological and symbolic aspects of death and immortality very seriously. He emphasized the enormous significance of the idea of immortality on the basis of the map of the human psyche, and especially of the unconscious, provided by mythology. But he also said: "As a physician I am convinced that it is hygienic to discover in death a goal toward which one can strive: and that shrinking away from it is something unhealthy and abnormal": and, "I . . . consider the religious teaching of a life hereafter consonant with the standpoint of psychic hygiene (Jung, 1936). In such statements it becomes unclear whether Jung is talking about the literal idea of a life after death or a more symbolic one. He surrenders much of the scientific viewpoint, however broadly defined, that humanity has struggled for so painfully over the last few centuries. We can thus call Jung's approach *hygienic-mythical.*

Both of these views are important: neither is completely satisfactory. Freud's attitude has the merit of unflinching acceptance of death as a total annihilation of the organism. Jung's view has the merit of stressing the symbolic significance of universal imagery around death and immortality.

A third perspective—which I shall call *formative-symbolic*—draws upon both Freud and Jung but takes into account the increasing awareness of symbol-formation as a fundamental characteristic of man's psychic life. I should emphasize that I am speaking of an ongoing *process of symbolization,* rather than of particular symbols (the flag, the cross, etc.). In classical psychoanalysis the focus tends to be on symbols as specific equivalents— pencil for penis, sea for mother, etc.—and much less on the more fundamental process of creation and recreation of images and forms that characterize human mentation.

SYMBOLIC IMMORTALITY

I would hold, in the context of this psychoformative view, that even in our unconscious lives we are by no means *convinced* of our own immortality. Rather we have what some recent workers have called "middle knowledge" of the idea of death (Weisman and Hackett, 1961). We both "know" that we will die, and resist and fail to act upon that knowledge. Nor is the need to transcend death *mere* denial. More essentially, it represents a compelling universal urge to maintain an inner sense of continuous symbolic relationship, over time and space, with the various elements of life. In other words, I am speaking of a *sense* of immortality as in itself neither compensatory nor pathological, but as humanity's symbolization of ties with both biological fellows and history, past and future. This view is consistent with Otto Rank's stress on humanity's perpetual need for "an assurance of eternal survival for his self." Rank suggested that "man creates culture by changing natural conditions in order to maintain his spiritual self (Rank, 1958). But this need for a sense of symbolic immortality, interwoven with biology and history, is for the most part ignored by individually biased psychological theory.

The sense of immortality can be expressed in five general modes. The first and most obvious is the biological mode, the sense of living on *through* and *in* one's sons and daughters and their sons and daughters. At some level of consciousness we imagine an endless chain of biological attachments. This mode has been a classical expression of symbolic immortality in East Asian culture, especially in traditional China, with its extraordinary emphasis on the family line: In Confucian ethics, the greatest of all unfilial acts is lack of posterity. But this mode never remains purely biological: it becomes simultaneously biosocial, and expresses itself in attachments to one's group, tribe, organization, people, nation, or even species. Ultimately one can feel at least glimmerings of a sense of immortality in "living on" through and in humanity.

A second expression of the sense of immortality is the theological idea of a life after death or, more importantly, the idea of release from profane life to existence on a higher plane. The literal idea of an afterlife is not essential to this mode, and such a notion is not present in many religions. More basic is the concept of transcending death through spiritual attainment. The power of spiritual life to in some way overcome death is exemplified in all the great religious leaders around whom religions have been founded: Buddha, Moses, Christ, Mohammed. Within each of the religious traditions there has been a word to convey the spiritual state in which one has transcended death: the Japanese word *kami;* the Polynesian term *mana;* the Roman idea of *noumen;* the Eskimo concept of *tungnik;* and the Christian doctrine of *grace.* All these words describe a state in which one possesses spiritual power over death, meaning, in a symbolic sense, that one is in harmony with a principle extending beyond the limited biological life span.

The third mode of symbolic immortality is that achieved through "works": the mode of creativity, the achievement of enduring human impact; the sense that one's writing, one's teaching, one's human influences, great or humble, will live on; that one's contribution will not die. The therapeutic efforts of physicians and psychotherapists are strongly impelled, I believe, by an image of therapeutic impact extending through the patient to others, including the patient's children, in an endless, potentially beneficent chain of influence. The "therapeutic despair" described so sensitively by Leslie Farber (1966) as an occupational hazard of the psychiatrist treating schizophrenic patients might well result from the perception that one's strenuous therapeutic endeavors are not producing these lasting effects, that one's energies are not animating the life of the patient and cannot therefore symbolically extend the life of the therapist.

A fourth mode is the sense of immortality achieved through being survived by nature itself: the theme of eternal nature. This theme is very vivid among the Japanese, and was one of the most important kinds of imagery for survivors of the atomic bomb. It is strong not only in Shinto belief but in the European Romantic movement and in the Anglo-Saxon cult of the great outdoors—indeed in every culture in one form or another.

The fifth mode is somewhat different from the others in that it depends solely upon a psychic state. This is the state of *experiential transcendence,* a state so intense that in it time and death disappear. When one achieves ecstasy or rapture, the restrictions of the senses—including the sense of mortality—no longer exist. Poetically and religiously this has been described as "losing oneself." It can occur not only in religious or secular mysticism but also in song, dance, battle, sexual love, childbirth, athletic effort, mechanical flight, or in contemplating works of artistic or intellectual creation (Laski, 1961). This state is characterized by extraordinary psychic unity and perceptual intensity. But there also occurs, as we hear described in drug experiences, a process of symbolic reordering. One feels oneself to be different after returning from this state. I see experiential transcendence and its aftermath as epitomizing the death-and-rebirth experience. It is central to change or transformation and has great significance for psychotherapy. Experiential transcendence includes a feeling of what Eliade has called the "continuous present" that can be equated with eternity or with "mythical time" (Eliade, 1959). This continuous present is perceived not only as "here and now" but as inseparable from past and future.

The theory of symbolic immortality can be used to illuminate changes in cultural emphasis from one historical period to another. We can think of historical shifts as involving alterations in the stress given to one or another mode or combinations of modes. The Darwinian revolution of the nineteenth century, for example, can be seen as entailing a shift from a predominantly theological mode to a more natural and biological one. The continuous transformation in China over the last few decades involves a shift from a family-centered biological mode to a revolutionary mode which I have written about elsewhere as emphasizing humanity's works but including also elements of other modes with periodic emphasis upon experiential transcendence.

Following the holocaust of World War II the viability of psychic activity within the modes has undergone something of a collapse, at least in the West. We exist now in a time of doubt about modes of continuity and connection, and I believe this has direct relevance for work with individual patients. Awareness of our historical predicament—of threats posed by nuclear weapons, environmental destruction, and the press of rising population against limited resouces—has created extensive imagery of extinction. These threats occur at a time when the rate of historical velocity and the resulting psychohistorical dislocation had already undermined established symbols around the institutions of family, church, government, and education. Combined imagery of extinction and dislocation leave us in doubt about whether we will "live on" in our children and their children, in our groups and organizations, in our works, in our spirituality, or even in nature, which we now know to be vulnerable to our pollutions and our weaponry. It is the loss of faith, I think, in these four modes of symbolic immortality that leads people, especially the young to plunge— sometimes desperately and sometimes with considerable self-realization— into the mode of experiential transcendence. This very old and classical form of personal quest has had to be discovered anew in the face of doubts about the other four modes.

DEATH IMAGERY

In postulating a theory of symbolic immortality on such a grand scale, one must also account for the everyday idea of death, for the sense of *mortality* that develops over the course of a lifetime. Freud's notion of the death instinct is unacceptable, and could in fact be viewed as a contradiction in terms in that instinctual forces are in the service of the preservation of life. Nor is death an adequate goal for life. Yet as is generally the case with Freud when we disagree with him, the concept, whatever its confusions around the instinctual idiom, contains an insight we had best retain concerning the fundamental importance of death for psychological life. Hence, the widespread rejection of the death instinct poses the danger of throwing out not so much the baby with the bath water but perhaps the grim reaper with the scythe.

Freud himself faced death heroically and understood well the dangers involved in denying humanity's mortality. But at the same time Freudian theory, insisting that death has no representation in the unconscious, has relegated fear of death to a derivative of fear of castration. Freud also seemed ambivalent about whether to view death and life within a unitary or dualistic perspective. His ultimate instinctual dualism opposed death and life instincts. Yet the notion of life leading inevitably toward death is a unitary vision, and it is this unitary element that I think we should preserve. This unitary perspective on death would insist upon its overall consistency as an absolute infringement upon the organism (as opposed to certain contemporary efforts to subdivide death into a number of different categories); and as an event anticipated, and therefore influential, from the beginning of the life of the organism.

I believe that the representation of death evolves from dim and vague articulation in the young organism's inchoate imagery to sophisticated symbolization in maturity. I rely partly here on Kenneth Boulding's work on the image, in which he has stressed the presence in the organism from the very beginning of some innate tendency or direction which I call an *inchoate image* (Boulding, 1956). This image is at first simply a direction or physiological "push." But inchoate though it may be, the image includes an *interpretative anticipation of interaction with the environment*. Evidence for the existence of innate imagery can be drawn from two sources: one is ethology and the other is observation of rapid eyeball movements (REM) in sleep studies.

Work in ethology has demonstrated through the study of *releasing mechanisms* the existence of what I am here calling an image. The newborn organism is impelled innately toward certain expected behavior on the part of older (nurturing) organisms, which when encountered, acts as a releasing mechanism for a specific action (such as feeding) of its own. Sleep studies also suggest the presence of images in some form from the beginning of life, possibly during prenatal experience, that *cause* or at least provide some basis for the rapid eyeball movements observed in various species. Rather than demonstrating the presence of pictorial images, these two areas of research suggest the presence at birth of primordial images or precursors to later imagery.

In the human being the sequence of this process is from physiological push (or direction of the organism) to pictures of the world (images in the usual sense) to symbolization. Within this theory of evolving imagery we can understand the elaboration of the inner idea of death from earliest childhood in terms of three subparadigms or polarities. These are: connection versus separation, integrity versus disintegration, and movement versus stasis. The inchoate imagery of the first polarity is expressed in a seeking of connection, what John Bowlby has described as "attachment behavior" around sucking, clinging, smiling, crying, and following (Bowlby, 1969). The organism actively seeks connection with the nurturing or mothering person. First this quest is mainly physiological, then it is internalized in pictorial image-formation, and finally it becomes highly symbolized. The organism's evolution is from simple movement toward the mother to a nurturing relationship with her, and eventually toward connection with other people, with groups, with ideas, with historical forces, etc. Where this striving for connection fails, as it always must in some degree, there is the alternative image of separation, of being cut off. This alternative image of separation forms one precursor for the idea of death.

In a similar way one can look at the idea of integrity versus disintegration. As indicated in the work of Melanie Klein on the infant's fear of annihilation, there is from the beginning some sense of the organism's being threatened with dissolution, disintegration (Klein, 1952). The terms of this negative image or fear are at first entirely physiological, having to do with physical intactness or deterioration; but over the course of time integrity, without entirely losing its physiological reference, comes to assume primarily ethical-psychological dimensions. At those more symbolized dimensions one "disintegrates" as one's inner forms and images become inadequate representations of the self-world relationship and inadequate bases for action.

The third mode, that of movement versus stasis, is the most ignored of the three; but it has great clinical significance and is especially vivid to those who deal with children. An infant held tight and unable to move becomes extremely anxious and uncomfortable. The early meaning of movement is the literal, physiological idea of moving the body or a portion of it from one place to another. Later the meaning of movement takes on symbolic quantities having to do with development, progress, and change (or a specific collectivity in some form of motion). The absence of movement becomes a form of stasis, a deathlike experience closely related to psychic numbing.

One could illustrate in detail the evolution of these polarities over the course of the life cycle. But it is clear that rather early, or earlier than is usually assumed, death achieves some kind of conscious meaning. By the ages of 3, 4, and 5 children are thinking and talking, however confusedly, about death and dying. And over the course of the next few years something in that process consolidates so that the idea of death is more fundamentally learned and understood. At every developmental level all conflicts exacerbate, and are exacerbated by, these three aspects of what later becomes death anxiety—that is, disintegration stasis, or separation. These death-linked conflicts take on characteristic form for each developmental stage and reach a climax during adolescence. During young adulthood there occurs a process partly described by Kenneth Keniston around the term "youth" (Keniston, 1968), and partly described in my own work around the concept of the "protean style" (Lifton, 1968, 1970, 1971). I see the continuing search characterizing the protean style as a constant process of death and rebirth of inner form. The quest is always for images and forms more malleable and inwardly acceptable at this historical moment than those available from the past. Sometime in early adulthood one moves more fully into the realm of historical action, and one then connects with the modes of symbolic immortality.

Later, in middle adulthood, one becomes impressed with the fact that one will indeed die. It becomes apparent that the limitations of physiology and life span will not permit the full accomplishment of all one's projects. But even with this fuller recognition of mortality, the issues of integrity, connection, and movement remain salient. Old people approaching death look back nostalgically over their whole lives. This "life review," as it is sometimes called, has to do with a process of self-judgment, of examining one's life around issues of integrity, but also around those of connection and movement, and is evidence of relationship to the modes of symbolic immortality.

APPLICATION IN CLINICAL WORK AND PSYCHOPATHOLOGY

I want to suggest the clinical applicability of this paradigm of death and the continuity of life to various categories of psychopathology. Psychiatrists have turned away from death, as has our whole culture, and there has been little appreciation of the importance of death anxiety in the precipitation of psychological disorder.

What I am here calling the sense of immortality is close to what Erik Erikson calls "basic trust" (Erikson, 1950). Erikson emphasizes the issue of basic trust as the earliest developmental crisis, and he sees the legacy of this earliest time as having vital importance for adulthood. But the establishment of trust itself involves confidence in the integrity, connection, and movement of life, prerequisites for a viable form of symbolic immortality. Where this confidence collapses, psychological impairment ensues.

The principle of impaired death imagery—or more accurately, impaired imagery of death and the continuity of life—is a unitary theme around which mental illness can be described and in some degree understood. I see this kind of impairment as being involved in the etiology of mental illness but not causative in the nineteenth century sense of a single cause bringing about one specific effect. Rather, impaired death imagery is at the center of a constellation of forms, each of which is of some importance for the overall process we call mental disturbance. Here I would point to three issues central to the process of mental illness. The first is death anxiety, which evolves in relation to the three polarities I have described. The second is psychic numbing, which I see as a process of desymbolization and deformation. The image which accompanies psychic numbing is that "if I feel nothing then death does not exist; therefore I need not feel anxious about death either actually or symbolically; I am invulnerable." A third principle is what I call "suspicion of counterfeit nurturance." This is the idea that if death exists then life is counterfeit. Ionesco's question—"Why was I born if it wasn't forever?"—illustrates the relation of this theme to the quest for immortality. But it is a very old question.

Death anxiety can be seen as a signal of threat to the organism, threat now understood as disintegration, stasis, or separation. All anxiety relates to these equivalents of death imagery, and guilt too is generated insofar as one makes oneself *responsible* for these processes. In other writing I have distinguished between static (either numbed or self-lacerating) and animating guilt, and have emphasized the importance of the latter in the process of self-transformation (Lifton, 1973).

One can take as a model for much of neurosis the syndrome which used to be called "traumatic neurosis" or "war neurosis." It is generally described as involving the continuous reliving of the unconscious conflicts aroused by a traumatic situation. More recently emphasis has been placed on imagery of death aroused by a trauma, rather than a trauma per se. Thus the syndrome has been called by some observers "death anxiety neurosis" (Teicher, 1953). I see this process in terms of the psychology of the survivor as I have elaborated that psychology in my work on Hiroshima and more recently with antiwar veterans. My belief is that survivor conflicts emerge from and apply to everyday psychological experience as well. When one "outlives" something or someone, and there are of course many large and small survivals in anyone's life, the specter of premature death becomes vivid. Simultaneously one begins to feel what I came to call in my Hiroshima work "guilt over survival priority"—the notion that one's life was purchased at the cost of another's, that one was able to survive *because* someone else died. This is a classical survivor process and is very much involved in traumatic neurosis. In describing traumatic neurosis, earlier observers spoke of "ego contraction." This is close to what I call psychic numbing, also very marked in the survivor syndrome and in neurosis in general.

A great number of writers (including Stekel, Rank, Horney, and Tillich) have emphasized patterns closely resembling psychic numbing as the essence of neurosis. Stekel, in 1908, spoke of neurotics who "die every day" and who "play the game of dying" (Stekel, 1923). Otto Rank referred to the neurotic's "constant restriction of life" because "he refuses the loan [life] in order to avoid the payment of the debt [death]" (Rank, 1950). The neurotic thus seeks to defend himself or herself against stimuli in a way Freud (1962) described in a little-known passage in *Civilization and Its Discontents*. Freud observed:

> No matter how much we may shrink with horror from certain situations—of a galley slave in antiquity, of a peasant during the Thirty Years War, of a victim of the Holy Inquisition, of a Jew awaiting a pogrom—it is nevertheless impossible for us to feel our way into such people, to divine the changes which original obtuseness of mind, a gradual stupefying process, the cessation of expectations and cruder or more refined methods of narcotization have produced upon their receptivity to sensations of pleasure and unpleasure. Moreover, in the

case of the most extreme possibility of suffering, special mental protective devices are brought into operation.

It is strange that Freud turned away from his own argument at this point and concluded that it was "unprofitable to pursue this aspect of the problem any further." For that argument contained the core of the idea of psychic numbing in extreme situations. The holocausts described by Freud have become almost a norm, a model for our times. But in lesser degree, what Freud called "narcotization" and I am calling psychic numbing is associated with the individual "holocausts" and survivals around which neurosis takes shape.

Let me now make some preliminary suggestions about the significance of these struggles around death imagery for the classical psychiatric syndromes. I am exploring these relationships more fully in work in progress, and my hope is that others will as well.

If we view neurosis in general as an expression of psychic numbing—shrinking of the ego and diminished capacity for experience—we can see in depression specific examples of the impaired mourning, impaired symbolization, and impaired formulation of the survivor. Where a known loss triggers the process, as in reactive depression, the depressed person acts very much like a survivor, and psychic numbing becomes very prominent. He often expresses the feeling that a part of him has died, and that he "killed" the other person in some symbolic way by failing to sustain the other's life with needed support, help, and nurturance. The idea of either having killed the other person or having purchased one's own life at the cost of another person's is fundamental. Such feelings are also related to Freud's explanation of guilt, in that earlier ambivalent feelings toward the other person included hate and death wishes, which now become attached to the actual loss. The whole issue of grief and its relation to mental disturbance is too complex to examine fully here. I can only say here that grief is of enormous importance in the experience of survival and in its residuum of mental and physical disturbance related to psychic numbing.

In character disorders, and in the related phenomenon of psychosomatic disorders in which one speaks through the "language of the body," there are lifelong characterological patterns such as deadening or numbing of various aspects of the psyche. This numbing may involve moral sensitivity or interpersonal capacities. However the numbing is expressed, there is a situation of meaninglessness and unfulfilled life, in which the defensive psychological structures built up to ward off death anxiety also ward off autonomy and self-understanding.

Turning to hysteria, the "psychic anesthesia" emphasized in early literature suggests the centrality of stasis, deadening, or numbing. Freud's case of Anna O., for example, is properly understood as a mourning reaction (Krupp and Kligfeld, 1962). The hysteria followed very quickly upon the death of Anna's father and had much to do with her reaction to that death. Her conception of being alive became altered in such a way that merely to *live* and *feel*—to exist as a sexual being—was dangerous, impermissible, and a violation of an unspoken pact with the dead person. Whether or not there is a mourning reaction directly involved, hysteria tends to involve either this form of stasis or its seeming opposite, exaggerated movement or activity that serves as a similar barrier against feeling and living. These patterns again resemble those I encountered among Hiroshima survivors.

In obsessional neurosis and obsessive-compulsive styles of behavior the stress is upon order and control. One tries to "stop time," to control its flow so as to order existence and block spontaneous expression, which is in turn felt to be threatening and "deadly."

Much of Freudian theory of phobia evolved from the case of Little Hans. In this case Freud interpreted castration fears as being displaced and transformed into a fear of horses—the inner danger being transformed into an external one (Freud, "Analysis of a Phobia in a Five-Year-Old Boy"). But I would say that Little Hans's experience could also be understood in terms of fear of annihilation and separation. His castration fear epitomized but was not the cause of his general death anxiety. Rather than viewing this death anxiety as secondary to castration anxiety, as psychoanalytic literature has done ever since, we do better to reverse our understanding and interpret the castration anxiety as an expression of more general death anxiety.

Finally I want to turn to psychosis and to an application of this theoretical position to schizophrenia. One is appalled by the degree to which death imagery has been observed in schizophrenic persons without being really incorporated into any conceptual scheme. As with more general psychiatric concern with death, the situation is changing. Harold Searles writes at some length about the problems a schizophrenic person has with the "universal factor of mortality." Searles says that the schizophrenic patient doesn't really believe he is living, doesn't feel himself to be alive, feels life passing him by, and feels stalked by death. Thus the patient employs a variety of techniques to defend against death anxiety, and yet in another sense feels already dead, "having therefore nothing to lose through death" (Searles, 1961). And what Ronald Laing calls the "false self" is very close to what I am calling a numbed or "dead self." Laing goes on to "translate" from what he calls "schizophrenese" and describes "the desire to be dead, the desire for a non-being" and "perhaps the most dangerous desire that can be pursued"; and the "state of death-in-life" as both a response to "the primary guilt of having no right to life in the first place, and hence of being entitled at most only to a dead life" and "probably the most extreme defensive posture that can be adopted" in which "being dead, one cannot die, and one cannot kill" (Laing, 1965). What Searles and Laing describe of schizophrenics is directly reminiscent of the process I observed among survivors in Hiroshima, and is similar to the *Musselmanner* phenomenon that occurred in Nazi concentration camps: so extreme was the state of psychic numbing that, as one observer put it, "One hesitates to call their death death" (Levi, 1961). These were people who had become robots.

The schizophrenic experiences a pathetic illusion of omnipotence, a despairing mask of pseudo immortality because he or she is blocked in the most fundamental way from authentic connection or continuity—from what I have been calling a sense of symbolic immortality.

But the productions of schizophrenics are infused with death: again like the Hiroshima survivors at the time the bomb fell, they see themselves as dead, other people around them as dead, the world as dead.

Wynne, Lidz, and others who have studied family process in schizophrenia emphasize the transmission of "meaninglessness, pointlessness, and emptiness," of "irrationality," of "schism and skew" (Jackson, ed., 1960). Bateson's "double bind" theory of conflicting messages received by the child also stresses the difficulty faced by the child in establishing a coherent field of meaning (Jackson, ed., 1960). All these theories represent a transmission of "desymbolized" or "deformed" images, which cannot cohere for the child and which leave him or her overwhelmed with death anxiety and suspicion of counterfeit nurturance. In the child's experience nurturance is dangerous: he flees from it into isolation, stasis, a "safer death" of his own.

It may require several generations to produce a schizophrenic person. But one can say that, however the inheritance mechanism may operate, whatever the contribution of genetic legacy, the early life of the schizophrenic is flooded with death anxiety, and the result is thought disorder and impairment of reality sense. The schizophrenic's behavior and symptoms represent alternate tendencies of surrender to death anxiety and struggle against it. The near total suspicion of counterfeit nurturance which characterizes the schizophrenic's emotional life renders his or her psychic numbing more extensive and more enduring than any other form of psychiatric disturbance. Although one sometimes sees in acute forms of schizophrenia an exaggerated response to stimuli, the general and long-range process is one of profound psychic numbing. To the schizophrenic as to certain survivors of mass holocausts, life is counterfeit, inner death predominant, and biological death unacceptable. Because the schizophrenic's entire existence has been a series of unabsorbable death immersions and survivals, he or she ultimately settles for a "devil's bargain": a lifeless life.

The paradigm of death and continuity of life I have elaborated here—together with psychoformative and psychohistorical perspectives—can help keep psychiatry and psychoanalysis close to their biological origins without imposing on them an instinctual determinism. The paradigm recognizes the scope of humanity's symbolization and provides a link between biology and history, a link essential to make if either is to be sustained.

I close with a few quotations. The first is a slogan from an eighteenth century guild—very simply: "Remember to die." Ostensibly it was a reminder to make advance funeral arrangements through the guild, but, however inadvertently, it conveys much more. The next is from the playwright Peter Weiss, who said: "Once we thought a few hundred corpses would be enough, then we said thousands were still too few; today we can't even count all the corpses everywhere you look." And the last is from Yeats:

Man is in love and loves what vanishes,
What more is there to say?

REFERENCES

Boulding, Kenneth, *The image,* Ann Arbor: Univ. of Michigan Press, 1956.

Bowlby, John, *Attachment and loss* (vol. I: Attachment), New York: Basic Books, 1969.

Cassirer, Ernst, *An essay on man,* New York: Doubleday Anchor, 1944; *The myth of the state,* New York: Doubleday Anchor, 1946; and *The philosophy of symbolic forms* (3 vol.), New Haven: Yale Univ. Press, 1953–1957.

Eliade, Marcea, *Cosmos and history: the myth of the eternal return,* New York: Harper Torchbacks, 1959.

Erikson, Erik H., *Childhood and society,* New York: Norton, 1950.

Farber, Leslie, The therapeutic despair, *The ways of the will,* New York/London: Basic Books, 1966.

Freud, Sigmund, Thoughts for the times on war and death, Standard Edition, vol. XIV, London: The Hogarth Press and the Institute of Psychoanalysis, 1957, p. 289.

Freud, S., *Civilization and its discontents,* Standard Edition, vol. XXI, 1962, p. 89.

Freud, S., Analysis of a phobia in a five-year-old boy, Standard Edition, vol. X, pp. 5–149.

Jackson, Don B. (ed.), *The etiology of schizophrenia,* New York: Basic Books, 1960. (See various chapters.)

Jung, Carl, *Modern man in search of a soul,* New York: Harcourt Brace, 1936, p. 129.

Kardiner, Abram, Traumatic neuroses of war, *American Handbook of Psychiatry,* 1959, vol. I, pp. 246–257.

Keniston, Kenneth, *Young radicals,* New York: Harcourt, Brace & Jovanovich, 1968.

Klein, Melanie, et al., *Developments in psychoanalysis,* London: The Hogarth Press, 1952.

Krupp, George R., and Bernard Kligfeld, The bereavement reaction: a cross-cultural evaluation, *Journal of Religion and Health,* vol. I, 1962, pp. 222–246.

Kuhn, Thomas, *The structure of scientific revolutions,* Chicago: Univ. of Chicago Press, Phoenix Books, 1962.

Laing, R. D., *The divided self,* Baltimore: Penguin (Pelican), 1965, p. 176.

Langer, Susanne, *Philosophy in a new key,* Cambridge: Harvard Univ. Press, 1942; *Feeling and form,* New York: Scribners, 1953; *Philosophical sketches,* Baltimore: Johns Hopkins Press, 1962; and *Mind: an essay on feeling,* Baltimore: Johns Hopkins Press, 1967.

Laski, Marghanita, *Ecstasy: a study of some secular and religious experiences,* Bloomington: Indiana Univ. Press, 1961.

Levi, Primo, *Survival in Auschwitz,* New York: Collier, 1961, p. 82.

Lifton, Robert J., *Revolutionary immortality: Mao Tse-tung and the Chinese revolution,* New York: Random House, 1968, p. 10.

Lifton, Robert J., *Death in life,* New York: Random House, 1968, pp. 540–541.

Lifton, Robert J., Protean man, *Partisan Review,* Winter 1968, vol. 35, 1:13–27; *History and Human Survival,* New York: Random House, 1970, pp. 311–331; and *Archives of General Psychiatry,* April 1971, **24**:298–304.

Lifton, Robert J., Experiments in advocacy research, *Research and relevance,* vol. XXI of *Science and psychoanalysis,* J. H. Masserman (ed.), pp. 259–271. Also in the academy newsletter of The American Academy of Psychoanalysis, Feb. 1972, vol. 16, no. 1, pp. 8–13.

Lifton, Robert J., *Home from the war: Vietnam veterans, neither victims nor executioners,* New York: Simon & Schuster, 1973.

Lifton, Robert J., *The broken connection,* ms., chapter on "Death and Psychiatry."

Rank, Otto, *Will therapy,* New York: Knopf, 1950.

Rank, Otto, *Beyond psychology,* New York: Dover reprint, 1958, p. 64.

Searles, Harold, Schizophrenia and the inevitability of death, *Psychiatric Quarterly,* 1961, **35**:631–665.

Stekel, Wilhelm, *Nervous anxiety states and their treatment* (trans. Rosalie Ga-

bler), New York: Dodd Mead & Co., 1923, as cited in Jacques Choron, *Modern man and mortality,* New York: Macmillan, 1964, p. 131.

Teicher, Joseph D., "Combat fatigue" or "death anxiety neurosis," *Journal
of Nervous and Mental Disease,* 1953, **117**:234–242.

Weisman Avery, and Thomas Hackett, Predilection to death: death and
dying as a psychiatric problem, *Psychosomatic Medicine,* May–June
1961, vol. 33, no. 3.

16

LAW FOR THOSE WHO ARE TO DIE

THOMAS L. SHAFFER

ROBERT E. RODES, JR.

Law serves order by serving people. Every living person will someday take his or her place among the dead. Law, in its service to those who are living, serves those who seek to take their place among the dead. The living have social and personal interests in living things. They are interested, for themselves and others, in life, liberty, and the pursuit of happiness. Arguments from (or for) the living will tend to appeal to social policy or personal comfort—the law should arrange people's affairs so that the suffering will suffer less, so that those who pursue happiness may pursue it more effectively, so that the broad enterprises of society will continue to serve citizens. One who prepares to take his place among the dead aims to appropriate death and to transcend it. He seeks postmortem influence, a place in history, an identity which death will not destroy. The law of inheritance repeatedly illuminates these differing human dispositions, but other sorts of law—corporation and family law, for example—contain the distinction as well.

THE PHILANTHROPIST AND THE SYSTEM

James B. Duke, as one of the living, brought heat and light to much of the southeastern United States and considerable personal comfort to himself. In his old age, he lent his fortune and his name to Duke University. It is probably fair to say that building an academic monument to himself was his way to seek a place among the dead—among those who are gone but not forgotten. He also left behind him a formidable industrial empire, part of which was the Duke Power Company. That, too, might be fairly regarded as promising him a place among the dead.

Mr. Duke sought to tie the two enterprises together by provisions in his will that trustees of a significant part of the funds for Duke University were required to keep most of their assets in stock of the Duke Power Company. We may suppose that his tying the power company and the university together in this fashion gave added assurance of his place among the dead by providing for the mutual health of his two institutions: the power company was to support the university and the university was to keep the power company in business.

The trust was established in 1924. By 1963, the trustees were moved to notice that the American economy, the state of electric power in North Carolina, the nature and size of Duke University, and many other things, had changed. They began to feel that the trust for Duke University would be more productive (and therefore better calculated to serve the purposes of the living) if it were invested more widely—especially if it were invested in business enterprises which would grow as the Duke Power Company had grown before World War II, but was no longer growing. They sought judicial permission to depart from the instructions in Mr. Duke's will. The court denied the petition, because Mr. Duke's instructions had not proved so perilous that the purposes of the trusts were threatened. Mr. Duke's place among the dead was entitled to reasonable protection, particularly if the purposes of the living were not clearly threatened by judicial respect for the purposes of the dead.

The court here balanced the interests of the living against those of the dead. This is the essential work of the law of inheritance (wills, trusts, death taxation, etc.), as it builds on and restricts the essential human instinct for resolving death through property. In our own system, we have chosen particular ways to go about this task. We support (as the living) a state of affairs in which we can benefit materially from the property of those who are no longer among us. We support (as the dead[1]) a system which survives because it exploits the property of dead citizens. The choice is not inevitable. There is an Indian culture in Arizona in which a dead man's possessions are buried with his corpse. In that culture, no one is wealthy. The living choose to begin anew with every generation, the dead to carry their effects into the next world rather than leave them as memorials.

In any event, the first purpose of a system of inheritance is order. It is a choice made by the living. Government seeks to impose order on the division of the things the law protected for the dead person while he or she was alive. Order is also a choice made by those who seek a place among the dead, because it implies perservation. Death and property are all tied up in this concern for order. Some of the most precarious moments in the order of a family (the living) or a nation (the dead) are provided by the crises that death brings to ownership and power. Such a crisis may involve a fight over grandma's china. Or it may involve a Hundred Years' War.

The second purpose of a system of inheritance is the support of the dead person's dependents. This is a purpose of the living, who have need of support, and of those who seek a place among the dead through their posterity. This purpose has deep psychological roots. You can feel the roots when you talk to an effective life insurance salesperson. The maintenance of a support relationship is of crucial human concern from a psychological, anthropological, or attitudinal point of view. Loss of the support relationship would diminish the life of the person lost. Maintaining the support

---

[1] Here and throughout this chapter, we are using the term *the dead* to refer not to dead people, but to living people concerned with their place among the dead—i.e., the place they will occupy in the world's life and thought after they die.

relationship after the death of a provider—either through carrying out the provider's wishes or through frustrating them—is a principal way in which the law promises reconciliation with unavoidable death.

There are two sides to the point. The indefinite provision of support, support which will continue even after the provider is dead, is a step toward immortality; it is a way to take one's place among the dead. (We say that somewhat tentatively, since we belive it is something more than that.) The provision of support is also a moral imperative. Moral bread-winners provide for their offspring; it is immoral to refuse to do so. (Mr. Duke should not have denied all benefit of his wealth to his own family, and he did not do so. He would not have been admired if he had tried.) This moral imperative about breadwinners, a purpose of the living, is therefore legally and *morally* applicable, even after the breadwinner dies. A primer for life insurance salespeople notes that "the prospect buys because he will feel guilty . . . if he doesn't buy."

The third purpose of a system of inheritance is to inhibit the growth of private wealth and to raise revenue for governmental purposes. It is a purpose largely of the living, since it tends to distribute wealth among citizens without regard for the ongoing projects of those who assembled it.

The fourth purpose of a system of inheritance is to encourage the aggregation of wealth and the growth and vigor of the private economy. One of the most significant inducements to investment in economic growth in the United States, for example, is the fact that the death of an investor defeats the income tax on capital gains. Until 1977, those who received the dead person's property took, as the tax lawyers say, a "stepped-up basis." A share of stock which cost the breadwinner of the family $10 passed to an offspring worth $200, and neither breadwinner nor offspring paid income tax on the gain.

This loophole encouraged the breadwinner to invest in parts of the economy which could grow (or shrink)—that is, in the more speculative quarters of the investment market. That is a purpose of the living. It encouraged them, as well, to retain their investment all their life, lending stability to the enterprise they invested in (also a purpose of the living) and providing fortune for their posterity (a purpose of the dead).

These four purposes of a system of inheritance—order, support, the inhibition of private power, and the encouragement of wealth—are not consistent, any more than a person who simultaneously rages against the dying of the light and lays himself down for a gentle sleep is consistent in his own purposes. The law serves both the living and the dead.

Of course, systems of property law take death into account in cultur-ally diverse ways. Property law sometimes regards death as cessation, as the end, and sometimes regards it as transition rather than cessation. The practical difference is that property systems which regard death as cessation tend to fail; they tend to be uncertain and evaded. Property law systems which regard death as transition tend not to fail: that is, they tend not to be evaded, and they tend to be predictable. The difference is therefore not fanciful, but neither is it eschatological (although systems of inheritance which regard death as transition are paralleled in poetry and myth on the one hand and in theology on the other). In social, economic, and therefore legal, terms, inheritance governs conduct toward death. Death has a universal effect on conduct. No one lives without reference to his or her death; no one lives without property; and therefore a jurisprudence which talks of property ownership in those who are to die talks as universally as the law is ever able to talk.

THE SPENDTHRIFT AND THE DEAD HAND

An example of this legal focus, and of the historical development of the law of testaments (wills, etc.), is the manipulation of the living through restrictions stated in a trust. The issue begins, as most American property law does, in England.

Saunders v. Vautier Richard Wright's will set up a trust for his minor grandson, Daniel Wright Vautier. Two thousand shares in East India stock were to be held by the trustee until Vautier's twenty-fifth birthday. Vautier was entitled to the dividends from the stock until the whole amount was to become payable to him. If he died before age 25, the stock was to be paid to his executor. No one else had a property interest in the stock. When Daniel reached the age of majority (21), he sued in the British courts to have the stock turned over to him. He argued that the stock was being held for him, that he was an adult, and, therefore, that he ought to have it. He said he *owned* the stock in the baldest test of ownership—no one else had or could have a claim to it which stood higher than his. Two levels of the English judiciary, in 1841, agreed with Daniel, and he was paid 4 years sooner than his grandfather meant for him to be paid. Daniel had, Lord Langdale said, "an absolute indefeasible interest" and therefore a right to waive protections instituted for his own benefit.

Broadway National Bank v. Adams The Supreme Judicial Court of Massachusetts decided to depart from the English rule. Charles Adams's brother left Adams's family $75,000. Trustees under the brother's will here were ordered to pay the income from that amount to Charles, and, after Charles's death, to continue the income payments to Charles's wife. The principal amount, after both died, was to be paid to Charles's children. One may suppose that the brother felt about Charles and his wife as Richard Wright felt about Daniel Vautier's first 4 years of majority. Adams in any case directed that Charles's income be "free from the interference or control of his creditors, my intention being that the use of said income not be anticipated by assignment." This is a classic version of the spendthrift clause. The English courts, loyal to the Saunders principle, held that such a clause in a will was void with respect to income payable to a beneficiary. But where the English judges talked of Daniel Vautier's "absolute and indefeasible interest," those in Massachusetts said that "the founder of the trust" (Adams's brother, long since dead) was "the absolute owner of his property," with an "entire right to dispose of it . . . as he saw fit."

As one might suppose, Charles Adams had apparently lived beyond his means. The plaintiff in the case was not Charles but a creditor of his, a bank. The bank argued in effect that no one should be allowed to own something (here Charles's right to income) his creditors could not reach (and that was the rule in England). The Massachusetts judges said Charles did not own anything creditors could reach, which, beyond begging the question, was to say that Adams's dead brother owned whatever it was that Charles's creditors might have reached, if Charles, rather than his dead brother, had owned it. Since someone has to own the "absolute and indefeasible" thing which creditors can reach, the dead brother must be seen to have withheld that thing, and, since he hadn't given it to anyone else, he must, even in death, have still had it. The judges said of the dead brother, using the present tense, "He has the entire jus disponendi . . . the creditor . . . cannot . . . take more than he was given. . . . The donor has not seen fit to give the property to the creditor, but has left it out of his reach."

There is in Anglo-American property law a dogma of electricity, a kind of flow-of-interest concept (the old cases called it "seisin"), which requires that answerability for property must always be somewhere. It is easy to take the tradition on its own terms and to say that the Massachusetts rule on spendthrift trusts turns on ownership by the dead. [There were a couple of instances in seventeenth century English property law in which seisin could not be accounted for, and the judges said that it must be "in nubibus" (clouds) or "in gremio legis" (the bosom of the law).]

The idea that the dead own property is a shade jocular or sarcastic, because we all suppose that you can't take it with you. Modern law students scoff in this vein at cases where the testator is allowed to require the legatee to marry a gentile Protestant, or to use the legacy only for a college education, and medieval English legislators were moved to denounce a "dead hand" in the control of property by ecclesiastical corporations. That the dead own is a concept born more of indignation than of analysis. It is supposed to be absurd to conceive of dead people owning things, and therefore the concept condemns itself.

It would be better for analysis to identify the concept accurately in the first place. The concept is one of *ownership in those who seek to prepare a place for themselves among the dead*. It is a concept of ownership which takes death into account and allows the person who is to die *to acquire* and *to plan* with reference to death. It is not altogether flamboyant to say that American trust law, as it was developed by nineteenth century Massachusetts judges, allows a person to own his or her death, to make of it an experience rather than an occurrence. It is possible to justify their rule (and it became the rule almost everywhere else in the United States) in behavioral and economic terms, some of which would have been abhorrent to them. One of these arguments is an argument for the dead and one an argument for the living.

A broadened experience for persons is a worthy objective of the law. Since we are all property owners, and are all among those who will die, the law might laudably encourage us to plan for death, to make death our own. It is reasonable of John Denver to sing, "I would like to be around when I die." Who wouldn't? And if law can give me a little of that experience, by letting me live on, for a little while, in my things, it should do it. Massachusetts property law, which still dominates the United States, tended in the era of *Broadway National Bank v. Adams* to allow a property owner to defraud his wife, starve his children, pollute the environment, and exploit those who worked on his land. It was a small thing, in that economy, to let the owner seem to retain a little of his Puritan clout when he went beyond the great divide. Planning for death—being able to plan with property—makes death less fearsome. That is reason enough for the development of American trust rules.

Most rationalizations of American capitalism tend to encourage acquisition. A traditional defense of acquisition would probably say that the soil's best fertilizer is the footstep of the person who owns it; that responsible civil discourse turns on the assumption of the burdens of ownership; or even that private ownership is required by something in human nature. A welfare-state defense might say that acquisition is what makes social welfare and distribution of wealth possible. Both rationalizations are arguments of the living. The law is inclined to encourage acquisition—either because it is good to get or because tax revenues from the getter are needed so that the state can do worthwhile things. It is reasonable to suppose that acquisition will be encouraged if the acquirer can direct what is to be done with his property when he dies. It is therefore better to have a legal policy which encourages acquisition than one which doesn't.

If not better, it is at least more consonant with what people seem to want. There is curious support for that conclusion in the fact that English lawyers commonly get spendthrift-trust results within the *Saunders v. Vautier* rule by using trusts which do not define ownership. (For example, one can say "principal to Daniel when he is 25," or "income to Daniel but he cannot assign it," and risk failure; or one can say "as much to Daniel as the trustees want to give him" and get the same result without risk. The English have solved consequent conceptual problems by making the trustee the owner of the property.)

It is also possible to fashion arguments against spendthrift trusts from purposes of the living. Money should be spent or retained by those who are able to benefit from it. If that is not done, there seems to be little reason not to bury wealth with the corpse. These arguments become especially compelling when the creditor laying claim to funds held for the beneficiary of a spendthrift trust is a public agency which has assisted the beneficiary, or the beneficiary's dependents, or one whom the beneficiary has injured. These pressures probably account for:

1. Case law which makes exceptions to the prevailing rules for special classes of claimants, or which construes the beneficiary to include dependents and those who provide minimal support

2. Case law which permits trusts to be limited to the provision of support or to amounts set in the discretion of the trustee, even where spendthrift trusts are not permitted

3. A statutory scheme in New York which makes spendthrift clauses ineffective as to dependents and certain other appealing creditors

4. A statutory scheme in Arizona which dissolves spendthrift restrictions, regardless of what the trust document says, when the beneficiary can demonstrate that he or she is no longer in need of protection

These resolutions of the tension between the living and those who plan their place among the dead suggest that ownership rests generally with the living, but parental concern (as opposed to a desire to control the living) may justify recognizing some measure of ownership in the dead.

THE COMPANY AND THE IMMORTALS

Somewhat similar tensions affect our law of corporations. In our day, the portraits of bygone leaders are apt to hang on the walls of corporate boardrooms rather than those of inherited mansions. Many a manager or even factory worker has sought a place among the dead in the continuing identity of Otto's Brewery or Acme Tool and Die. The business corporation was developed to enable people to amass capital for economic development—a purpose of the living. People invested in it to make money—another purpose of the living. But it began early to attract transcendent loyalties, and to serve the Fords and Carnegies as vehicles for writing their particular vision large on society—purposes of the dead.

As early as 1919, the Ford Motor Company was making vats of cash, most of which Henry Ford wanted to spend on expanding production and lowering prices, on putting more and more people in Fords. One of his stockholders, Dodge, wanted to take it all home in the form of dividends. Dodge's desire was surely a purpose of the living. Ford had an altruistic motive, no doubt, but it was the continuation of *his* altruism he envisaged—a purpose, in great part, of the dead. Dodge, after losing a lawsuit, sold out and brought out his own car; his name lives on among the good guys in white hats. But it is apparent that Dodge and his successors ultimately subscribed to Ford's instincts about family destiny; assuring the continuity of the enterprise in generations to come continues to be a valid purpose of corporate management, and one for which corporations can legitimately withhold dividends from stockholders now living.

Continuity means growth, and growth means expansion. In our mature economy, expansion often means absorbing other enterprises. This kind of expansion furnishes one of the great debates in modern corporate law. Should the famous names and local landmarks of the past century of entrepreneurship be permitted to merge their identities into the great corporate blobs of Associated Industries or I.T.T.? Many people feel the larger unit makes for greater efficiency—a purpose of the living. Others feel that there is no compensation for the loss of units which several generations of hard work—on the part of the dead—have gone into building up. The argument is curiously like that over the absorption of feudal authority into the absolute monarchy of eighteenth-century France. When the kings had shown that there was no need for counts and barons, the people had little trouble showing that there was no need for kings. When the multiplicity of business entities are absorbed into one great conglomerate, it will be hard to argue that that conglomerate should not be the state.

The point is illustrated by a law office example of corporate planning, called among teachers of lawyering skills "The Case of the Frustrated President":

Sidney spent 30 years of time and energy building a prosperous manufacturing business. As he grew in age and became nostalgic about his disappearing leisure, he decided to collect his gains and retire. His first idea was to sell his business to charity, but his lawyers—members of a large, business-oriented firm—advised him that the federal income tax consequences of that choice were bad; two other schemes for sale of the business also failed to work out, both because legal advice was discouraging. Sidney finally decided to accept an offer from a larger concern. The plan was that his company would be acquired, in an attractive stock-trade scheme, by a national concern of good reputation. Having agreed in principle with officers of the larger business, Sidney brought his lawyers into the case.

They tried to cool the negotiations with three warnings: (1) Sidney, even though he planned to remain nominally at the head of his own company, would become an employee of a largely impersonal concern; (2) he was too young and active (at 55) to retire; and (3) he did not really know much about the business organization he was joining; he knew its commercial reputation, but he did not know how he would feel as part of it.

Sidney had ample early opportunity to back out, but he did not take advantage of it. He had a second opportunity when tax rulings proved to take a long time, but his choice survived the delay. Finally, at the eleventh hour, the deal had to be renegotiated because of a fall in value of the acquiring stock, but Sidney endured the renegotiation. His company was, after 3 years, acquired, and Sidney became the president of a wholly owned subsidiary.

Sidney then learned that the acquirer had also taken over one of his local competitors; the head of the competitor became Sidney's superior. The management of the large company ignored Sidney's ideas about the business; although he was a director, he found that he had no power. Although the national company did well, Sidney's old company lost money and was not regarded as a significant part of the national enterprise.

Sidney's lawyer, looking at his client about 3 years after the acquisition, felt vindicated in warning Sidney not to make the deal. And he felt this even in the face of the fact that Sidney came out of it with $3 million in cash and few serious business responsibilities. Sidney, the lawyer said then, "is basically an unhappy man. . . . The best explanation he can give . . . is that his old business is the one that he had built up from the start, and it's like a child that is dying or has died. A parent just does not like to see this sort of thing happen." Sidney even came to his lawyers to see if they could negotiate his reacquiring his old company; they talked him out of it. The child could not be brought back to life.

The old company was finally closed down and liquidated. Sidney, as a director of the national company, voted with the majority on that decision. He later invested his money in a series of unsuccessful ventures, and lost most of it. He died recently, unhappy and broke. From the perspective of the living, Sidney seems largely to have made the right decisions, but he lost his place among the dead.

Sidney could have retained his company and enlisted lawyers and insurance underwriters to do estate planning for him. They would have devised stock purchase agreements and similar things to assure the continuation of the company after Sidney's death. The law, especially the Internal Revenue Code, encourages that sort of enrollment by those who are to take their place among the dead. Sidney could not, though, (as an English testator once tried to do), have ordered his wealth reduced to paper money and burned. The voice of the living, who seem always to need the money, would have drowned out Sidney's attempt at that kind of immortality.

Between burning money and Sidney's indestructible corporation there are cases in which the courts either redefined a dead man's eccentric purposes or frustrated them:

Pulitzer Joseph Pulitzer left ownership of his newspapers in two trusts. Both trusts were to pay income and principal to the Pulitzer family. One of them, the principal asset of which was *The New York World,* was (unlike the other, which owned *The St. Louis Post-Dispatch*) subject to unusual restrictions on sale. The trustees were forbidden to sell *The World,* and, for all that appears in the case reports, this was the only difference between the two trusts. *The World* trustees obeyed the charge until *The World* was within 3 months of folding, and then petitioned a New York court for relief from the restrictions; the court granted their petition.

Brown Robert K. Brown, who had managed to acquire most of downtown Waterbury, Connecticut, provided by trust in his will that none of his land could be used for buildings more than three stories high, and that those which were higher than that "shall not be repaired above the third story, but all stories above the third shall be condemned and removed." His trustees petitioned the Connecticut court for relief from the restriction; their petition was granted.

Although the courts in *Pulitzer* and *Brown* reached similar results, they reasoned differently. The difference is one of candor. The New York court pretended that Pulitzer had not foreseen that *The World* would fall on evil days. The judge said that the purpose of the separate trust for *The World* shares was to provide money to the family; he pretended he was merely carrying out Pulitzer's purposes when he frustrated Pulitzer's wishes: "A man of his sagacity and business ability could not have intended that from mere vanity, the publication of the newspapers, with which his name and efforts had been associated, should be persisted in until the entire asset was destroyed or wrecked by bankruptcy or dissolution." The Connecticut court did not try to argue that Brown had not meant what he said; it simply held that he had gone too far: "The restrictions militate too strongly against the interests of the beneficiaries and the public welfare to be sustained, particularly when it is remembered that they are designed to benefit no one, and are harmful to all persons interested, and we hold them invalid as against public policy."

"Wills are noxious things," Rex Stout's Nero Wolfe said. "It is astonishing, the amount of mischief a man's choler may do long after the brain cells which nourished the choler have rotted away." The likelihood is that Joseph Pulitzer did want his trustees to ride *The World* all the way down, and a modern observer, nostalgic for cities where the sun shines on the streets, might find more public benefit than the Connecticut judges did in Brown's will. But in both cases the welfare of the living was seen as unduly restricted by the purposes of the dead. Both cases call to mind the testator in Pittsburgh, who, fearing that no one would care for his beloved dogs as well as he had, ordered the dogs destroyed at his death. The probate judge forbade the executor to carry out that order.

THE FAMILY AND THE FUTURE

In what we call family law, the purposes of the living in providing comfort, companionship, economic security, and sexual satisfaction (themselves not always compatible) have clashed from time immemorial with the purposes of the dead in securing a posterity, carrying on the family name, increasing the family wealth, continuing the family business, or whatever. Out of this clash grow a number of the policy questions with which the law deals. How far do we allow parents to control their children's education? A great deal, because they have their thoughts and values to hand down? Or very little, because after all the children have their own lives to live, and their own world to live them in? How seriously do we take marriage settlements? Seriously, because the parties are providing for the indefinite future? Or lightly, because the future is unpredictable, and the present is what matters? On what grounds do we allow divorce? Disloyalty of one party to the dynastic purposes of the other? Or failure of the parties to get along?

An example is the case where divorce is sought, or defended against, because one of the spouses has refused to have children. In states where divorce is still based on the "fault" of one of the parties, "desertion" is generally recognized as one of the kinds of fault for which a divorce can be had, and an unjustifiable refusal of sexual intercourse is recognized as a form of desertion, even though the offending spouse continues to live in the house, cook the meals, bring home the paycheck, or whatever. With the law in this condition, a case occasionally comes up in which a husband or wife is willing to have intercourse, but insists on using a contraceptive every time. Is this a refusal of intercourse, and so desertion, and so ground for divorce?

It depends, obviously, on what you think of marriage. Mutual comfort, companionship, sexual satisfaction, the shared expression of love—all the customary purposes of the living—can be served about as well with contraceptives as without. If you enjoy children, having them may itself be a purpose of the living, but no more an essential one than living near the sea, going to the theater, or any of the other interests you would like to share with your spouse.

It is as a purpose of the dead that procreation enters into the very essence of the marriage relation. You see your children not only as a continuation of your physical being but also as a continuation of your activities and outlooks, and a fulfillment of your long-range aspirations. A court looking at these purposes might well feel that frustrating them constituted a total abandonment of the marriage. As one might expect, considerations of this kind were more persuasive to the Victorians than they are to us. Old cases tend to hold that the refusal to have children amounts to desertion; recent ones tend to hold that it does not.

One of the things you have children for is to teach them what you believe in, so that things you consider important will not pass from the scene when you do—a purpose of the dead. But your children will have their own lives to live, and must be prepared to live them in their own way—a purpose of the living. There is a certain tension between these two purposes, and if you resolve that tension in a different way from the rest of society, you are apt to hear about it from the Welfare Department, the truant officer, or the police.

So it was that the decision of the Old Order Amish not to send their children to high school ran afoul of the compulsory education laws in most states. The Amish felt that a high school education had nothing to offer a person who was to live in the Amish manner, and might well turn him or her to live in some other way. Of course, they were right: The American high school plays a central part in the acculturation process of the mainstream. Accordingly, a number of civil liberties advocates were not willing to support the Amish claim that their freedom of religion was violated when they were required to send their children to school. They were concerned about the right of the children to grow up with open options—a purpose of the living—whereas the Amish were claiming the right of parents to pass on their own life-styles to another generation—a purpose of the dead.

The Supreme Court, in *Wisconsin v. Yoder,* decided in favor of the parents, without going too far into the theory. A majority seemed to think high school was not as important as it was cracked up to be. Justice Douglas suggested that the children did not much want to go to school either. This generation of judges, preoccupied as most of us are with purposes of the living, is not apt to take a firm stand on parental rights. A couple of generations ago, it would have been generally recognized that part of everyone's constitutionally protected freedom was the freedom to decide what his or her children were to grow up to be.

THE WRITER AND THE TRUTH

A final example is freedom of expression. Do we allow people to express their thoughts freely because they need to give permanent form to their ideas (a purpose of the dead), or is it because we wish to insure the prevalence of good ideas (a purpose of the living)? Whenever we pass on questions of who is entitled to say what, and through what media—a good deal of a constitutional law course is devoted to these questions—we have this underlying dichotomy in the back of our minds. The issue tends to come up in the current debate over a reporter's right to protect his or her sources.

Grand juries, courts, legislative committees, and a good many other public agencies are entitled to ask ordinary citizens what they know about matters of public concern, and where they learned it. These persons can get into no end of trouble if they fail to respond. Hence, if a vigorous public servant reads in the newspaper that his favorite columnist has just had a guided tour of a letter bomb factory, or knows the names of eight police captains that are on the take, he is apt to call in the columnist and ask questions. The columnist will point out, reasonably enough, that he would not learn all these interesting facts if he could not be relied on to keep certain crucial details to himself. Then the ordinary citizen would never find out about the scope of crime and subversion in the community. The judge or office-holder, unimpressed with this argument, then begins to rattle the keys of the jailhouse, and speak of contempt. The columnist appeals for protection to the constitutional guarantee of a free press.

There is a certain intellectual leap in this argument. The freedom to publish information in your possession does not inescapably entail the freedom to assemble further information in order to publish it. But the columnist argues from the purpose of the constitutional provision. We protect a free press, he says, in order to safeguard "the public's right to know." Hence, the protection must extend to the whole process by which the public is informed.

This argument conceives a free press as a purpose of the living. Wisdom will be reached by an informed citizenry fortified by a thorough airing of public problems and proposed solutions to them. There is an alternative view of what a free press is for. It might be considered as aimed at protecting the right of a person to objectify, communicate, and, to some extent, perpetuate, what is on his or her mind. This can be considered a purpose of the dead. It is a matter of launching your thoughts as a projection of yourself, thoughts being less ephemeral than individuals.

The law of freedom of the press tends to favor the interpretation of it as a purpose of the dead. The columnist is not allowed to refuse to answer questions (though some legislatures are in the process of changing the law on this point). Similarly, constitutional protection is not extended to commercial advertising as it is to other publication—presumably because it is your pocketbook, not your mind, that is involved. And again, the Supreme Court cases on obscenity seem to envisage a right to communicate what is on your mind, even if sex is, rather than a serious concern with making the latest sexual data available to a waiting public. There is talk, to be sure, about "redeeming social importance," but it tends to be secondary to talk about "serious artistic purpose."

Only in libel cases do purposes of the living seem to predominate. You can say almost anything you wish about a politician, and the court will protect you from libel suits—because the courts feel that the broadest scrutiny will insure the best possible candidates for office. This purpose outweighs the politician's interest in his reputation, which tends to be a purpose of the dead. But you cannot make so free with a totally private person, for there is no public interest beyond mere curiosity in bringing his foibles to light.

SYNTHESIS: THE LAW OF THE DYING

These examples—from the Amish farmer who seeks to perpetuate a way of life to Duke who desired to maintain the association between his business self and his philanthropic self—present a fundamental tension between living and dying within the context of human relationships. The relationships themselves, in our view, suggest a synthesis for the cases and a principle upon which the law can decide issues presented by people wo are to die.

One who buys life insurance for the care of his dependents seeks to provide in death what he provides in life—willingly seeks that result, out of care and out of a joy in a companionship neither he nor his closest companions in life would care to do without. So of the Amish parent, whose love for his child causes him to wish for the child a life in association with what the parent, as one of the living, wishes for himself. So of James B. Duke, who sought health in his business and in his university with the same breath which he sought health for himself.

We see this as a *law of the dying*. It is a legal synthesis in terms of other people and their companionship in life and in death. In each of the areas of the law which we have considered here, it offers a characteristic approach. In inheritances, it gives primary consideration to the decedent's last gestures of affection for those who have accompanied him on his journey, and to the arrangements for discharging the moral obligations left behind. In the corporation, it supports neither a dream nor a meal ticket, but a matrix of personal relations among people engaged in a common enterprise, and between members of the community and those who serve them. It conceives of free speech and a free press as vehicles for mutual encouragement and support among those who go through life and face death together, and as a means for their sharing of experiences. In the family, it looks for a mingling of life stories, begun in dialogue and ended in company, and for a context in which new life stories can begin.

John Hersey's novel, *The Wall*, presents an example: An old married couple are in a queue before a Nazi officer who is dividing Jews from the Warsaw Ghetto into two groups—one bound for the work camp and one for the furnaces. The old couple bicker with one another, even in these circumstances, as they have bickered for years. When they reach the officer, the old man is sent to the work group and the old woman to the death group. They stop bickering because they are no longer together. After several moments, the old man looks, from his status of salvation, at his condemned wife. And then he walks over and joins her, and they resume bickering. They end their lives in dialogue and in company.

At this point, let us put in a tabular form the three approaches we have taken up, (Table 16-1) and then let us show how our own approach, the law of the dying, would deal with the specific cases we have looked at.

THE DUKE TRUST CASE

The Duke trust case would seem to have been resolved correctly. Much of the court's rationale—and ours—turns on the fact that Duke is not long dead, that his investment restrictions proceeded from business experience gained in relationships he sought to preserve—his family, his business associates, and those who, at his philanthropic behest, gathered to begin a university. As the family descends and both business empire and university become more clearly public institutions—in other words, as human relationships which once included Duke grow dimmer—the trust should no doubt grow more impersonal. It should become a public enterprise which serves public purposes of both the living and the dead. But the purposes of the dying—of James B. Duke—remain to be carried out; they survive in living people.

Spendthrift Trust Law

The spendthrift trust law seems to us to constitute a law of the dying when it fastens on paternal purposes more than on purposes of dominance. The two are no doubt difficult to distinguish in many cases, but the trend in Arizona and in legislative and common law definitions of beneficiary seem to us to represent the right trend. The trust proceeds, however restricted, should be available to those to whom the decedent *or the beneficiary* have obligations of support (including those the beneficiary purposely or negli-

TABLE 16-1

	Law of the Living	Law of the Dead	Law of the Dying
Inheritance	Supports uses of decedent's property for maximum benefit to living persons and present social needs.	Supports uses of decedent's property to insure survival of his memory and continuity of his projects	Supports uses of decedent's property to insure maintenance of personal relations and discharge of moral obligations.
Corporations	Support industrial and commercial development and efficient distribution of goods and services.	Support continuing identity of roles and projects for those who devote themselves to business.	Support continuity of interpersonal relations with business and within community served by business.
Family Law	Supports economic benefit, companionship, and sexual satisfaction for marriage partners, plus education of children to take places in society.	Supports continuing physical, cultural, and social identity through having and rearing children.	Supports interrelation of life stories of husband and wife, and initiation of life stories of children.
Free Speech and Press	Support dissemination of ideas in hope that good ones will gain acceptance and bad ones will be less dangerous. Support dissemination of information for informed action. Support communication as essential element in social relations.	Support externalization, and hence survival, of particular individuals' thought.	Support mutual encouragement and sharing of life experiences.

gently injures), and the trust restrictions should dissolve when legitimate purposes of support are fulfilled (as in the Arizona statute).

Frustrated Presidents and Corporate Profit

Here the law should encourage and protect productive human relationships. These occur in business and appear to occur most positively in associations which are small enough to foster a person's influence over others. Mergers of small businesses into large ones no doubt carry with them an immediate economic gain—as was true in Sidney's case—but they do it, as we are finding out, at the price of creating corporate states and, very possibly, even economic decadence. Business enterprises should be encouraged to foster what people can do together, to define efficient production in moral terms, and to serve the legitimate interests of groups of persons in the community. This means that the remorseful Sidney, and Henry Ford, were right and that Sidney's lawyers and Dodge were wrong.

Eccentric Purposes

There is very little in either the candid *(Brown)* or not so candid *(Pulitzer)* judicial opinions to suggest a consideration of the human relationships which Joseph Pulitzer sought to honor and perpetuate among those who produced *The World,* or which Robert Brown valued in striving to keep the sunlight on the streets of Waterbury. A modern court would doubtless place more value on the fourth estate and on sunshine. In both cases, we think, judges considered too narrow a group of people (beneficiaries of monetary income rather than beneficiaries of the enterprise), and saw obligation as purely a matter of the support of dependents. Modern judges might more readily consider that a businessperson's obligations run as well to employees and to neighbors.

Family Cases

A family comes to be because two persons seek to write their life stories together—to make two stories mesh, as much as they can, into one. And a family grows because this new story is initiated in new lives. The initiation of the new story is a legitimate purpose of the enterprise, and therefore legitimately seen as implicit in marriage and legitimate in child rearing. We are inclined to sympathize with the spouse who, giving all consideration to changing circumstance, nonetheless seeks to have children. And we agree with the Supreme Court's decision in the Amish case—not so much because children are a means to immortality (every parent knows they are not) as because a person's most fundamental philosophy of life is likely to be the best he or she has to give children, the best a parent can do to satisfy an obligation to initiate a new life story with honesty and with hope.

Free Press

We live among cataclysmic metaphors on reading—among knowledge "explosions" and "deluges" from the media. The assumption, which may be true, is that a person is what he reads, sees, and hears. Assuming all of this, the law should, we think, encourage what people can do to support one another and to foster hope together. (It is evident that people are more hopeful together than they are apart.) The best reason for free speech is neither political progress nor self-expression but the fact that people grow better and grow together when they communicate. The best reason for a free press is that it can assist in the enterprise and that its suppression tends to suppress the enterprise. A theory of personal liberty focused in this fashion would probably not disagree with modern free speech decisions very much, but it would emphasize, more than they have emphasized (in, say, controlling obscenity), the fact that personal growth is difficult and each of us needs all the help he can get.

CONCLUSION: BIRCH TREES

Robert Frost looks at a birch tree and associates his boyhood joy in climbing such a tree with his adult need to climb up to simplicity. "It's when I'm weary of considerations," he says, ". . . I'd like to get away from earth awhile." But that thought suggests a more permanent separation than he has in mind:

> *May no fate wilfully misunderstand me*
> *And half grant what I wish and snatch me away*
> *Not to return. Earth's the right place for love;*
> *I don't know where it's likely to go better.*

Earth is the right place for love, but love—unlike the joys of ownership, perhaps—tends to transcend time. Love has a way of needing an immortality which poses no tension between the purposes of the living and the purposes of those who are to die. Love, as the late Judge Roger Kiley (paraphrasing Aquinas) said, is helping someone else to grow, and the demands of growth are insistent to the lover as living and as dead.

Life is a lonely and difficult journey for most of us. Its comforts are for the most part in accepting other people and having other people accept us. Acceptance comes hard, though—so hard that the occasions when we accept and are accepted at the same time are probably the best life has to offer. Such occasions give joy to the living and hope to those who are to be dead. And the result makes all of the world, and all of life, better. Law cannot create these occasions, but it can encourage, protect, and cherish them. In doing so, it is a law for the dying. As John Denver's song says:

> *I hope that you will think of me in moments*
> *when you're happy and you're smiling.*

> *That the thought will comfort you on cold and*
> *cloudy days if you're crying,*

> *That you'll love to see the sun go down*

> *And the world go around. . . .*

REFERENCES

Branzburg v. Hayes, 403 U.S. 665 (1972).

Briggs, J., The psychology of successful persuasion, *Chartered Life Underwriter Journal,* April 1967, p. 49; July 1967, p. 59; April 1968, p. 51.

Broadway National Bank v. Adams, 133 Mass. 170 (1882).

Cantrell v. Forest City Publishing Co., 43 *United States Law Week* 4079 (1974).

"The Case of the Frustrated President," in Freeman, H. (ed.), *Legal interviewing and counseling,* St. Paul, Minn.: West Publishing Co., 1963.

Cocke v. Duke University, 131 S.E.2d 909 (North Carolina 1963), noted in 1964 *Duke Law Journal* 184.

Colonial Trust Co. v. Brown, 105 Conn. 261, 125 Atl. 555 (1926).

Denver, J., "Around and around," recorded on the album "Poems, prayers, and promises," R.C.A. Records (Cherry Lane Music Co.), 1971.

Dodge v. Ford Motor Co., 204 Mich. 459, 170 N.W. 668 (1919).

Dunne, J., *A search for God in time and memory,* New York: Macmillan, 1969.

Frost, R., "Birches," in *The pocket book of Robert Frost's poems,* New York: Pocket Library, 1956.

Goody, J., *Death, property, and the ancestors,* Stanford, Cal.: Stanford Univ. Press, 1962.

Gray, J., *Restrictions on the alienation of property,* 2d ed., Boston: Boston Book Co., 1895.

Hersey, J., *The wall,* New York: Knopf, 1950.

Judge Kiley's remark is oral history—from the eulogy at his funeral mass, September 9, 1974, in Chicago.

Mandlebaum v. McDonell, 29 Mich. 77 (1874).

The marriage cases: *Rosner v. Rosner,* 108 N.Y.S.2d 196 (1951); *Penovic v. Penovic,* 387 P.2d 501 (Calif. 1955); *Kober v. Kober,* 16 N.Y.2d 191, 211 N.E.2d 817 (1965); Annot., 25 *American Law Reports (second series)* 928.

Paris Adult Theatre I v. Slaton, 413 U.S. 9 (1973).

In re Pulitzer's Estate, 29 N.Y. Supp. 87 (Surrogate 1931).

A rationale for the spendthrift trust, 64 *Columbia Law Review* 1232 (1964).

Rodes, R., Jr., *The legal enterprise,* Notre Dame: Univ. of Notre Dame Press, 1976.

Saunders v. Vautier, 4 Beav. 115, 49 English Reports 282 (1841).

Shaffer, T. *Death, property, and lawyers,* Cambridge: Dunellen, 1970.

Shaffer, T., *Planning and drafting wills and trusts,* note 32, pp. 242–245 (sources on spendthrift trusts); Appendix two, pp. 260–262 (New York and Arizona statutes), Mineola, N.Y.: Foundation Press, 1972.

Shaffer, T., *Legal interviewing and counseling in a nutshell,* St. Paul, Minn.: West Publishing Co., 1976.

Shaffer, T., *Law for the innocent: On being a Christian and a lawyer* (in press).

Shneidman, E., Orientations toward cessation: a reexamination of current modes of death, *Journal of Forensic Sciences,* **13:**33, 1968.

State newsman's privilege statutes, *Notre Dame Lawyer,* **49:**150, 1973.

Stout, R., *The red box,* New York: Farrar and Reinhart, 1937.

Tannenbaum, R. and S. A. Davis, Values, man, and organizations, *Industrial Management Review,* **10:**67, 1969.

Valentine v. Christenson, 316 U.S. 52 (1942).

Wisconsin v. Yoder, 406 U.S. 205 (1972).

17

DEATH AND MODERN POETRY

MICHAEL A. SIMPSON

I n the first part of the twentieth century during a period of un-
precedented carnage, humanity devoted much of its spare time to
diligently overturning manifestations of the previous era's taboos
regarding sex. In the latter part of the century amid relatively
unbridled expression of sex, we have been busily demystifying
and trying to find ways of coming to terms with the twin taboo—death. As
once with sex, so now with death, we laboriously rediscover that everyone
else seems to do it, too, and that it feels better if we can talk about it. The
trend is now well established in many countries, though especially prominent and well organized in America. Death, once almost an un-American
activity, has emerged as a minor industry. This does not mean that we are
necessarily becoming more accepting of death, but that as counterphobic
defenses become relatively more popular than straightforward denial, it is
becoming increasingly profitable to cater to the current counterphobic
interest in the subject. The growth of a death literature in recent years has
been a phenomenon unequalled in recent literary or publishing history.
Similar in quantity (though not, in the main, in quality) to the death
genres in medieval and Victorian literature, several dozen books a year
have been produced in the last few years, until a Thanatology Book Service or Death-Of-The-Month Club seems menacingly likely. In modern
poetry, too, death has become a more insistent motif. Yet although death
has been a continuing theme in literature, there have been relatively few
formal studies of this (Griessmair, 1966; Fiedler, 1960; Hoffman, 1964;
Valdez, 1964; Weber, 1971), and such as exist are often so obscure and
self-absorbed as to border on the mercifully incomprehensible.

DEATH AND THE POET

Death and love are probably the two most consistent themes in poetry
through the ages. From the very earliest times, poets of every race and
nation have dealt with aspects of death—indeed, some of the very earliest
known poetry, such as the various Creation myths (be they African, Mel-
anesian, Norse, or Eskimo) seek to explain how death came to earth.

In the period up to the Middle Ages the great romances and *chansons
de geste, La Chanson de Roland, Tristan et Iseult,* and the *Morte d'Arthur,* or its
earlier form, *La Mort d'Artus,* exemplified the proper way to die. "Know ye
well," said Gawain, "that I shall not live two days." Knowing and calm,
he prepared for death according to custom, and in a manner not unlike
the recently lauded ideal of acceptance. One removed one's weapons, lay
down with crossed hands—*gisant*—and awaited death. One expressed appropriately one's recollection of people and things one had loved—Roland

"was seized by several things to remember." During this mannered lamen-
tation, the companions would gather round the deathbed. The dying person, presiding over the ritual, would pardon them, make confession, and
after a final prayer would wait silently and patiently—and "never again
uttered a word."

By the fifteenth or sixteenth century (Dubruck, 1964; Spencer, 1930),
the poet had become more concerned with the distasteful maggotry of
physical death and decomposition, as in de Nesson's verse:

> *O carrion, who are no longer man,*
> *Who will hence keep thee company?*
> *Worms engendered by the stench*
> *Of thy vile carrion flesh.*

Two further distinctive treatments of death emerge in the works of
the early poets. An erotic relationship to death is seen intermittently, as
Eros and Thanatos meet. Just as in Bernini's *St. Theresa,* the distinction is
blurred between the swoon of orgasm and the traditional agony of death—
so erotic-morbid themes are seen in poetry as well. "The grave's a fine and
private place," and none, Marvell thought, did there embrace. Yet there's
a comfortable and easy sensuality in some of these early poets' dealings
with death.

The more common approach that began to dominate increasingly
from the seventeenth century on was rhetorical romanticism (Rehm, 1967;
van Ingen, 1966; Ayuso Rivera, 1959; Alonso, 1971; Fougeres, 1974).
Elaborate expressions of grief stated with baroque courtliness and elegance
could be of great length, but seldom conveyed any sensation of genuine
depth of emotion. Later still, this developed into the gloomy and smug
melancholy of the romantic cult of the dead. Thomas Gray's all too familiar "Elegy Written in a Country Churchyard," widely translated and imi-
tated, established the genre.

In almost every period, all the major moods are reflected in the poetry of death: grief, desolation, hope, resignation, bitterness, exhilaration,
and courage. Probably all mature adults consider the question of whether
there is any conscious existence beyond death. In the West there has been
official allegiance to the idea of personal immortality, though quite recently—as relatively few people, faced with severe crisis, act as if they were
indeed assured of an eternal life—the belief has come increasingly to represent a formality or cliché rather than a deeply felt guiding principle.
Poets have often explored this theme, arriving at widely varying conclusions. They often emphasize the enduring things which will survive—
sometimes stressing biological immortality through one's children and descendants; sometimes the social immortality derived from the continuing

impact of one's work, one's ideas, or one's writings; and occasionally immortality through a more modest acceptance of the chemical and physical survival of our bodily elements. Poets, unable to deny their own mortality, have often dwelt on the immortality of their verse. This is a recurrent claim of Shakespeare in the Sonnets, for example:

> So long as men can live or eyes can see,
> So long lives this, and this gives life to thee
>
> *(Sonnet 18)*

> Your monument shall be my gentle verse
> Which eyes not yet created shall o'er-read
>
> *(Sonnet 81)*

> Not marble nor the gilded monuments
> Or princes shall outlive this pow'rful rime
>
> *(Sonnet 55)*

Another popular mode has been to mourn the deaths of fair young ladies, wives and lovers. There is little humility in evidence: each poet has loved most perfectly the most beautiful, most sweet, most pure, and glorious woman. All very well and true, perhaps, though there are few signs of recognition that anyone else might love as deeply. Few living lovers are described as so perfect as the dead, or at least the unobtainable.

Apart from formal art forms such as the epitaph and the elegy, many poems of death through the centuries lament the death of a loved or admired person, expressing sorrow over the passing and tribute to his or her life's work. While, in a sense, all deaths may be considered premature, the death of the young is seen as especially tragic and purposeless, and has inspired some of the bitterest verse.

The universality and inevitability of death is handled with satisfaction, as poets take heart at the realization that even the tyrants and oppressors will die in time. Only in the grave, so far, have all men truly achieved equality; only there does a classless society ultimately exist.

A type of boastful acceptance of death, stressing its attractiveness and almost a longing for it, became a literary conceit adhered to over several centuries. Pierre de Ronsard wrote a poem entitled "Hymn to Death": "I salute you, blissful and profitable death"; and Henry Vaughn spoke of "dear, beauteous death, the jewel of the just." To William Wordsworth, it was "the great haven of us all"; to Stephane Mallarme, "la balsamique mort." The Romantic poets, Byron, Shelley, Novalis, and the younger Goethe exemplified this convention (Koch, 1932; Rehm, 1950; Schmidt, 1968; Unger, 1968). Shelley (Kurtz, 1933), for example, wrote a vast version of "Queen Mab" (never published) when he was 18, and dealt with death in Stanza IX:

Mild was the slow necessity of death:
The tranquil spirit failed beneath its grasp. . . .

Just five years later, by the spring of 1815, his doctors pronounced him to be dying of consumption. Though severely ill, he improved during the summer. Several of his poems of that year, like "Spirit of Solitude" and "Alastor," allude to death. "Daemon of the World" opens with:

How wonderful is Death,
Death, and his brother Sleep!

He revised a section of "Queen Mab," but changed the tense from past to the more personally apt present, and added a line on resignation, so it read:

Mild is the slow necessity of death:
The tranquil spirit fails beneath its grasp,
Without a groan, almost without a fear,
Resigned in peace to the necessity,
Calm as a voyager to some distant land,
And full of wonder, full of hope as he. . . .

John Keats, similarly ill, considered his death with more apparent regret and forlornness:

When I have fears that I may cease to be
    Before my pen has glean'd my teeming brain,
Before high-piled books, in charactery
    Hold like full garners the full ripen'd grain;
When I behold, upon night's starr'd face,
    Huge cloudy symbols of a high romance,
And think that I may never live to trace
    Their shadows, with the magic hand of chance;
And when I feel, fair creature of an hour,
    That I shall never look upon thee more, . . .
            . . . then on the shore
Of the wide world I stand alone, and think
Till love and fame to nothingness do sink.

Goethe, in "Herman and Dorothea" for instance, kept to the traditional approach

> *The touching image of death*
> *Presents no horror to the wise*
> *And does not appear as the end*
> *To the devout believer.*

By his own definition, then, he must have been neither wise nor devout, for he avoided any contact with death, and is reported to have refused to attend funerals, to have kept away from his mother and his wife when they were dying, and to have approached his own death with notable anxiety.

In the last part of the nineteenth century, as Sylvia Anthony pointed out (1973), there was a period in which adults seemed to enjoy watching a child play with the idea of death, and children were taught to recite poetry in which death was the principal theme. The English schoolchild's repertoire might include Macaulay's "Horatius" ("And how can man die better than facing fearful odds"); Byron's "The Destruction of Sennacherib" ("The Assyrian came down like a wolf on the fold") or "The Burial of Sir John Moore at Corunna" ("Not a drum was heard, not a funeral note, / As his corpse to the ramparts we carried"); and of course the sublimely silly "Casabianca" by Felicia Hemans ("The boy stood on the burning deck / Whence all but he had fled"). Many such macabre and mawkish monstrosities were incorporated in such perennial anthologies as F. W. Palgrave's *Golden Treasury,* first published in 1861, and inflicted upon generations of schoolchildren for nearly a century.

Not only clandestine parodies of these awful works but more frankly ribald verses on death were produced in the early years of the twentieth century, as taste swung away from the sentimentality of Little Nell and Little Eva and the portentously zany Gothic horrors of *Struwwelpeter* to Hilaire Belloc's *Cautionary Tales* and Graham's *Ruthless Rhymes.* All this verse, whether treating death with solemn sentimentality or satire, coincided with a very high child-mortality rate. As that rate declined, so did the theme of death in children's literature, rhymes, verse, and tales.

In Emily Dickinson (Anderson, 1960; Cody, 1971; Patterson, 1973), one begins to see the development of a more personal and distinctly modern approach to death, which is a predominant theme in her poetry. During her lifetime, she lost most of those she loved, friends and kin, and had great difficulty coping with the frequent bereavements. When she was 13, a close friend, Sophia, died. Emily was a frequent visitor during the illness, and after the death she "gave way to a fixed melancholy" and had to be sent away to relatives for a long recuperation. She seems to have repressed this experience, for when another close friend died when she was 19, she wrote of it as her first bereavement; also three years later, hearing of another death, she wrote, "Oh N. is dead—the first of my friends." Throughout her life she showed an avid curiosity about the deathbed. She sought out the most detailed account obtainable of the final moments of her friends, badgering her correspondents for the minutiae of the event. "You must tell us all you know about dear M.'s going," she would write. "Was M. willing to leave us all? I want so much to know if it was very hard." What did they say? What did they do? In "Promise this, when you be dying," she beseeches her friend to summon her to the bedside at the last.

In her poetry she approaches the subject in various ways. In "There's been a Death in the Opposite House," she describes the whole sequence of formalities from death to burial in her New England town, observing it as if peeping from behind the net curtains—and in fact her house was next to the cemetery, and she would sit and watch the funerals. In another verse, she describes with irony the smooth funeral parlours, the satin caskets, the corpses conjured by embalming into "people of pearl," the anguish muffled in the cushioned carriages. In fact, she records the progression in America toward increasing professionalization and denial of death, as the undertaker, who undertook to bury the dead, became the mortician, whose function (like the beautician) was specifically to obscure the facts of death from a society that, having lost its belief in the soul and immortality, could not bear too much reality. The mortician, in turn, became the funeral director, who (like a film director) directed a production, a basically secular ritual which might use religious trappings and decorations, but lacked in most part the beliefs that originally made the rituals meaningful and comforting.

Death as the great leveler, the ultimate democrat, was already a well-established cliché, yet Dickinson applied it, with more novelty, to the then current controversy over the emancipation of slaves. The racial distinctions, she said, are "Time's Affair" and will disappear in death, as the Chrysalis of Blonde or Umber becomes "Equal Butterfly." Several poems center on the moment of death and the deathbed scene. Indeed she is one of the last poets to accept the convention that one should gather round the dying to learn from them, perhaps to be afforded some glimpse of the life beyond.

Despite the religiosity and devoutness of her upbringing, her beliefs were severely shaken by her experience of bereavement. Sometimes she takes the traditional viewpoint. Experiencing "Death's bold Exhibition" at the graveside, she claims, helps us to realize both what we have been and what we will become. In another verse, she suggests that knowing that we shall soon cease to exist can humble us appropriately, while the knowledge that we shall exist again can exalt us—if we can believe in it, of course. Immortality and an afterlife are what she longs for, but ultimately doesn't believe in or trust. One of her most comfortable treatments of this theme is in "Because I could not stop for Death." Though she was too busy with life, Death kindly stopped for her. She takes a leisurely drive in his carriage, and recognizes that they are heading for eternity and that in a way she had always known this.

The cumulative effect of her multiple losses came when, after the loss of a friend of great importance to her, she considered that she too had died, and described her continuing existence as death in life. In "So give me back to death," she explains that she had feared death because it would deprive her of her beloved—now that life has thus deprived her, she is in the grave already. Elsewhere she writes, "My life closed twice before its close" and in another poem, "The grave my little cottage is," she lays out the "marble tea" and waits for real death and final reunion with her loved ones.

Some of the poems anticipating her own death are marred by an excess of self-pity, and elements of a more spiteful, "you'll be sorry when I'm dead" attitude. There's also the vindictive, "Mine enemy is growing old" attitude in which she rejoices in the aging of a onetime friend. One can appreciate that as a woman and as a poet she must have been deeply frustrated, writing poetry she could not publish and loving without fulfillment. Having ceased expecting much from life on earth, she came to hope for eventual gratification in a life to come. Her love poems deal mostly with celestial betrothals, and the metaphor of the funeral as a wedding to eternity occurs. In the poem that follows she uses another telling metaphor:

> *Death is the supple Suitor*
> *That wins at last*
> *It is a stealthy wooing*
> *Conducted first*
> *By pallid innuendos*
> *And dim approach*
> *But brave at last with Bugles. . . .*
> *It bears away in triumph*
> *To troth unknown.*

Perhaps the most succinct statement of her loss comes in one of her finest poems:

> *The Bustle in a House*
> *The Morning after Death*
> *Is solemnest of industries*
> *Enacted upon Earth -*
>
> *The Sweeping up the Heart*
> *And putting Love away*

We shall not want to use again
Until Eternity.

Walt Whitman (Carlisle, 1973) provides a distinct bridge between the typical approaches of nineteenth and twentieth century poets, and manages to show more consistent comfort in dealing with the facts of death. In the final section of *Leaves of Grass* he gathered poems written throughout his life dealing with parting, death, and the uncertainty of what follows. In many of them he expresses a positive belief in death as a passage or journey to a transcendental life, as in "Heavenly Death provides for all." In others, such as "Of Him I Love Day and Night," he sees death as more of a completion and an essential part of life, and finds all places to be "burial places," all "fuller of the dead than of the living." In "As the Time Draws Nigh" he speaks of his own death, when his voice will suddenly cease; he expresses some dread of the unknown, but satisfaction because he has existed positively. While in "Yet, Yet, Ye Downcast Hours" he shows a failure of confidence and frank fear. The problem of loss and bereavement is explored in "When Lilacs Last in the Dooryard Bloom'd," written on the occasion of Lincoln's death. At first he finds the death incomprehensible and threatening, and complains of the inadequacy of the routine gestures of mourning—the processions and lying in state, the dirges and flowers. They may serve to demonstrate grief and love, but they don't comfort him. Later, however, he comes to express an acceptance of death, regarding it as a bearer of peace and rest to the dead.

THE POET AT WAR

Though poets had always tended to take notice of wars, often writing suitably heroic verse to celebrate the local victor, the two world wars of this century were the first to produce distinctive groups of poets and new poetic approaches to the subject. Up to 1914, the traditional format tended to be watery and naïve romantic heroism, which was full of classical unreality, or the equally unreal, hairy-chested heartiness of the early Rudyard Kipling or W. E. Henley, redolent with an optimistic chauvinism that one could hardly get away with nowadays. Consider, for example, Henley's "Song of the Sword":

The Sword
Singing —
His high, irresistible song.
Making death beautiful.

or Rupert Brooke's famous piece, "The Soldier":

> *If I should die, think only this of me:*
> *That there's some corner of a foreign field*
> *That is forever England. There shall be*
> *In that rich earth a richer dust concealed;*
> *A dust whom England bore, shaped, made aware.* . . .

More recent generations have been less generously enthusiastic about enhancing foreign ecology. Rather than dealing directly with the horrors of war, Brooke portrayed more of a nostalgia for the coziness of the white teacups and tastefully trimmed gardens that the battlefront lacked.

The First World War evoked its share of the *Dulce et decorum est pro patria mori*—the belief in the sweetness of a patriotic death for the glory of the fatherland and in the expectation of eternal justice and a fit reward. Some of the early poems, like Brooke's "Peace"—"Now, God be thanked who has matched us with His Hour"—expressed exhilaration at the chance of exposure to war, as if it were some super Sunday school outing, and simply bound to be wizard fun. Such martial imagery as trailed across the fields of hyperbole was usually medieval—warriors and fair maidens, swords and shields. The precise mechanisms of poetry were perverted to hide the horrid realities of death, and indeed to transubstantiate them, to fit them into some grand Hegelian motif and pattern. Grossly overpraised, these early poets of the Great War achieved popular sales equalled by few poets at any time. One saw the poet as a recruiting sergeant urging youth to volunteer and celebrating the utility of human sacrifice. Their unreality, as Mersmann (1974) has pointed out, was essential to maintaining "the heroic complacency" that led a generation far too cheerfully into the holocaust.

But a second wave of young soldier poets—men like Wilfred Owen, Robert Graves, Siegfried Sassoon, and Edmund Blunden—produced true war poetry, very different from that of Brooke, Grenfell, or Nichols. Their literary reputation has grown steadily, although some lesser rivals like Yeats rejected them for the most petty reasons. They failed to keep to properly *poetic* subjects, or to treat them with properly *poetic* anemia. They wrote no long, overworked odes—there wasn't time in the trenches. They invoked pity for the dead, finding the deaths ugly and stupid, wasteful, pointless, degrading, and unheroic. War was dealt with realistically, with crisp anger, bitterness, and sorrow.

> *The place was rotten with the dead; green clumsy legs*
> *High-booted, sprawled and grovelled along the saps.*
> *And trunks, face downward in the sucking mud,*

Wallowed like trodden sand-bags loosely filled
And naked, sodden buttocks; mats of hair,
Bulged, clotted heads, slept in the plastering slime[1]

Even Rudyard Kipling, who had written some of the most sanguine imperialistic verse before 1914, did not produce the crudely patriotic verse one might have expected. Especially after his only son was killed in action, he produced surprisingly bitter poems, stressing the wastefulness of the carnage, and condemning the generals, profiteers, and politicians who so lightly directed the slaughter.

The Second World War produced a different poetry, building on the experience of the realism of the First World War's poets in a society in which the sublime romantic unreality of Brooke was less viable. Death itself was rather different—men were less often lodged in the static horrors of the trenches; technology had made it easier and more distant, less personalized, less angry, and more often concerned with the general corruption of society. Randall Jarrell, for example, was struck by the ease with which human beings—playing with their pets and watering the flowers as they heard the news of atrocities—could fail to empathize with those they considered enemies. He was also intrigued by the loss of innocence, and often compared the soldier to a child, as in "Absent with Official Leave." Yet his examples tend to be abstract rather than real people—"The Ball Turrett Gunner," "The Wingman," "A Pilot from the Carrier."

POETS AND SUICIDE

The personal dimension inherent in death by suicide has long concerned poets, as Alvarez (1971) has explored with great accomplishment. Many poets have killed themselves, such as Cesare Pavese, Paul Celan, Randall Jarrell, Yesenin, Tsvetayeva, Mayakovsky ("In this life, it is not difficult to die," he wrote, "It is more difficult to live"), and others.

One particular group of modern poets, whom some have named the "Confessional Poets" (Philips, 1973), has become increasingly distinctive in recent years not only for the urgent exposure of their most personal feelings but for the morbid fascination with death and the high suicide rate shown by members of the group.

The Confessionals certainly represent a substantial and refreshing change from their predecessors, whose sometimes self-conscious avoidance

---

[1] Siegfried Sassoon, "Counter-Attack," 1919.

of the direct expression of personality and emotion tends to be dictated by Eliot's bank clerk asceticism. Eliot has indeed insisted that poetry should represent not a turning loose of emotion, but an escape from emotion. Even the breed of Audenesque academic poems, though witty and scattered with erudite references from Homer to the *New Yorker,* tends to be as arid as a tea biscuit, and sometimes deliberately obscure. John Crowe Ransom, perhaps, typifies the dry aestheticism—the denial of strong emotion and the striving for *objectivity* (in poetry, there is no objectivity; only some statements which are less subjective than others)—that preceded the Confessionals—he could describe death euphemistically as "a brown study," or at worst "vexacious."

The Confessional School (if such they be, and they show more cohesion and more claim to such a title than any comparable group of modern poets) is usually deemed to have started with the publication of Robert Lowell's *Life Studies* in 1959, although Anne Sexton, W. D. Snodgrass, and Theodore Roethke were already writing similar verse. Although most of these poets have insisted that they were not strictly writing about themselves, the autobiographical flavor to their work has been notable.

In *Life Studies* Lowell turned to his private life as a source of poetry with what was thought at the time to be startling candor. His nervous breakdown, his marital problems, were exposed and explored. In one of the poems, "Uncle Devereux is dying," he experiences the death of the first person to die in his household in his lifetime and considers that he grew up and came of age as a result of the experience. Later poems deal with his father's death. He cringes at his father's ordinariness and failures, his "unhistoric" soul, his last words—the inelegant "I feel awful." Finally, materialistic to the last, he's buried under the slice of pink-veined marble and the business-like motto he chose. Other poets may have found death terrifying, even devastating—Lowell seems to have found it embarrassing, awkward, gauche.

W. D. Snodgrass published one especially interesting series of poems, *Remains,* under the pseudonym "S. S. Gardons" on the occasion of his sister's death (ironically, on Independence Day). Only through death, he implies, could his mousey and drab sister achieve some independence—from her sickness, from her lackluster life, from her dominant mother. In "Viewing the Body," he contrasts this pallid life with her gaudy death—the red satin folds surrounding her in the coffin, the flowers "like a gangster's funeral," and the eye shadow "like a whore." Now people say, "Isn't she beautiful?" though she never dressed like that before.

John Berryman's *Dream Songs* are especially filled with accounts of friends' suicides and deaths—Randall Jarrell, Sylvia Plath, Yvor Winters, William Carlos Williams, and Delmore Schwartz. Death and the contemplation of suicide spill right through his verses, as if stalking the poet to the end.

In only one, "Dream Song No. 259," does he seem to express some hope in life, admitting that his desire for death, though strong, was never strong enough, and concluding that he can bear it. The obsession with death which his father had shown haunted him from a very early age, and the theme of his father's suicide recurs frequently, as in "Dream Song 145":

> he only, very early in the morning,
> rose with his gun and went outdoors by my window
> and did what was needed.

From that moment, he tried again and again to read his father's mind, to understand that act, searching, as Plath was also to do, to find some way to forgive his father for leaving him to live on alone. For him, as he describes in "Dream Song 241," *father* was the loneliest word in the language. In "Dream Song 235," written after hearing of Hemingway's suicide in the sixties, he writes:

> Mercy! my father; do not pull the trigger
> or all my life I'll suffer from your anger
> killing what you began.

He made pilgrimages to his father's grave in Oklahoma, and in one of his bitterest songs, "No. 384," fantasizes murdering the suicided father, or joining him, in an explosion of the bitterness of desertion and loss. He threatens to spit upon "this dreadful banker's grave," as he'd like to dig down and axe open the casket to see "just how he's taking it, which he sought so hard." The desire for death grew stronger until, on January 7, 1972, spectators watched Berryman jump from a high bridge onto the Mississippi River's ice, where, "in modesty of death," he could join the father who had left him so long ago.

Theodore Roethke (Hoffman, 1970), too, shared both the self-exposing quality and the continuing interest in death of the others in this group. He returns to death as a puzzle, less concerned with the expectation of it than with a contemplation of its odd nature, and attempts to define it in general terms. In the sequence, "Meditations of an Old Woman," including the line "What Shall I Tell My Bones?" the old lady comes to accept the whole spectrum of life, celebrating the naturalness of its variety.

Of Sylvia Plath (Newman, 1971; Melander, 1972; White, 1974), archpriestess of the current genre of poetic *Liebestod,* Alvarez (Holbrook, 1971) has said: "The achievement of her final style is to make poetry and death inseparable." As expressions of hate, especially of self-hate, her poems are unique. They are often astonishing, even impressive, though not necessarily always good. The enormous popular romanticization of her suicide has spoiled the critical perspective with which her work has been assessed, and she runs a severe risk of becoming a premature icon.

The theme of death is less prominent in her earlier verse, and she reveals no particular sense of personal commitment to the subject in these apprenticeship pieces. "All the Dead Dears" is an exception. Her inspiration was a stone coffin, dating from the fourth century A.D., in the Cambridge Archeology Museum. It contained the skeletons of a shrew, a mouse, and a woman, the woman's anklebone having been slightly gnawed. All things, it seems, take part in the "gross eating game" of mortality, and she recognizes her kinship with the skeleton. There's a growing sense of a relationship to the dead, even a threatening one, as when she writes that the generations of dead women "reach hag hands" to haul her in. But at this stage she still handles life and death with some matter-of-fact naturalness. The motif of death by drowning begins to appear more frequently, and is often regarded as a means to achieving peace, as in "Lorelei," "Mussel Hunter at Rock Harbour," "Full Fathom Five," and "Suicide Off Egg Rock," in which she considers a man's state of mind—feeling "dead in life"—before he jumps to his suicide. She contrasts the landscape made hideous by man with the man who waits to die. She shows no pity for either.

"Two Views of a Cadaver Room" contrasts medical students nonchalantly dissecting corpses with the lovers in a Breugel painting oblivious to the "carrion army" at their elbow. In "Last Words," she considers the sort of burial she would like. She wants, not the plain box, but a grand sarcophagus with symbols of power and rebirth and real domestic things like her copper cooking pots and her pots of rouge about her. "Cut" describes her reaction to cutting her thumb—a reaction very much like that of the wrist-cutter, who cuts so as to break back into reality, and to lose "the thin papery feeling" of depersonalization. It has a characteristically striking opening with strong and memorable phraseology, both vivid and morbid. But she can do nothing more with the theme than continue to rub her wound in our eyes, again displaying her weakness for excess.

Other themes recur. Love is dangerous, a fruit that's "death to taste," and in "Electra on the Azalea Path," she insists to her father that it was her love that "did us both to death." Bees, closely associated with her dead father, the gentle Otto Plath and author of *Bumblebees and their Ways*, recur in the later poems, like "Electra," "the Beekeeper's Daughter," "The Bee Meeting," "the Arrival of the Bee-Box" and "Stings." By "Stings," it seems that only in death, if even then, will the queen bee (with whom she identifies) achieve self-realization. There is still some ambivalence toward death in The Bee poems, though, for there is still some fear of death along with the wistful conviction that it is a potential liberator from the drudgery of life. Gradually, more explicit expressions of a death wish without fear emerge, as in "I am Vertical," where she admits that she would "rather be horizontal." "Death & Co.," in which she pictures herself reposing in death, shows a duality between death's fearfulness and sensuality.

"Daddy" deals with the pain of her father's premature death, and her feeling that he betrayed her by dying. This soon becomes one of the most strongly voiced hate poems in the language. One critic has called it "the Guernica of modern poetry," a vivid, if unearned, accolade. She wrestled with the internalized image of her Bad Father on whom she could comfortably place the blame for all her faults and problems, and justify her unremitting, unforgiving hate—ironically, the purest emotion she seems to have ever achieved. Here we see one of the last outwardly directed sputters of the powerful hate that later turned in upon herself so destructively. Finally, by "Edge," close in time to her suicide, it is all calm. As she contemplates the finality of death with the emotionless calm of hopelessness, she concludes that to die is to be perfected.

> *The woman is perfected.*
> *Her dead*
> *Body wears the smile of accomplishment, . . .*

These final poems also contain her striking and chilling declaration:

> *Dying*
> *Is an art, like everything else*
> *I do it exceptionally well.*
> *I do it so it feels like hell.*
> *I do it so it feels real.*
> *I guess you could say I've a call.*

By the time of "Lady Lazarus" and "Edge," she speaks as one who only feels real by meeting the test of suicide. Some critics, like Alvarez, have incorrectly imputed to Plath an objectivity she never achieved. She does not, as he suggests, give her suffering a broad, general meaning by assuming the suffering of all other victims and declaring herself a she-Christ or at least an honorary Jew. On the contrary, while she can describe her own unhappiness with impressive clarity, she indulges in it, revels in the pain through which she can at least temporarily feel real, and claims a vicarious legitimacy by borrowing the features of other, more heroic, sufferers—a gratuitous Jew using the litany of Dachau and Auschwitz to render her own desperation more respectable. Yet the regressive reasoning by which she backs herself into her own final solution bears no rightful comparison with the suffering of the wartime millions whose support she seeks. At no time does she reveal a glimmer of compassion for anyone else's suffering.

Anne Sexton discussed with riveting directness her unhappy life, the deaths of friends and parents, and her psychiatric hospitalizations. In "Some Foreign Letters," she is reading the correspondence of her great-aunt, whom she only knew as a deaf and dying crone, and is surprised to find she too had a young life. At times she seeks to free herself from the weight of guilt and mortality, as in "The Truth the Dead Know," in which she walks from the churchyard, refusing to join in the procession to the graveside, with the declaration, "I am tired of being brave," and turns to her own life and a day at the Cape instead; or in "A Curse Against Elegies," in which she proposes that one should indeed live for the living and not for the dead. But she cannot long accept death, "that old butcher," who hacks at her dear ones, and she describes her breakdowns and hospital experiences with extraordinary clarity, as in the superb "You, Doctor Martin, walk / from breakfast to madness." In "The Double Image," she ostensibly describes a pair of portraits that hang side by side in the family home, one of her and one of her mother. But though she begins by mourning her mother's death, she sees her mother's portrait as "my mocking mirror" and begins to mourn for herself as well, "who chose two times / to kill myself."

Sexton, like Plath, returns to the theme of her father's death, and, in one verse, uses a quote from a psychoanalytic article as an epigraph: "Young girls in old Arabia were often buried alive next to their dead fathers, apparently as a sacrifice to the goddesses of the tribes."

Sexton and Plath reputedly spent hours together "talking death" and sharing details of their suicide attempts. By her third volume, *Live or Die,* Sexton was dispassionately arguing the case for suicide, as seen in her central poem "Wanting to Die." Although she has "nothing against life," there are times when "the almost unnameable lust returns":

> *But suicides have a special language.*
> *Like carpenters they want to know* which tools.
> *They never ask* why build.

On the occasion of Sylvia Plath's suicide, she expressed a sort of jealousy:

> *Thief!*
> *how did you crawl into,*
> *crawl down alone,*
> *into the death I wanted so badly and*
> *for so long. . . .*

And finally, in 1974, Ann Sexton did kill herself, and the only shocking thing about it was that no one was surprised. She had promised it to us for so long. Her final poems appear in her posthumous volume, *The Awful Rowing Toward God.* With more wit and human warmth than Plath allowed herself, Sexton explores and explains her emotional state. Though she has shown, as Plath certainly did, an overvaluing of her personal sorrows to the detriment of appreciation of the rest of the world, she, unlike Plath, has verbalized it, though she lacked the capacity to change.

Denise Levertov has expressed concern over the effect that Sexton's death may have on others, and usefully stresses the distinction between creativity and self destruction, for the two have been confused too often, especially in recent years. Sexton, like Plath and Berryman before her, seems to have suffered from a failure to appreciate the distinction. Levertov claims to have heard many accounts of attempted and sometimes successful suicides by students who, loving Plath's poetry, assumed that they needed to reenact in their own lives the gory details of hers. In the same way, some admirers of Lowell felt, with pathetic hubris, that drinking was a prerequisite to writing well, just as earlier generations of poetasters had become alcoholics emulating Dylan Thomas or Brendan Behan. While they might well have matched their masters gill for gill, and tot for tot, they somehow never got down to the writing they promised. Neither, in the end, did the "masters" they emulated. There is no evidence to suggest that artists and poets are any more vulnerable than the rest of the population, even if some are given to more picturesque problems. Certainly the creative impulse and the self-destructive impulse can coexist, and they not infrequently do, but there is no causal relationship. Depression and suicidal ideation, like most psychopathologies, hinder art—they do not nurture it.

L'ENVOI

As we have seen, death has been an enduring theme in poetry. Although individual poets have described it in their own ways, broad and generally recognizable styles of approach have been strongly favored during different historical periods. One of the clearest contrasts between the treatment of death in modern poetry and the manner in which earlier poets used the theme lies in the use of personal, literal experience. Whereas previous generations of poets tended to depict their personal experiences in terms of universals, today's poets describe universal verities in terms of their personal experiences. Instead of calling upon classical, public, and collective mythologies to express their own distress, they offer their own private mythology to illustrate the universal experience.

In recent years, indeed, the trend has been toward more intimate expression of personal distress, to the point of direct poetic revelation of frank psychopathology. Finally, we should also consider the intensely personal uses of poetry by the suffering, who use it as a means of exposing the dimensions and nature of their suffering, either for private record or for constructive sharing in the cause of therapy. This final poem was written for me by a young man in prison. He had just turned 21, and wanted to express his guilt, self-hate, and the horror of being evil and unable to control it. Shortly after sending it, he poisoned himself, for death was the conclusion he drew.

> *Dear Doctor,*
> *Evil Evil evil evil*
> *World is evil*
> *Life is evil*
> *All is evil*
> *if I ride the horse of hate*
> *With its evil hooded eye*
> *turning world to evil*
> *Evil is death warmed up*
> *Evil is live spelled backward*
> *Evil is me*
> *Evil is lamb burning bright*
> *Evil is love fried upon a spit*
> *And turned upon its self*
> *Evil is sty in the eye of the witness*
> *I am that sty*
> *hung upon a coughing horse*
> *That follows me at night*
> *Thru a hollow street*
> *Wearing blinkers*
> *Evil is running after me*
> *With glue feet*
> *I'm running*
> *Evil is screwing strangers*
> *friends*
> *Poor dear flesh not evil*
> *Lonely meat is not evil*
> *But evil is looking*
> *at me*
> *in my window*

I am paranoid about evil
Evil is 21 years old
and in my wrong mind
Evil is being out of my head
asleep or awake
Evil passes blind
thru filtertips of mind
in pot visions
where a horse walks
A horse that wants to eat me
Horse eats consciousness
I am afraid of it.
I am running
I hate you Evil
mad horse
We all go mad when we die
but to ride mad horse alive
is a form of dying
each mad day a death
I am paranoid about it
Evil has caught me
Horse is humping me
Wearing blinders
Horse wants me to mount
Horse wants me to ride
without a halter
I am running from it
with two feet
I'm afraid
I don't want to die
mad,
mad is
mad is me
mad is me riding
mad is me riding. . . .

REFERENCES

Alonso, F., Del Rosario, M. *Una Visión de la muerte en la lírica española; la muerte comp amada.* Madrid: Gredos, 1971.

Alvarez, A. *The savage god.* London: Weindenfeld & Nicolson, 1971.

Anderson, C. R. *Emily Dickinson's poetry: Stairway of surprise.* New York: Holt, 1960.

Anthony, S. *The discovery of death in childhood and after.* Harmondsworth, Maryland: Penguin, 1973.

Ayuso Rivera, J. *El Concepto de la muerte en la poesía romántica española.* Madrid: Gredos, 1971.

Black, E. L. *1914–18 in poetry.* London: University of London Press, 1970.

Carlisle, E. F. *The uncertain self: Whitman's drama of identity.* East Lansing: Michigan State, 1973.

Cody, J. *After great pain: The inner life of Emily Dickinson.* Cambridge: Harvard, 1971.

Dubruck, E. *The theme of death in French poetry of the Middle Ages and the Renaissance.* The Hague: Mouton, 1964.

Fiedler, L. A. *Love and death in the American novel.* New York: Criterion Books, 1960.

Fougeres, M. *La Liebestod dans le roman francais, anglais, et allemand au XVIIIe siècle.* (Prof. de Jean-Pierre Moúnier.) Ottawa: Naaman, 1974.

Griessmair, E. *Das Motiv der Mors immatura in den griechischen metrischen Grabenschriffen.* Innsbruck: Universitats-verlag Wagner, 1966.

Holbrook, D. Out of the ash. *The Human World,* November 1971, **5**, 34.

Hoffman, F. J. *The mortal no: Death and the modern imagination.* Princeton: Princeton, 1964.

Hoffman, F. J. *Theodore Roethke: The poetic shape of death.* In (J. Nazzaro (Ed.), *Modern American poetry.* New York: McKay, 1970, pp. 301–320.

Koch, F. *Goethe's Stellung zu Tod und Unsterblichkeit.* Weimar: Verlag der Goethe-gesellschaft, 1932.

Kurtz, B. P. *The pursuit of death: A study of Shelley's poetry.* New York: Oxford, 1933.

Levertov. D. Ann Sexton: Light up the cave. *Ramparts,* December 1974–January 1975, **13** (5), 61–63.

Melander, I. *The poetry of Sylvia Plath: A study of themes.* Stockholm: Acta Universitatis Gothoburgensis/Almquist & Wiksell, 1972.

Mersmann, J. F. *Out of the Vietnam vortex.* Lawrence: The University Press of Kansas, 1974.

Newman, C. *The art of Sylvia Plath.* Bloomington: Indiana, 1971.

Patterson, R. *The riddle of Emily Dickinson.* New York: Cooper Square Publications, 1973.

Phillips, R. *The confessional poets.* Carbondale: Southern Illinois, 1973.

Rehm, W. *Orpheus, der Dichter und die Toten: Selbst-deutung und Totenkult bei Novalis, Holderlin und Rilke.* Dusseldorf: L. Schwann, 1950.

Rehm, W. *Der Todesgedanke in der Deutschen Dichtung van Mittelalter bis zur Romantik.* Tubingen: Niemeyer, 1967.

Sassoon, S. *The war poems of Siegfried Sassoon.* Wondon: William Heinemann, 1919.

Schmidt, G. *Die Krankheit zum Tode: Goethe's Todesneurose.* Stuttgart: F. Enke, 1968.

Spencer, T. *Death and Elizabethan tragedy: A study of convention and opinion in the Elizabethan drama.* Cambridge: Harvard, 1930.

Unger, R. *Herder, Novalis und Kleist: Studien uber die Entwicklung des todes Problems in denken und dichten von Sturm und Drang zur Romantik.* Darmstadt: Wissenschaffliche Buchgesellschaft, 1968.

Valdes, M. J. *Death in the literature of Unamuno.* Urbana: University of Illinois Press, 1964.

van Ingen, F. *Vanitas und Memento Mori in der Deutschen Barocklyrik.* Groningen: J. B. Wolfers, 1966.

Weber, F. P. *Aspects of Death and Correlated Aspects of Life in Art, Epigram and Poetry.* (Reprint) College Park, Maryland: McGrath, 1971.

White, C. A. *A developmental study of the art of Sylvia Plath.* Unpublished masters thesis, McMaster University, 1974.

18

DYING TO POWER: DEATH AND THE SEARCH FOR SELF-ESTEEM

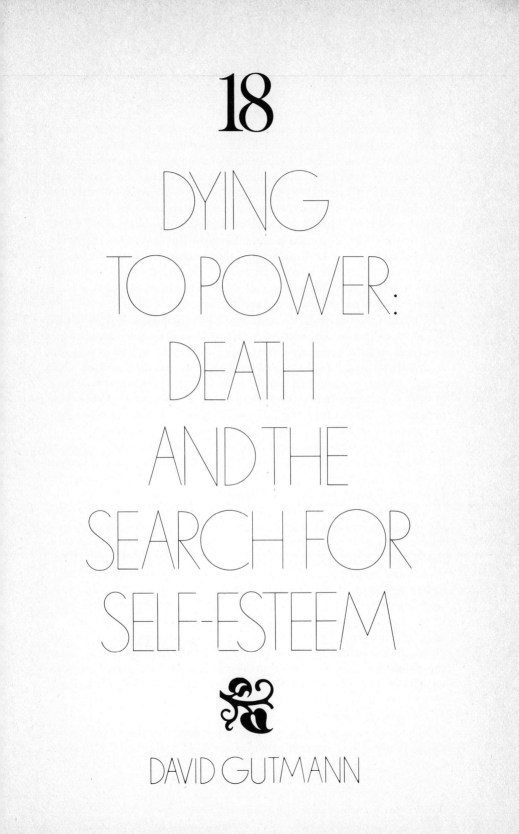

DAVID GUTMANN

P
MODERN CONSUMERSHIP
OF LIFE- AND DEATH-STYLES

op psychologists have reduced their production of books on achieving the good orgasm; instead, they are now telling us how to compose an aesthetic decomposition—a graceful death. Thus, there sits on my desk a publisher's announcement of a recent work, *Coming to Terms with Death,* proclaimed as a "do it yourself book on how to die gracefully" (Cutter, 1975). It adds, "This book offers some remarkably cheerful ideas on what is usually perceived as a grim subject. Maybe it is the perfect gift for Mom." The current interest in morbidity goes beyond such trendy trivia: death has become the growth industry of serious publishing, and the volume which includes this chapter is only one small entry in a rapidly expanding scholarly literature. Death gurus also proliferate, as do their followers—sometimes called "death groupies"—and any seminar on dying is guaranteed a full registration.

There are some obvious reasons for this lively interest in dying. In an age in which productive efforts have turned inward toward the cultivation of a perfect self, "hang-ups"—including the craven fear of death—are regarded as psychic blemishes, irrational curbs on personal freedom. Thus, certain lumpen psychologists celebrate death, proclaiming this feat a proof of their inner liberation, precisely because the unenlightened public fears to die. In the words of the blurb referred to above: "Death is a taboo topic in current America. . . . This book should be the perfect gift for any parent, but if you're uncomfortable with that notion, you bear witness to the pernicious influence of the taboo." In these instances, the psychologist functions as a secular theologist, reversing the moral charge from negative to positive, turning violations of taboo into virtuous acts.

But the exhibitionism and provocativeness of trendy psychologists is not in itself sufficient to account for our recent cultural necrophilia. Like most symptoms, it is overdetermined—fed by many sources, some of them much more irrational than the necrophobia that they seek to undo. Thus, while taboo subjects are explored, the previously dehumanized members of society are at the same time rehumanized, sometimes even sentimentalized: blacks, women, homosexuals, the insane, and the aged. Along with these, the dying have entered the Third World, acquiring the kind of respectful awe that up to now was mainly reserved for successful murderers. Furthermore, as earnest theology students flock to their bedsides, the dying are treated to the kind of intensive and often intrusive care which, if it does not hasten their demise, may at least make them welcome it.

The dying have always been strange, eerie, and hence feared; but our omnivorous society routinely converts the strange into the exotic, and by the same token, into items of consumption. Leafing through the "how-to" books on dying, one gathers that death, as an experience, has entered the ranks of exotica—much like Mandarin cooking. The younger members of United States society have become experts in the "consumership of experience": the consumption of life-styles has replaced the previous generation's concern for the consumption of material goods. Exotic experiences, even those which are intrinsically painful, take on the glamour of a strange drug, or foreign cuisine, and have to be sampled at least once. Thus, I learned recently that the members of a California commune kidnapped a dying hospital patient so that they could vicariously "experience dying." This story may well be apocryphal, but as such it tells us something about the culture that spawns such fantasy: "Don't knock it until you've tried it" becomes a guiding principle, even in regard to death.

ANIMISTIC VIEWS OF DEATH AND POWER

But death is after all transcultural; and humans have always fled death, fought death, or sought death for reasons that may have to do with its universal rather than its parochial meanings. Thus far, I have been considering the current fascination with mortality in our society as though it were only one transient fad among many; but if we look at the wider, transcultural implications of death, we may better understand why it has suddenly become fashionable for our particular time and culture. Perhaps death, like other elemental experiences—hunger, pain, fear, rage, and orgasm—overrides any particular cultural idiom and defines for all people, regardless of their origins, the ways in which it will be commonly experienced and understood. Thus, transhuman generalizations about death may tell us much about our own contemporary fascination with this topic.

The most obvious though persistent theme that we can draw from a comparative review of the beliefs and attitudes that cluster around mortality is this: Death invariably leads not to an end of existence, but to a change of state from one form of collective participation to another. Humans readily concede the end of their corporeal existence; but they will not admit the cessation of communal, collective, existence. In spirit form, the dead either remove themselves to a separate community or some remote plane of existence or, usually as ghosts, maintain—though in some altered form—the social bond to their original community. In some cultures the dead are viewed as benevolent protectors of the living; in others, the dead are aggrieved litigants, demanding reparation for their murder—death. In either case, whether they use if for good or for evil purposes, the dead dispose of great power, far beyond anything available to them in their earthly existence. Indeed, the dead are so strong that even to dream of them risks infection from their malign power. Thus, among traditional Navajo, dreams and persistent thoughts concerning the dead are not regarded as symbolic events, but as evidence of the ghost's presence within the dreamer. The Navajo assume that the dream image and the reality that it connotes are one and the same; thus, the dead person is assumed to be concretely located within the dreamer's head, and the Navajo assume that it has entered there by force to cause mischief.

Thus, an aged Navajo medicine man, specialist in the ceremonial for ghost sickness, tells me that this infection is a side effect of the ghost "wind": "The soul of the person resides in his wind, and this goes out of him when he dies to become the ghost, the Ch'indi. The Ch'indi wind gets on them. Maybe sometimes it just brushes them, but that makes them sick. The wind that the dead person had becomes Ch'indi, it might be a relative's wind, like his mother, but it comes back to bother him." The "evil-way" ceremony for exorcising the spirit has two major goals—to contain the power of the ghost, and to pay the ghost off. The Navajo curing ceremony is rather like a bargaining session in which a case is settled out of court: the ghost is drawn to the treatment site, he is restricted to a defined area and offered payment, the "ghost bribe."

The same informant explained this automatic malice of the dead toward the living: "It's like when you owe somebody money. He keeps coming around and coming around until you pay him off." In the Navajo case, as in other preliterate cultures, the ghost has two kinds of power: the moral advantage of the unpaid creditor, and the *mana* that automatically attaches to the ghost status, as manifested in the spirit wind. Again, the social bond between the living and the dead is not ruptured by death, which instead brings about a reversal of previous emotional signs: a mother's love is changed by death into lethal hate. Apparently, then, the malign power of the dead may be predicated on the strength of social bonds among the living; but to the Navajo mind at least, even the dead of alien folk have great power and inclination to harm them. Thus, the Navajo maintain to this day, in their traditional camps, the ritual of "enemy way" for protection of those who have been in contact with non-Navajo populations or corpses. Accordingly, Navajo veterans who may have killed enemy soldiers, and even Navajo nurses who have been in contact with enemy (white man) dead, are still subjected to the enemy way ritual on their return to the reservation. Again, the Navajo believe that it is the unharmonious social relationship between the subject and the enemy dead that makes the power of the enemy malignant. The ritual, which has the aim of restoring the lost harmony, consists of the ceremonial reenactment of a battle in which both sides fight over some ceremonial token, achieve possession of it in turn, and finally make peace. The peace established between the warring factions is supposed to bring harmony between the Navajo patient and whatever piece of enemy spirit power the victim has been at odds with.

THE DEAD AS POWER BRINGERS

Clearly then, for the Navajo—as for many other groups—the dead are upwardly mobile: when they shuffle off this mortal coil, when they leave the pragmatic community, they intersect a domain of great power, and they enhance their own. Either they themselves become charged with power or they represent an interface, a *cusp,* through which the potentially destructive power of the supernatural realm can penetrate into the vulnerable community of ordinary humans. In the Navajo case, that power can only be deflected or blunted through a ceremony of propitiation.

The adversary stance of the dead toward the living is highlighted when the deceased is an enemy killed in war. Until the "bad" power has been drained off or neutralized, the slain enemy is a greater threat to the adversary community than a living foe. Thus, animistically conceived, war is the practice or set of practices whereby the community beats back bad enemy power, captures that power, and converts it to the collective store of "good" or community power. Considering the Papago Indians of Arizona, Redfield (1962) wrote: "All acts of the community at war—not just the war party—tended towards one goal: success of the war party and then the draining off of the supernatural power acquired through the slaying into a safe and usable form."

Paradoxically, the successful warrior gains the power of his victim by submitting, in his turn, to some relic of the slain enemy: among the headhunters of New Guinea the successful warrior was for a time shut out of the community and confined to a hut beyond its borders, where he lived alone in a special, dyadic relationship with the head of his victim. There he would propitiate the trophy: he would pray to it, and bring it gifts of food. After the required term of peace making between the slayer and the slain, the successful warrior would reenter the community, and the trophy would be adopted into his clan. The once destructive power embedded in the trophy had by then become an integral part of the clan's store of prowess and courage. Along the same lines, Wallace (1960) tells us that any scalp taken by the Iroquois would be put through an adoption ceremony and would become in effect, with its power, part of the Iroquois nation.

In all these cases the dead, as vessels of awful power, are not occasional or even unwanted intruders into the human realm. Rather, they are *vital* to the continued existence of the daily, pragmatic world. The idea that

Hades, the spirit realm, is a place of wailing shadows is relatively recent, a modern notion that came in with the Greeks, perhaps appearing first in the poetry of Homer. The "civilized" idea that locates essential power and substance in the living rather than in the dead goes against our species consensus, developed in human prehistory, which asserts the opposite: that this, our daily world, is insubstantial, ultimately a place of shadows, and owes its transient vitality to totemic, ancestral, or ghostly sponsors, and to the magicians and warriors that capture and import supernatural power for the sake of their community.[1] By and large then, simple communities—though their conceptions of power and the routes to power might vary—exist as islands in the sea of energy that beats upon the shores of the known, comprehensible world but that stretches into the disquieting reaches of the unknown. Power gets into the mundane world to sustain ordinary individuals as well as forms of nature, but it does not originate there; in concert with other supernatural sponsors, the dead provide a pivotal link between the essentially powerless mundane community and the centers of vitality that lie beyond its borders. According to this prevalent view, the dead do not feed off the living; rather, the living are chronically in debt to the deceased for their own vitality, and they pay interest on that debt through continual ritual and sacrifice.

DEATH AND REVELATION

The same dialectic between death and vitality directs the search, by the living, for personal power, for the sense of self-esteem. Like Hart Crane's hero, men, across time and cultures, have decided that they must go face the Great Death so as to earn the Red Badge of Courage. Individual candidates must endure at least some simile of death so as to acquire a personal core of power, registered in the subjective sense of solidity, of "thereness" as a self, and in the feeling of self-worth. Consider Róheim's (1930) description of the magician's initiation among the Australian bush tribes. The candidate goes to the place of the spirits; he lies down passive-

---

[1] An 83-year-old Navajo medicine man, close to death, told me that he was passively concerned because young Navajo did not try to learn the "rain songs, the livestock songs, the grass songs" that he knew. His songs literally brought in the power that sustained these forms in nature. If they were not sung, sheep, rain, and grass would disappear, and the people would starve. In effect, the world would end with his death. There is probably a note here of "Après moi, le déluge," but his was a cultural idea rather than personal megalomania. He and his medicine songs were not themselves the sources of vital power but only the incidental bridgeheads through which that power moved to revitalize the daily world. In his view, any man who knew the chants could restore the crucial connection to supernatural power.

ly, facing toward their cave; he is taken into their cave, cut to pieces, eaten, and put together again with a new set of organs by the same spirits that first destroyed him. The candidate emerges from the cave reborn, imbued with the power of the dangerous spirits who now have become his sponsors. In effect, the magician has voyaged through death in order to reach the terrain of power that is unavailable to ordinary, uninitiated humans.

Across the planet the future medicine man of the Sioux moved, via his *token* death in the vision quest, to medicine power. The Sioux candidate went into the desert without food, clothing, or arms. Carrying none of society's protections, he starved, froze in the night, and sang his death song. Finally, as he approached his final delirium, his totem animal appeared to him in a vision and revealed the future source of his medicine power. Free then to return to his tribe, the candidate knew his totem lodge, and the appropriate rituals that would link him with the power of his totemic sponsor. Again, the self must risk total dissolution before it can lay claim to the vital energy that will be its core and center. There appears to be a human consensus: Rebirth brings a renewal of vitality; but death is the precondition for rebirth.

THE POWERS OF THE PREMORBID AGED

The face to face, preliterate folk society is generally a male gerontocracy. Any senior man who has led an exemplary life according to the local mores will normally become one of the guiding elders of his society. Anthropologists usually explain such participatory gerontocracy in a matter-of-fact, concrete manner: Power accrues to age as barnacles accrue to hulls—older men are powerful because they have lived long enough to garner the land, the wealth, the trophies, and the knowledge on which prestige and the reputation for wisdom are based. But this is a materialistic explanation, a kind of ethnographic Marxism; it accounts for the old man's wealth in goods, but not for his wealth in the less visible mana on which his prestige and awesomeness are ultimately founded. Thus, questioned about the power of their elders, native informants do not dwell on wealth, the badge of secular power; they are more impressed by the ties that old men can uniquely maintain with extrahuman power sources. Paradoxically, the old man in the folk society acquires power by virtue of physical and psychological qualities peculiar to the aged that cause him to lose status in a secular society. The primitive gerontocrat's power stems as much from physical weakness, *from closeness to death,* as from the particular wisdom or skills that he may have acquired over time. Precisely *because* of their frailty, the aged are moving into the country of the dead; they take on some of the fearsome aura of the corpse that they will soon become. Furthermore, in many cultures the aged blend with the deified figures of those already dead—the ancestors. Thus, Shelton (1965) finds that the revered tribal elders of the Nigerian Ibo are closest to the spiritualized forefathers, who are closest to the gods.

Here again, the aged merge with the mythic time when the people emerged from the sacred into the banal world; thus, they carry around them the power that moved through events in those special times. In effect, the traditional aged are anchored to the awesome vitality of the dead at two points: in their early life, and in their oncoming future. They intersect the ancestral past, and they overlap the spirit world which they will soon enter. As they blend with that world, they acquire its essential physiognomy and powers. Along these lines, Mead (1967) found the Balinese life cycle to be circular: both the child and the grandsire are at the "highest points" of life, because each is closest to the other world.

MURDER: THE ROUTE TO BAD POWER

There appears to be another general rule linking death to power: Good, benign power is acquired passively and masochistically—through dying, or through suffering age and weakness—but bad, malevolent power is acquired actively and sadistically, usually through some taboo act of murder: the slaying of a parent, a sibling, or a child. Typically, the sorcerer is one who has violated society's firmest taboos against incest and/or the murder of a close relative. In effect, the myth of Oedipus tells the story of a de facto sorcerer posing as a king. Unknowingly, he had violated the ultimate taboo: having killed his father and lain with his mother, he automatically became the entering wedge of bad influences—manifested in plagues and famine—within his kingdom.

Alternatively, the sorcerer wins destructive power not by an act of murder, but by violating the firm taboos hedged around the already dead. For example, the Wimbaio sorcerer of Australia reputedly digs up a corpse, and eats its bones. In effect, he reverses the procedures described earlier, whereby a "good" Australian magician acquires his power. Instead of being killed and eaten, the sorcerer kills and then eats. In the equation of power, he has refused the place of the victim, and has boldly taken the place of the god. Likewise, in the Banks Islands, the sorcerer eats a morsel of corpse flesh, and thereby allies himself to the ghost who will from then on direct destructive powers against any target indicated by the sorcerer. Closer to home, the Navajo have great fear of the dead, and avoid any precincts associated with them. However, the Navajo witch relies heavily for his evil magic on corpse powder—the ground up flesh of the dead— taken from the graveyards where proper folk will not go.

These examples, from the chronicles of sorcery, lead us to qualify the generalization, emerging from this comparative review, concerning the intimate relationship between death and power: Vitality comes to the person who dies or to the person who causes death. In effect, the sorcerer gains his power by making someone else do the dying for him. But in all these instances—the ghost, the magician, the gerontocrat, or the sorcerer—death is the doorway to vital power, the doorway to enhanced life. Psychologists usually contend that contemporary religious beliefs in the afterlife, in a heaven and a hell, represent a denial of death, a refusal of the religious individual to acknowledge termination. But again, this brief review suggests that the psychologist rather than the believer is the true deviant, for the latter—regardless of who is right or wrong—restates the overriding human consensus on the nature of death. The religious believer looks to death as a *rite de passage,* rather than as a final termination; it is the temporary trial through which one passes—as in all initiations—on the way to a more elevated and expanded existence.

THE MODERN LINKAGE OF DEATH AND POWER

My argument is essentially this: The archaic, "vitalistic" view of death as the precondition for renewal and expansion is no longer confined to the religious sectors of our society, but has reappeared in the secular consciousness as well. Furthermore, our widespread fascination with death does not point to some lethal impulse of our society, but is only one symptom of a wider, frantic, and often misdirected search for the headwaters of self-esteem. I have argued elsewhere (Gutmann, 1973, p. 571) that our culture suffers from a

> Pathology of subjective power, endemic to secular post-industrial society whether it is organized by capitalist entrepreneurs or by socialist visionaries. In our case, the American tragedy seems to be that democratic, egalitarian society, founded on the concept of the free individual, does not maintain the inner sense of vitality, the inner sense of power, that individualism requires; and that as a consequence, the forms of power awareness, acquisition, and maintenance that were the rule in pre-industrial and autocratic societies are again making their appearance among us.

Death is one such metaphor of power.

The sense of internal vitality, of self-esteem, coheres within the individual as the conjoint product of culture and its subjective metaphor, the superego. If the superego is weakened, but culture remains strong, (upheld by its traditions and the priests who conserve them) then the individual can still, though vicariously, gain a sustaining sense of solidarity and worth through cultivating conformity rather than autonomy. Instead of identifying with their superegos, individuals gain self-esteem through their identification with, and service to, the leaders, mores and symbols of their culture. However, when superego and culture are both weakened, then individuals typically become disconnected, "alienated," from both the internal and external storehouses of self-esteem. The result—as we see in the alienated members of our own society—is a frantic, magpie search for alternate, ad hoc sources of psychic power, where power and its dispensers are conceived in the most archaic and concrete terms. In order to reduce their sense of emptiness, the alienated masses become catholic in their quest for the ultimate sources of certainty. Any substance, practice, or leader that seems to promise resource and integrity will be uncritically taken up and just as uncritically abandoned. Thus, Rennie Davis switches from the leadership of the peace movement to become the proselyte of a 15-year-old "perfect Master." Others migrate restlessly among encounter groups, revolutionary movements, drug and food cults, totalitarian leaders, and mystical religions.

Finally, they are energized by death. Because of the power meanings latent within it, the death experience now grips the contemporary imagination. As part of the hectic search for psychic nutriment, death has been discovered, even erotized, as the latest power trip. Thus, precisely because they entail a reversible death experience, the hallucinogenic drugs have been eulogized as the doorway to new life. Among LSD users that I interviewed, the acquisition of omnipotent power was a central theme. And their narcissistic fantasy was made real for them *via* the sequence of death-rebirth experiences provided by LSD and similar drugs. Thus, they reported vivid, drug-induced experiences of disintegration, of dying as a self and subsequently coming together as a new and stronger person, armed with a superior insight.

Schizophrenia, the metaphor of ego death, has been turned up as another anodyne against alienation. Thus, schizophrenia has recently been romanticized—much like the drug trip—as a bold, mythic adventure, in which the individual decomposes artificial, arbitrary distinctions— between self and other, between present and past, between "here" and "there"—that prevent most individuals from experiencing their essential linkage to the totality of the universe and its centers of vitality. In effect, the Langian psychologists, the PR agents of schizophrenia, have given up on the quest for an integrated, autonomous self, and have decided that coherence and vitality can only be found in a mythic universe, whose essential unity and power will be discovered—*consumed* might be the better word—*via* the death of the self and its artificial boundaries. Again, a token death, this time in madness, is the precondition for rebirth on some higher, more enriched plane of existence.

THE DEATH OF A POET

For others, the trip into death—and through it, into perfection—is conceived and enacted in a more direct manner. Thus, Sylvia Plath (1965, 1971), a poet who committed suicide (and became thereby the priestess of her own postmortem cult), expressed the closeted meanings of the death trip in these images, abstracted from poems written shortly before the ending that so obsessed her. In the excerpts that follow, she rephrases the ancient notion that the risen dead have a terrible, but admirable, power that frightens even God and Lucifer:

> *Dying*
> *Is an art, like anything else.*
> *I do it exceptionally well.*
>
> *I am your opus,*
> *I am your valuable,*
> *The pure gold baby*
>
> *Herr God, Herr Lucifer,*
> *Beware*
> *Beware.*
>
> *Out of the ash*
> *I rise with my red hair*
> *And I eat men like air.*
>
> (from *"Lady Lazarus"*)

> *Now she is flying*
> *More terrible than she ever was, red*
> *Scar in the sky, red comet*
> *Over the engine that killed her -*
> *The Mausoleum, the wax house.*
>
> (from *"Stings"*)

Plath also stated, quite baldly, an elitist view of death—the idea that the dead, as a kind of artistocracy, have real *class:*

The Woman is perfected.
Her dead

Body wears the smile of accomplishment,
the illusion of a Greek necessity

Flows in the scrolls of her toga,
Her bare

Feet seem to be saying:
We have come so far, it is over.

Each dead child coiled, a white serpent,
One at each little

Pitcher of milk, now empty.
She has folded

Them back into her body as petals . . .

(from "Edge")

The meaning is plain: To be dead is, finally, to be perfect. The dead are glacial and remote; they are the tenement of an awesome presence; and, most importantly, they are without need. Self-sufficient at last, folded back into themselves, the dead have found the essential pivot of self-esteem. Death is not the ultimate insult to the self, but the final confirmation of narcissism. The solipsistic fantasy, "I could live in a nutshell and be king of infinite space!" is confirmed by the quiet message of the dead: "To be nothing is to be everything."

The danger is that those who entertain this potent fantasy will also believe it; and that, urged by the hectic spirit of these times, they will quest after incorruptible perfection and instead find the ultimate drabness: death.

REFERENCES

Cutter, F. *Coming to terms with death.* Fresno: California School of Professional Psychology, 1975.

Gutmann, D. The subjective politics of power: The dilemma of post-superego man. *Social Research,* 1973, **40,** (4), 570–616.

Mead, M. Ethnological aspects of aging. *Psychosomatics,* 1967, **8,** 33–37. (Supplement)

Plath, S. *Ariel.* New York: Harper & Row, 1965.

Plath, S. *Crossing the water.* New York: Harper & Row, 1971.

Redfield, R. The folk society. In M. P. Redfield (Ed.), *Human nature and the study of society: The papers of Robert Redfield* (Vol. 1). Chicago: University of Chicago Press, 1962. Pp. 231–253.

Róheim, G. *Animism, magic and the divine king.* New York: Knopf, 1930.

Shelton, A. Ibo aging and eldership: Notes for gerontologists and others. *Gerontologist*, 1965, **5**, 20–23.

Wallace, A. The institutionalization of cathartic and control strategies in Iroquois religious psychotherapy. In M. Opler (Ed.), *Culture and mental health.* New York: Macmillan, 1960.

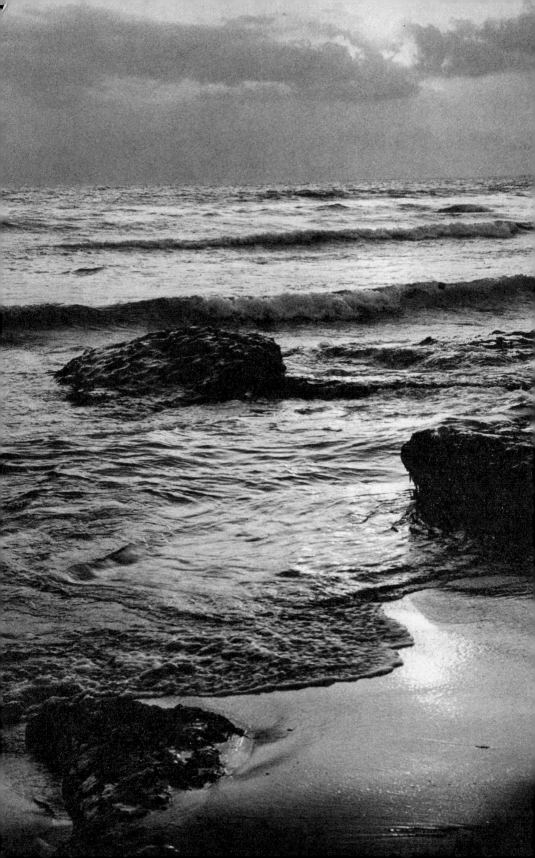

PART
SIX
EPILOGUE

19

EPILÓGUE

HERMAN FEIFEL

A number of authoritative themes emerge from efforts thus far in the thanatological sphere:

Death has many faces and meanings, and perceptions of it vary in diverse cultures and in differing eras. Further, divergent views of death, at times, may mirror dissimilar frames of reference rather than necessarily basic discord.

Death is "all the time" and is lodged in our bowels. It is not just fortuity, mischance, or an exclusivity of the old and moribund. We are all observer-participants with respect to death.

The tradition and modes of current medical care are overly geared to treating acute pain. One of the changing realities of modern medicine is emergence of the patient who suffers from chronic pain as the result of a long-term illness or terminality. Too often the patient who fails to meet the success calculation of the acute care hospital finds himself in a therapeutic limbo, a nether world of no expectancy. The challenge is to broaden our efforts in controlling chronic pain and to provide greater relief and well being for the chronically ill. In this regard, it appears appropriate to reaffirm a legitimate role for the helping professions—that when cure is not possible, concern and comfort are just as fitting and valid in meeting authentic needs of the patient.

We must guard against deifying the physical saving power of modern medical technology. It is the *living* rather than the *dying* of the person sick-until-death which requires prolongation. The quality of life, not mere insentient survival, stands in need of our worship.

Increasing privatization of death needs to be undercut. It is evident that ritual can be liberating as well as enslaving for survivors in their grief. Death is the occasion, furthermore, when the community needs to expand its current network of care and appreciation of the requirements of the bereaved.

Man has a legitimate need to face away from death. None of us can tolerate incessant exposure to death. And, in truth, who is to say that under certain conditions repression of the notion of death may not even be salutary? Studies of airplane pilots in World War II, for example, revealed that those who performed best in combat tended to retain in moments of most extreme danger the illusion of invulnerability. The clinical work of Avery Weisman and Laurens White likewise discloses that use of denial can nullify the threat of impending death in a way to help us cope better with reality. Unfortunately, too many of us resort to inordinate expulsion of the actuality of death, resulting in self-estrangement and social pathology. To face death is the beginning of mastery over life's terrors. We must be at home with death's mystery and fear if we are not to become alienated from our nature and destiny, lose basic contact with who we are. If we

352

accept death as necessity rather than strive to demote it to the level of accident, energies now bound up in continuing strivings to shelve the idea of death will be available to us for the more constructive aspects of living, perhaps even fortify our gift for creative splendor against our genius for destruction.

Some mandates and implications are also in order:

1. Twentieth century physics has become aware of the way in which the specific methodology we use to gain information can determine our conception of reality. One is reminded of the English astronomer Eddington's parable of the investigator who studied deep-sea life by means of a net of ropes of a two-inch mesh and who afterward concluded, "There are no fish smaller than two inches in the sea!" In this frame, vital grasp of the significance of death requires that we see each human being not principally as a perceiving consciousness nor as an epistemological subject as do Descartes and Hume but as a person, self-aware, involved with others, and concerned with salvation. I do not mean to be misunderstood as pleading for a return to unreined impressionism, or as oblivious to the considerable contribution of "method." I ask, rather, for a field of regard committed to purposive and striving man: one whose scope will not be made parochial by a limiting philosophy of science; one whose concepts will not be essentially derived from methods of study but rather from the functioning of human life, embodying courage, love, tragedy, will, and delight as well as memory capacity, pulse rate, blood count, and socioeconomic level. Too often have we worked with portions of the human individual and tried to make a virtue of this. The challenge is to enlarge horizons without sacrificing our gains.

With regard to method itself in the thanatological sphere: We are learning that in order to optimize knowledge concerning the influence of death upon behavior we must probe, more penetratingly than we presently do, the oscillating and fluctuating meanings of death within as well as between individuals and groups; unravel more intelligibly existing bonds among verbally expressed opinions, fantasy musings, and unconscious ideas about death; and strengthen our bridges to personality theory and social structure.

2. The time is ripe for "death education" to assume a rightful role in our development. Its pertinence is not only for those in the helping professions who deal with dying, death, and bereavement but for all of us—in the home, school, and in our general cultural upbringing. Proper resolution of such thorny issues as the current ongoing reassessment of euthanasia and organ transplanting, appropriate evaluation of the notion of a national health-care and delivery system, and deeper comprehension of the human predicament demands not only reconstruction of training cur-

ricula in medical, nursing, social work, and seminary schools, not only engagement of those responsible for developing social policies in health, but, more fundamentally, complementary dialogue between professionals and an informed general community.

3. Perspectives about death evolving from findings in the area of death not only have applicability to such a dilemma as euthanasia but also possess potential for helping clarify such social issues as abortion, capital punishment, and war. Additionally, there is increasing recognition that such disparate behaviors as alcoholism, drug abuse, personal violence, and other destructive acts have links to overt and latent meanings which death has for the individual.[1] All life-threatening behaviors involve confrontation, in one way or another, with the threat of possible injury or ultimate death to self and others. Manifestly, life can be menaced and compromised in many ways short of death and on varying levels of experience. In this context, such notions as "partial death," "subintentioned death," "student suicidalism," "symbolic death," and grief over loss other than life such as a limb, job, or old neighborhood, will also profit from a more comprehensive theory of death.

A caveat. The current state of knowledge in the field is such that the age of the prophets is far from over, and we should beware of becoming priests prematurely. The spotlight in the field of death, too often, tends to be overly focused on the dying person. I do not mean to minimize the positive influence this has had in fostering a more appropriate and dignified dying. Indeed, my own efforts in this regard have contributed to this civilizing development. Behavioral scientists, however, need to respond more robustly to findings which disclose that the steering force of consciousness of death is active at all age levels, and in areas of life that are ordinarily not viewed as death-related situations.

A final thought. We live in an age of history dominated by the conquests of science. Yet, science equips man but does not guide him. With due deference to the vista-expanding, judicious, and practical advice offered the reader and others in the field in this book, as well as to findings that will emanate from future studies, one wonders whether, in the last analysis, it is only a compelling vision of man and his role in the universe that can prepare us to face and integrate the certainty of death and its sequelae.

---

[1] A research program, the Role of Death Attitudes and Value-Belief System in Alcoholism, Drug Abuse, and Violent Behavior, supported by the Veterans Administration and directed by the editor, is approaching completion and will be reported on in the near future.

Man of the late Middle Ages and early Renaissance participated in his own death. It is fitting that we in the late twentieth century recapture our sovereignty over death and, hence, life. In responding to our temporality, we shall find it easier to define values, priorities, and life goals, and move toward a more common sharing of our humanity—all too eroded in the present world.

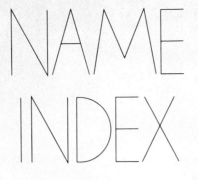

NAME INDEX

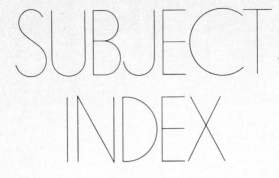

SUBJECT INDEX